ADVANCE PRAISE FOR THE AGELESS BOOMER

"The Ageless Boomer is an extraordinary tool that will guide you in your journey to health and vitality."
—Joel Fuhrman, M.D., bestselling author of *Eat to Live*, *Super Immunity*, *The End of Diabetes*, *The End of Dieting*, *The End of Heart Disease*, and numerous other titles

"Rod Fisher has created a resource guide that should be part of every home library. While exposing the thieves that would rob us of our greater health potential, Rod expounds the virtues and practices that will enable us to enjoy healthier, happier, and more fulfilling lives. In a world of misinformation and confusion, he provides the lenses that offer clarity. Truly this is a book for all ages, families, and libraries."
—Dave Hall, inventor of the Cellerciser and speaker on Cellercise rebounding

"Rod can speak from experience, and he provides a solid example that healthy aging does not come from genetics and luck. It comes from making healthy choices over the long term."
—Brendan Brazier, bestselling author of the "Thrive" series of books and ironman athlete, from his foreword to *The Ageless Boomer*

"The book that you're holding in your hands is the answer to all your nutritional and exercise questions. You will become leaner and healthier for now and always! We all need to follow the simple and sound advice Rod gives within these pages, because it works and just makes sense."
—Jon Hinds, founder of the Monkey Bar Gym, from his preface to *The Ageless Boomer*

"The realm of diet & exercise books is a jungle of confusing and conflicting information. As the author of seven books on natural strength and fitness, I've seen it all: diet fads, weight loss schemes, exercise systems that cause more pain than gain, and celebrity-promoted 'miracle' drop-the-pounds programs based on promotional hype rather than real nutritional sense.
"That's what makes this book by Rod Fisher so refreshing. It's not about hype. It doesn't feature an airbrushed photo of a big-name celebrity on the cover. And it doesn't promise any miracles other than the ones your body is capable of producing naturally when given the right ingredients and raw materials.
"Enjoy this valuable collection of nutritional and physical culture wisdom! Your body—and your mind—will thank you for it."
—John Peterson, author of *Pushing Yourself to Power*, *The Miracle Seven*, and numerous other titles

"Medically sound and universally relevant, this book traces the most comprehensive path I have yet discovered to that elusive fountain of youth."

—Greg Tayler, M.D. (family medicine), a fitness fanatic who, at age 49, competes with top-tier athletes in triathlon and cycling races

"Rod Fisher has combined his sparkling intelligence with his passion for healthy living into a book, The Ageless Boomer, a highly readable and informative work. Mr. Fisher offers an alternative to the endless cycle of quick-fix diets and the dreary and numerous articles on the physical and mental degeneration of people of a certain age. His book is written in a style that is clear and accessible. My advice is to hang on to it so that you, the ageless boomer, can refer back to it for the next 60-plus years of your life!"

—Claire Morrison, Ph.D.

"As an avid runner who logged more than 40 miles a week and made consistent, good food choices, I considered myself to be very healthy. Upon reading *The Ageless Boomer*, I made a significant change to my daily routine and am now over 70% raw and food combining. In the first two weeks, my running performance increased and my recovery time post-race is strikingly shortened. I have never felt better."

—Sara Borchers Marino

THE AGELESS BOOMER

LIVING YOUNG FOR THE REST OF YOUR LIFE

Rod Fisher

"The Ageless Boomer is an extraordinary tool
that will guide you in your journey to health and vitality."

—Joel Fuhrman, M.D.,
bestselling author of Eat to Live

The Ageless Boomer

Published by RopeTree Press
www.theagelessboomerlife.com

First Edition
ISBN: 978-0-9981079-1-2

This book contains the opinions and ideas of its author. It is intended to provide helpful general information on the subjects that it addresses. It is not in any way a substitute for the advice of the reader's own physician(s) or other medical professionals based on the reader's own individual conditions, symptoms, or concerns. If the reader needs personal medical, health, dietary, exercise, or other assistance or advice, the reader should consult a competent physician and/or other qualified health care professionals. The author and publisher specifically disclaim all responsibility for injury, damage, or loss that the reader may incur as a direct or indirect consequence of following any directions or suggestions given in the book or participating in any programs described in the book.

Cover art by Ivailo Nikolov (tree) and Claude Monet (still life)
Cover photos by Daniel Haney and Suzanne Fisher
Cover design by Patrick Patno
Interior illustrations by David Moeller

To my children and grandchildren

TABLE OF CONTENTS

| PREFACE

By Jon Hinds, Founder of the Monkey Bar Gym

At this moment in history, Americans are the sickest, fattest, and weakest we've ever been. Many of us depend on synthetic drugs to make us feel better, but we continue to overeat and avoid exercise at all costs. But what if someone told you that you didn't have to depend on a drug to feel better and you could control overeating? *The Ageless Boomer* does exactly that. It takes the misinformation that we all hear and unscrambles it into useful information.

I've been a strength coach for over 35 years, and I've seen it all—the Zone Diet, the Atkins Diet, the South Beach Diet, the bodybuilders' diet, and now the irritating conglomerate, the Paleo Diet. But even still, with all our good intentions in trying to avoid our ascent as the most obese country in the world, we are failing. We overeat, we eat foods our bodies instinctively don't recognize, and we eat processed foods daily. We sit too much and move too little.

Jon Hinds is the former strength and conditioning coach for members of the LA Clippers and numerous other NBA players, many MLB players, and high-profile celebrities. He opened his first Monkey Bar Gym in 2000 with the motto, "No mirrors, no machines, and leave your egos at the door." Jon is an Ageless Boomer with two gold medals in Brazilian jiu jitsu, one from the Pan America games and one from the Rickson Gracie International BJJ World Championships.

Rod's book shows you how to move around these obstacles and get on the right path. He gives you the tools that will reconnect you with what's instinctual and natural for you to eat, and he's living proof! "The proof is in the pudding," I often say when I am training people. If I were an out-of-shape trainer telling you what you need to do to get in shape, how much credibility would I really have? That's why *The Ageless Boomer* is so great. Rod's not giving you information that he himself has not done or tried. He has used his own body as a laboratory to figure out what works and what doesn't, what feels good and what doesn't, and what makes sense and what doesn't. Learning from someone who has the ability to listen to the body and ignore the stimulus of our society is powerful.

Throughout this book, Rod will give you pearls of wisdom that make transitioning and succeeding at eating a more plant-based diet attainable. He'll give you results, he'll give you the truth, and most importantly he'll give you a plan in a simple, straightforward, no-nonsense style.

The book that you're holding in your hands is the answer to all your nutritional and exercise questions. You will become leaner and healthier for now and always! We all need to follow the simple and sound advice Rod gives within these pages, because it works and just makes sense. Anyone can benefit from this book … but truth be told, you owe it to yourself to read it!

FOREWORD:
THE THRIVING BOOMER

By Brendan Brazier, author of the *Thrive* book series

Most of you don't know Rod Fisher yet, but I can tell you that he's a remarkable person. He's seventy, but he has strength, flexibility, mental acuity, and unbelievable energy that people of all ages wish they had. For me, he's a living affirmation of the principles I've been practicing and teaching for the past two decades—eat whole, plant-based foods and get adequate physical activity if you want to achieve optimal health.

When Rod first told me about this book, I thought it had the potential make a big impact on a lot of people. Healthy living at any age is important to all of us, but it's difficult for someone like me, who's just turned 40, to talk about aging from a personal perspective. Rod can speak from experience, and he provides a solid example that healthy aging does not come from genetics and luck. It comes from making healthy choices over the long term.

Brendan Brazier is the best-selling author of the "Thrive" book series, co-founder and editor-in-chief of *Thrive* Magazine, and the creator and host of the Thrive Forward web series. He is recognized as one the world's foremost authorities on plant-based nutrition and is the nutrition consultant for the Garmin-Sharp pro cycling team as well as several NHL, MLB, MLS, UFC and Olympic athletes. He is a former professional Ironman triathlete, two-time Canadian 50km Ultramarathon champion and the creator of Vega, the award-winning line of whole food nutritional products.

The Ageless Boomer offers you a road map to healthy aging. And while it's written with Baby Boomers in mind, its lessons and suggestions apply to younger generations who want to be "ageless" for the rest of their lives. If you want to be ageless, now is the time to start.

OUR HEALTH CRISIS

During the past two decades, I have reached people all over the world, helping them improve their health by teaching them about whole-food, plant-based (WFPB) nutrition. It has been gratifying to see so many people make this positive change, but at the same time, many others still need to hear the message.

Record numbers of North Americans are facing chronic diseases like cardiovascular disease, diabetes, and cancer. Research leaves no doubt that the diet most people eat, which is rich in saturated fats, refined sugar, refined grains, and animal products, is the major contributor to the terrible state of health in which we find ourselves. The sedentary lifestyle of most North Americans compounds these problems. And the saddest part of this situation is that these conditions are preventable.

The Ageless Boomer targets the Baby Boomer generation, and with good reason. This demographic group includes approximately 76 million Americans between the ages of 52 and 70. Baby Boomers as a group are facing chronic health problems on a massive scale: 40 percent of men and 34.4 percent of women age 40-59 have cardiovascular disease; about 16 percent of Boomers have diabetes and 39 percent are obese. High cholesterol and high blood pressure are on the rise among Boomers as well.

The tragedy behind this health crisis is also a source of hope: these diseases are preventable. People who don't suffer from these conditions can avoid developing them, and for the vast majority of those who have already developed chronic diseases, they can get better. All they have to do is make proactive changes to improve their nutrition and exercise habits. Rod explains in detail what to eat, what not to eat, and how to get off the couch and get healthy. His approach is simple and it mirrors what I've told my readers for years.

KNOW BETTER, EAT BETTER, FEEL BETTER

In my Thrive Forward program, which offers people an individualized plan to revamp their nutrition habits, I say "Know Better, Eat Better, Feel Better." You can't feel better until you eat better, and you can't eat better until you know better. The media is awash in news about the latest findings and fads in diets, but research consistently shows that eating whole, plant-based foods results in the best health outcomes. And when you start eating WFPB nutrition, you will see the difference.

I encourage people to pursue mindful, purpose-driven eating. North Americans, by and large, eat mindlessly, choosing food because it tastes good or satisfies a craving. Most of them are not choosing whole plant foods, which do taste good—they choose refined, high-sugar,

high-fat foods that have been engineered to make them want more and more. At the same time, these foods deliver so little nutritional value that they leave consumers constantly hungry.

But you can't stop this cycle until you know how to eat better. My nutritional philosophy, which Rod shares, comes down to three primary objectives:

- Eat high net-gain foods
- Eat alkaline-forming foods
- Eliminate biological debt

Eating whole plant foods carries out all three of these objectives. It's not complicated, but the results are very impressive.

You can't feel better until you eat better, and you can't eat better until you know better.

Eat high net-gain foods. Rod and I recommend whole plant foods because they give you significant nutritional benefit while minimizing digestive stress. Digestion is an energy-intensive process, and refined foods and animal foods require more of your digestive energy than whole plant foods. That's why eating a meal filled with heavy fats and refined starches leaves you feeling tired and sluggish. Whole plant foods digest quickly with minimal digestive stress, creating a net gain in energy. **The less energy you spend on digestion, the more energy you have.**

Eat alkaline-forming foods. As you'll discover when you read this book, different foods produce acidic or alkaline conditions in your body. Foods that form acidic conditions include animal products, grains, and refined carbohydrates, while alkaline-forming foods include most whole plant foods. Acid conditions can lead to the development of kidney stones, loss of bone mass, reduced growth hormone (which controls the development of muscle mass), increased amounts of free radicals, and reduced cell energy production. All of these adverse effects can be avoided, however, by choosing alkaline-forming foods.

Eliminate biological debt. "Biological debt" is the term I use to describe the energy-depleted state of most North Americans—using stimulants to delay chronic fatigue while ignoring their lack of healthy energy from food and sleep. The human body can get two types of energy: energy from stimulation and energy from nourishment. Stimulation, which can come from caffeine, sugar, and even from stress (thanks to adrenaline) provides a boost of energy in the short term, but then leads to an energy crash—biological debt. Like credit card debt, biological debt needs to be paid back. Biological debt creates a crash that leads to fatigue, which many people counter with more stimulants. Fatigue causes stress, which results in elevated cortisol—leading to inflammation, storage of visceral fat, premature aging, and more. Energy from nourishment, however, provides sustained, long-term energy. Sound nutrition and healthy sleep address the root cause of fatigue. Eating a nutrient-dense diet with a balance of healthy fats, carbs, and plant-based protein is an investment in long-term vitality—without debt.

"Biological debt" is the term I use to describe the energy-depleted state of most North Americans — using stimulants to delay chronic fatigue while ignoring their lack of healthy energy from food and sleep.

By making mindful choices about your nutrition, you can multiply your energy, minimize or eliminate fatigue, improve your immune system, and strengthen every system in your body at the cellular level. Rod is going to teach you what you need to do so that you can know better, eat better, and feel better. And honestly, you're going to feel amazing.

THE POWER OF MOVEMENT

Eating a WFPB diet will transform your body, but nutrition alone isn't enough to create the ageless state Rod is trying to help you develop. Physical activity is crucial to your health as well.

The program works for exercisers of any age or fitness level because Rod provides options to adjust the exercises to fit your needs.

My second Thrive book, *Thrive Fitness*, came about when I had to take a break from training and I discovered how fortunate I was to be highly fit. From the time I was a teenager I had spent my time around other endurance athletes; they were my "normal." As I spent more time with people outside this athletes-only circle of friends, I discovered that my normal—a high energy level, healthy sleep, and sharp mental focus without caffeine or sugar—was an oddity. I set out to create a book that addressed the holistic components of nutrition, exercise, sleep, and stress reduction.

Rod has done something very similar in this book, and he's done it with a focus on the physical challenges you may face if you are over 50 and starting to exercise regularly for the first time. The program works for exercisers of any age or fitness level, however, because Rod provides options to adjust the exercises to fit your needs.

It's a simple, well-rounded program. It emphasizes strength training, which is a critical component of any fitness program, and it's especially important as we age. Rod devotes two chapters to strength-training exercises, and the result is a wealth of choices that will prevent boredom. He also includes chapters on walking and rebounding, two forms of exercise that are ideal for both beginners and advanced exercisers.

EVERYTHING YOU NEED TO LIVE AGELESSLY

The Ageless Boomer also includes chapters on hydration, sleep, stress management, and sun exposure. Rod explains how all these factors—nutrition, exercise, sleep, stress, and more—interact with each other, and each chapter gives you sound advice about how to get the greatest benefit for your overall health.

Life is the ultimate endurance sport—its demands are difficult and constantly changing, and there is no time limit or finish line. If you want your body and mind to perform well for you, give them the right fuel and care so that you can live a healthy, vibrant life now and for many decades to come.

PART 1

CHAPTER 1

GIVE YOURSELF THE GIFT OF HEALTH

■■■

Living healthy is a joyous celebration of life. It's time for baby boomers to stop thinking about wellness with a grudging "it's good for me" attitude and start embracing wellness as the greatest gift we can give to ourselves.

The goal of this book is to make you excited about living in your 60s, 70s, 80s, 90s, 100s, and beyond. I want to dispel your fears about living in pain and frailty and give you a path to living in strength and comfort, no matter your age.

START THE REAL
FIGHT AGAINST AGING

Americans are obsessed with hiding the signs of age.

Hair dye, hair restoration treatments, wrinkle creams, age-spot creams, Botox, filler injections, face lifts, lasers, implants, and more fuel a multi-billion dollar industry. BCC Research estimates the total global market for the anti-aging industry at $262 billion dollars last year, and North America is the leading market.

Isn't something wrong with this picture? We're so afraid of age that we will spend billions of dollars hiding its signs on the outside; meanwhile our insides are getting weaker and sicker. Is it worth it to hide the effects of aging when what we really want is to feel younger inside and out?

I believe we need to flip our paradigm about aging. A wrinkle or two is much less important than your ability to fight cancer. Gray hair is nothing if you have a fit, energetic body. And baldness is not a big deal compared to a healthy heart and lungs. We need to stop thinking about fighting age from the outside and start focusing on changing our bodies from the inside.

AGE IS INEVITABLE — "OLD AGE,"
AS WE KNOW IT, IS **NOT**

We associate old age with aching muscles and joints, flagging energy, increased risk of disease, memory loss, weight gain, and many, many more conditions that range from inconvenient to life-threatening. If our parents are still alive, we see them struggling with these "miseries," as they might say in the South. And some of you are starting to experience them yourself.

All this would be terrible news if there weren't an alternative—but there is. All these miseries can be mitigated or, in most cases, eliminated, by changes within your control. Adapting your sources of nourishment, like nutrition and sleep, and your level of exercise will yield amazing, energizing, rejuvenating results.

"What is the power of youth? The power of youth is vigor. It's the power of boundless energy and stamina; the power of emotional resilience and optimism; the power of agile reasoning, creative thinking, and comprehensive memory."

— Kenneth Cooper, M.D.,
Regaining the Power of Youth at Any Age

I am living proof that at 69 years old, a person can have youthful energy, flexibility, strength, and mental clarity. I have been cancer-free despite a genetic predisposition toward that disease. These are the best years of my life, and I am living them to their full potential.

I'm Rod Fisher, and I'm an Ageless Boomer.

MY STORY:
AN INVESTMENT IN HEALTH

During my annual checkup when I was forty, my doctor told me very plainly that if I didn't want to succumb to cancer at a young age as my parents had, I should seriously consider becoming a vegan. This was an alien concept in one way, but it was almost déjà vu in another: I had adopted a plant-based diet as a high school athlete.

When I was preparing for the 20-foot rope-climbing event as part of the high school gymnastics team, I noticed that diet actually effected my times. I discovered that if I ate meat and drank milk, I would not perform at my peak

Whole food plant-based (WFPB) diet:
A diet solely of foods derived from plants, without refinement or processing of those foods.

for the next meet. So I started experimenting, and after a great deal of trial and error, I found that if I went on a vegan diet (though I'd never heard the term vegan) for the entire gymnastics season, I performed at a much higher level. It was indisputable. My times proved it.

I came from a typical three-times-a-day meat-eating family, and my parents were shocked. They claimed this no-meat, no-dairy business was unhealthy and even called my coach to express their concern. But the results and the records spoke for themselves. I performed better when I was on a vegan diet. In the off-season, I'd go back to our meat-and-dairy diet. Years later, I

realized that the only time I ever got sick was during the off-season, never when I was part of the gymnastics team.

So early on, I discovered that balancing exercise and nutrition—and understanding how integral proper nutrition is to athletic performance—was vital to achieving peak athletic performance. But I never took it any further than that. Why? Because I didn't realize that there were other benefits to be gained from a whole-food plant-based lifestyle beyond increased athletic performance. Could it be that I had discovered not only the secret to super performance but also super health totally by accident when I was a gymnast?

At the time my doctor told me to consider going vegan, I had a young family, and I wanted to watch them grow up and enjoy grandchildren of my own. Was this doctor on to something—a preventative diet that would not activate the family gene that causes cancer? Better still, did I have it right all those years ago?

The answer to both questions is yes. Study after study has confirmed that every major

"I am convinced that the way we eat as a society has led us astray over the past decades, and that many of the current epidemics are surely due to our changed diet: increased preservatives, additives, and undernourishing foods."

—Actor Hugh Jackman's foreword to Brendan Brazier's Thrive

disease of aging—cancer, heart disease, dementia—is reduced in risk when you eat a diet dominated by fresh fruits and vegetables. Studies by Lester Morrison and John Gofman, Nathan Pritikin, Caldwell Esselstyn, Jr., and Dean Ornish have all shown how this kind of diet can dramatically improve heart health. In his groundbreaking work, *The China Study*, T. Colin Campbell explains the results of his study of 6,500 individuals in the 65 counties of China: the study found that as individuals' consumption of animal protein decreased, so did their rates of heart disease and many types of cancer.

I was right about the value of a vegan diet for athletic performance, too. Brendan Brazier's *Thrive* books, magazine, and related products are convincing a new generation of performance athletes that a plant-based diet can help them reach peak achievement. Actor Hugh Jackman, who has played the ageless character Wolverine for 15 years now, credits Brazier's advice on diet and fitness for helping him achieve the physique he needed for that role. When I was forty, I was much more concerned with the health benefits of the plant-based diet, but I can also attest that it provides great benefits for athletic performance and overall fitness.

"By getting healthier, you might save a lot of money over the course of your lifetime by eliminating costly medical bills for conditions you as a healthier person won't have. A couple retiring at age 65 could potentially save $100,000 or more. …You might also extend your lifespan by five to seven years. If that doesn't inspire you, think about how you'll feel if you have the energy to do what you want — like keeping up with your grandkids!"

— *Steve Vernon,*
CBS Moneywatch columnist and retirement advisor

I decided to follow my doctor's advice and adopted a WFPB diet that very day at my 40-year checkup. A month later, I was shocked by how different I felt—more energetic than I had been in years and healthier than ever. In fact, I felt my strength surging as it did when I was a gymnast. It seemed like a miracle; after all, once you've hit forty, it's all supposed to be downhill, right? Wrong! I went back to the doctor for a blood test and every single vital sign had improved—cholesterol, blood pressure, and more. I couldn't believe it.

And now, almost three decades later? I hardly ever go to the doctor because I'm never sick, but a few years ago my children insisted I go in for a checkup, just to be sure. I went to UCLA, where the medical team drew 19 vials of blood. They tested me for everything. After the doctor looked at my results, he joked, "You're going to live forever." He went on to say, "There's nothing wrong with you. Your blood tests came back better than an Olympic athlete's."

I wrote this book because I want other people to share this amazing experience. I want you to have the kind of optimal health I have, no matter what age you are.

You might be wondering why you should trust my advice. I'm not a dietician or a doctor—I'm a self-taught health expert. I had a great incentive for thinking about health because both my parents died very young of cancer. My mother died of lymphoma, and my father died of colon cancer. He was the last of 16 kids, and any who weren't killed by the Nazis were killed by colon cancer. That's powerful motivation. If I hadn't taken control of my health, I would have felt out of control, and I didn't want that.

The fact that healthy choices saved my life has helped turn my interest into my passion. My incentive now is making other people aware that they don't have to resign themselves to an early death or decades of illness. We have the power to change genetic and environmental fate with simple solutions in nutrition and exercise.

Before I retired and dedicated myself to this project, I worked on Wall Street. I wasn't an investment banker, I was a salesman—at least, I started as a salesman. I worked for a company called Telerate, which sold information. We sold terminals that broadcast certain information to our subscribers. Most of the information was about ski conditions. However, we also had three pages of live information on bids and offers in government security markets, and that was the only information our customers really cared about.

So I looked for ways to add more really critical information to our terminals, and that

was the start of a decades-long journey that eventually led me to form my own company, Market Data Corporation (MDC). By the time I left the company, we had hundreds of pages of critical information that empowered businesses at every level, not just the handful of the most powerful firms. We had thousands of viewers around the world.

My career taught me the value of information very early. My passion for great health has reinforced it. We swim in a sea of information about diet and exercise, but sometimes that information is as useful to us as ski condition information is to financial institutions. I want to zero in on the information that produces the greatest results for the greatest number of people. That's the kind of information I'm presenting to you in this book.

By far the best investment I ever made was investing the time and energy to optimize my health. I believe the same is true for everyone.

Investing in your health pays you back in many measurable ways. You'll reduce your medical costs, from prescriptions to hospital visits. You'll spend less on adapting your home to accommodate increasing frailty.

Are you still working? Most Boomers are. According to the Transamerica Center for Retirement Studies, 65 percent of Boomers plan to work past age 65 or don't plan to retire—ever. The AARP asked workers over 50 what was important to them in their jobs; 95 percent said they needed the money, and 60 percent said they were working to fully fund their pensions. If you're still working the investment in health has a huge dollar value. Not only will you miss fewer days in the immediate future from illness or injury, you'll also have many, many more productive years ahead.

"Nearly half (49 percent) of boomers still working say they don't expect to retire until they are 66 or older, including one in ten who predict they will never retire."

— Gallup Polls, January 2014

AGELESS LIVING: WHAT'S THE DIFFERENCE?

I call this book "Ageless Boomers" because it's about lifestyle practices that help us live in vigor and health. It's about bringing greater definition to our minds and bodies. It's about filtering out the negative influences that compromise our energy. It's about maximizing the quality of our nourishment and exercise so that our minds and bodies have optimal health.

It's also about challenging definitions. We grew up with definitions about nutrition, exercise, health, and age that don't hold up in light of modern evidence. Even though people across the Boomer generation are very different, we all understand the importance of challenging accepted ideas and re-evaluating what we think we know.

So what's the difference between Ageless living and traditional aging? Nourishment, exercise, and results. If you give your body the

Most importantly, the return on your investment in health is more than monetary. You're improving your quality of life dramatically. In this extended third trimester of life, we generally have greater freedom from family responsibilities and financial debts. Our children are grown and our mortgages are diminishing. It's time to enjoy life, travel, and check things off our bucket lists.

If you don't have optimal health, you can't enjoy these things to their full potential. But you can make your golden years really shine if you're willing to adopt a nourishing, active lifestyle.

best nourishment and perform basic exercise to keep it in good condition then you will achieve optimal results. This pattern is true in any time of life, but it's vital to understand as you reach your later years.

"The joy is that we can take back our bodies, reclaim our health, and restore ourselves to balance. We can take power over what and how we eat. We can rejuvenate and recharge ourselves, bringing healing to the wounds we carry inside us, and bringing to fuller life the wonderful person that each of us can be."

— John Robbins, author of Healthy at 100: The Scientifically Proven — Secrets of the World's Healthiest and Longest-Lived Peoples

When we were young, up until about age 30, our bodies gave us good results even if we ate nutrient-poor food and didn't exercise. As we reached middle age, our bodies started to react more noticeably to bad nutrition and sedentary lifestyle, but if we were busy working or raising kids (or both), we didn't give it much attention. Now, though, in our golden years, our bodies do not forgive neglect. One of the inescapable realities of aging is that poor nourishment and lack of movement leads to bad results: disease, frailty, pain, and shortened life span. You can change this pattern! You control your nourishment and exercise, so you control your results. Isn't that great?

The lifestyle I'll discuss in this book is not painful to adopt. The exercise will not injure you—it will make you feel better. The nutrition will not starve you—it will nourish you. The hard part is changing your habits, and for people in the extended third trimester of life, learning new habits can be very challenging. But the dramatic results will help motivate you to embrace the change.

LOOK AHEAD: WHAT YOU'LL FIND IN THIS BOOK

This book is designed to give you a lot of information in one volume. We have access to a wealth of knowledge about health and longevity, and I want to give you as much as I can. At the same time, I don't want you to feel buried in details without a clear path forward. I've tried to fill each chapter with clear, simple advice to get your transformation underway.

Here's an overview of what you'll find as you read on.

Part 1: Becoming an Ageless Boomer. This section will introduce you to the basics of the Ageless Boomer lifestyle. It will answer some of your initial questions about what you need to do to embrace the lifestyle and what the lifestyle will do for you.

Part 2: Nourishment. This section is the heart of the book because changing your diet is the single biggest thing you can do to transform your body. I'll tell you everything you need to know about adopting a whole-food plant-based (WFPB) diet. And trust me, you're going to savor the change! I'll also discuss some of the other nourishment you need to optimize your health.

You don't have to be healthy to start, but you have to start to be healthy.

Part 3: Exercise. This section will explain the very simple, accessible forms of exercise you can do to keep your body in peak condition. I'll talk about the cardio we all do—walking—as well as strength-training regimens that any person can do. I'll also talk about what I call "push-ups for the brain"—meditation. Your brain is part of your body, and it requires conditioning too.

As we go forward, challenge your own definitions of age. Challenge your belief that it's all downhill from age 40 on. Challenge the ideas you've always accepted about nutrition and exercise. And above all, challenge the voice that tells you "I can't." You can. And you will.

CHAPTER 2

REVISIT YOUR IDEAS ABOUT AGE

■ ■ ■

It's a sad reality, but many of us fear growing old more than we fear dying. Based on current trends, fear of aging is understandable—millions of Boomers are on track to suffer heart disease, cancer, frailty, and dementia. It's important to remember that we have a huge say in the way we age, and we don't have to be afraid.

BOOMERS:
LOOKING GOOD, FEELING BAD

We Baby Boomers, as a group, are a contradictory bunch. The name "Baby Boomers" conjures up a specific story—soldiers coming back home after World War II and starting families en masse, leading to the biggest increase in babies in American history. My own story is a twist on this one: I was born in 1946 to refugee parents who escaped Nazi Germany—my mother in 1938 and my father in 1939. As you might guess, my mom and dad arrived in the United States with nothing more than their lives, the clothes on their back, and the dream of living in freedom and raising a family in America.

Baby Boomers are Americans born between 1946 and 1964, a span of nearly two decades. Given that range, not all Boomers relate to the same events and experiences, even though popular media lumps them all together.

According to people who study demographic trends, though, Baby Boomers include everyone born between 1946 and 1964. Some of the experiences of my youth were history by the time later boomers were born. I grew up in Manhattan on 218th Street along the Harlem River, and I loved to climb trees more than anything. We would literally spend entire days in the treetops in the park across the street from my apartment. So much so that my mom never looked for me in the park; instead, she looked up into the trees. My passion for climbing trees was actually a comfort to her, because after seeing how I climbed, not only did she not worry about me falling, but she always knew where I was and where to find me. My dad had been a fencing master in Germany and an athlete all his life. He was really strong and had trained Charles Atlas style.

For older Boomers like me, this story is probably very familiar. Playing outside from dawn to dusk, walking to school, and following daredevil inspiration from the movies was part of growing up. But younger boomers, sometimes called the "Boomer Reboot" generation, grew up in very different circumstances. As Richard Pérez-Peña noted in a *New York Times* editorial in January 2014, "The gap between the two halves of the baby boom might be best summed up by some of the staples of radio and TV when we were kids. The classic boomers had 'Mr. Sandman' and 'Leave It to Beaver'—in my case, it was actually "Hopalong Cassidy," "The Lone Ranger," Gene Autry, and Roy Rogers—"We rebooted boomers? 'Sympathy for the Devil' and 'All in the Family.'"

Younger Boomers were kids while older Boomers were living through some of the defining experiences of our adult lives: the assassinations of John F. Kennedy, Martin Luther King, and Robert Kennedy, Woodstock, the Vietnam War. When we look at the full range of Boomer experience, the idea that we have a common cultural story falls apart.

When it comes to health, however, people aged 50-68 have a lot of common concerns. The biggest difference between younger Boomers and older Boomers in terms of health is how many of us are already experiencing age-related decline. And unfortunately, because many Boomers are getting sicker at younger ages, there isn't that much difference.

In March 2013, the *Journal of the American Medical Association* (JAMA) published the findings of Dana King and colleagues that Baby Boomers, as a group, were less healthy than the previous generation at the same age. The "previous generation" was the group aged 46 to 64 (average 54.1 years) during the years 1988-1994, so the average person in this group was born in 1934. These people fall into the group often labeled the "Silent Generation," people who were born during the Great Depression or World War II.

The second group, the Boomers, included people aged 46 to 64 (average 54.5 years) during the years 2007-2010, so the average person in that group was born around 1952. High blood pressure, diabetes, and obesity were higher among Boomers; the prevalence of high cholesterol was more than double the percentage among Boomers compared to Silent Generation members. Only about 13 percent of Boomers considered themselves to be in excellent health, compared to 32 percent of Silent Generation members at the same age.

This kind of health profile wasn't always the norm for Boomers. As Sarah Mahoney reported in *AARP Magazine*, Boomers used to be one of the fittest generations. We "felt the burn" with Jane Fonda and sweated along with Richard Simmons. In 1968, fewer than 24 percent of American adults exercised regularly—by 1984, 59 percent of us were regular exercisers, and by 1987, the peak, *that number was 69 percent*. But today? Only 35 percent of Boomers are regular exercisers.

To me, this is crazy. And it's totally unnecessary. We have the power to reverse this trend, to get back to feeling great regardless of age. As Mahoney writes, "… while many boomers will likely find their way back to fitness under a doctor's orders, what we really need to do is rediscover one of the first tenets of fitness—what millions of us learned from Hula-Hoops [and] roller skates…: It's supposed to be fun."

Fitness and fun have always gone together for me. Growing up, I played stickball (I was a "two-sewer" hitter, meaning I could drive the ball past two drain covers), curb ball, and sandlot baseball. In stickball, when we had enough change we'd use a Spaldeen ball (25 cents)—if we didn't we used a Pinkie (15 cents)—and they'd only last a day. Because it was only a matter of time before a speeding car would run over the ball and you'd hear a loud pop. And then there

"We really need to rediscover one of the first tenets of fitness — what millions of us learned from Hula-Hoops [and] roller skates: It's supposed to be fun."
— Sarah Mahoney,
AARP Magazine

was ringolevio, a very rough New York City game. If you knew how to play ringolevio well you were going to do well in life. And we played all of them in the street, so we got adept at dodging cars.

What about you? Maybe your passion was roller skating, maybe it was kick the can, maybe it was stickball or street hockey. Whatever game you played that made you run, dodge, and laugh like crazy, find that energy and tap into it, because it's still fun.

Another huge contributor to Boomers' declining health is poor nutrition, or "dysnutrition," as it's called by Carol Wolin-Riklin, MA, RD, LD, a bariatric nutrition

"It is the negative lifestyle habits — lack of exercise [and consuming] processed foods, fast foods, high carbohydrate snacks and meals — that have caused the rise of metabolic syndrome comorbidities: hypertension, hyperlipidemia, and diabetes."

— Carol Wolin-Riklin, MA, RD, LD
Aging Well, Spring 2011

coordinator at the University of Texas Medical School at Houston. In an interview with Maura Keller in *Aging Well*, Wolin-Rilkin explains that dysnutrition "leads to the need for weight management, glycemic control, cardiac health through diet management, and concern for older boomers plagued by high blood pressure and obesity."

Bad dietary choices are every bit as changeable as exercise choices—more so, in many cases, because physical limitations can slow (but not stop!) the rate at which you adopt exercise habits. But if you can lift a fork, you can change what you eat and change your life.

YOUTH THAT'S SKIN DEEP

According to the American Society for Aesthetic Plastic Surgery, 2013 was a banner year for plastic surgeries and procedures. The number of procedures increased 12 percent over 2012, making 2013 the biggest year for procedures since the Great Recession began in 2008. Patients spent 12 billion dollars on surgeries and non-invasive procedures. The most popular surgery was liposuction—the fast-track path to fat loss—performed more than 360,000 times. Botox injections were America's favorite non-invasive procedure, with more than 3.7 million injections performed in 2013 alone.

It amazes me that Americans will pour money into shooting a toxin into their faces while ignoring the consequences of toxic lifestyle decisions, that they spend billions having doctors suck away fat and then continue eating the foods that will bring that fat right back. Americans obsess about looking young but ignore the mounting evidence that so many of our choices,from constant screen watching to mindless candy munching, are literally aging us from the inside out.

I know I'm not the first person to tell you that eating healthy foods and conditioning your body will keep you younger longer. In fact, one of the authors I admire and the father of modern aerobics, Kenneth Cooper, published *Regaining the Power of Youth at Any Age* more than 15 years ago. Dr. Cooper is a great example of an Ageless Boomer, and he has been giving people advice about lifestyle choices that will keep them young for decades. About five years ago he and his son released a book called *Start Strong, Finish Strong* that covers many of the same topics as Cooper's previous book, updated with new information and additional advice. And the Coopers aren't alone—even the FDA and NIH, which are conservative about nutrition claims, recognize and promote the benefits of healthy eating for aging adults.

As Ageless Boomers, we may want to look our best, but the youth we want comes from the inside out. Our lives have brought us rewarding experience, and we appreciate it. We're not ashamed of our age.

So why do I need to tell you again? Because so many people haven't listened—just look at how many sick Boomers we have. I'm adding my voice to this conversation for two reasons: one, we still need to get the message out; two, and I say this with genuine humility, because I'm a

great example. I mean example in the sense of a pattern or a model, and when I describe Ageless Boomer practices it's so that you have a map to follow that will make you an example too.

As Ageless Boomers, we may want to look our best, but the youth we want comes from the inside out. Our lives have brought us rewarding experience, and we appreciate it. *We're not ashamed of our age.*

John Robbins, in *Healthy at 100*, examines four cultures where people live to remarkably old ages and, more importantly, experience great health for their entire lives. These cultures are very different from western cultures in many respects, and we'll look at some of those differences later in this book. Among the characteristics he identifies is a habit of celebrating and embracing age. Elders in these cultures are respected, engaged, and accepted as an integral part of the community.

Changing our culture so that all members respect the oldest among us is a big challenge. We can start by giving ourselves respect as older adults and extending that respect to all of the elders in our lives. We can respect ourselves enough to give ourselves nourishment that strengthens our bodies and exercise that conditions them. We can, as many have said, be the change we want to see in the world.

REASON TO WORRY:
BOOMER HEALTH CONCERNS

The National Health Interview Survey, 2004–2010, identified the following ten conditions as the top health problems among adults 40–64:

1. Arthritis/rheumatism
2. Back/neck problems
3. Other musculoskeletal conditions
4. Fracture/bone/joint injury
5. Depression/anxiety/emotional problems
6. Weight problem
7. Lung/breathing problem
8. Nervous system condition
9. Heart problem
10. Diabetes

Adults aged 40–64 identified these ten problems as most likely to "cause difficulty with physical function." They identified the same ten concerns, in a different order, as most likely to "cause them to need help with daily activities or personal care."

As I just pointed out, more Boomers experience these kinds of health concerns than earlier generations did at the same age. It's absolutely tragic that all of these conditions, which can be prevented by healthy lifestyle choices, afflict so many people.

I recently visited a display of photographs from 100 years ago at the Laguna Beach Art Museum. I was struck by the photos of the town's elders, the people who had reached advanced age 100 years ago. All of them were trim, all were in great shape, and all appeared healthy and vital. They didn't need a book like this to maintain a healthy lifestyle, but we do.

According to the CDC, in America, about 73 percent of men and almost 80 percent of women aged 45-64 are overweight.

"I was first exposed to leafy greens as a young boy through the cartoon character Popeye the Sailor. He would open a can of spinach, pour it in his mouth and then be able to beat up every bad guy in the place. So I ate my spinach on a regular basis so I, like Popeye, could be big and strong. I now mix spinach leaves with romaine lettuce as a base for my salad-a-day ritual.

"I laud Dr. Joel Fuhrman, a family physician who specializes in preventing and reversing disease through nutritional and natural methods for introducing me to the concept of a salad a day."

— Casey Dowd,
The Boomer, Fox Business News

This section breaks down some of the biggest health concerns among Boomers. My list looks a lot like the list above, but I've added cancer and dementia to that list, because many Boomers worry about them even if they haven't experienced them yet. I've collapsed a lot of the other issues together into more general categories such as obesity or bone and joint deterioration.

In 2011, heart disease was the leading cause of death of Americans, claiming 597,689 lives (according to the CDC). The statistics among Baby Boomers are not good: the 2013 Update from the American Heart Association (AHA) tells us that among 40- to 59-year-olds, 40 percent of men and 34.4 percent of women have cardiovascular disease (CVD). "Approximately 150,000 Americans died of CVD in 2009 who were less than 65 years of age," the AHA fact sheet explains.

No matter who you are, your risk is high: the AHA explains that even among people who are disease-free at the age of 45, two out of three men and around one out of two women will develop CVD. If you make it to 50 without developing CVD your odds are a little better: around 52 percent for men and 40 percent for women.

Unfortunately, most Boomers aren't doing the one thing that can radically cut their risk of heart disease: eating a healthy diet. While 73 percent of Boomers are non-smokers—a terrific trend—*less than one percent of us are eating a healthy diet!*

Imagine if we all started to look at unhealthy foods the same way we look at cigarettes. Imagine if we started to view refined sugar, saturated fats, and processed carbohydrates the same way we view tobacco smoke. If we did, we'd all take leaps and bounds forward in health. I know I did, and I hope you will too.

Boomers are booming in the obesity department. The CDC reports that during the years 2009-2012, adults age 45 to 64 had the highest rates of obesity—40 percent. That's not adults who are overweight—about 73 percent of men and almost 80 percent of women in that range were overweight.

Many Americans have resorted to drastic measures to reduce weight: the American Society for Metabolic and Bariatric Surgery estimates that 220,000 people had weight-loss surgery in 2008.

The Harvard School of Public Health points to obesity as the number two cause of preventable death in the U.S. (tobacco being number one). And, they note, that as tobacco use drops in the U.S., obesity will probably take the number one spot. "Obesity causes or is closely linked with a large number of health conditions, including heart disease, stroke, diabetes, high blood pressure, unhealthy cholesterol, asthma, sleep apnea, gallstones, kidney stones, infertility, and as many as 11 types of cancers, including leukemia, breast, and colon cancer."

Keep in mind that obesity, as defined by the CDC, is measured by body mass index (BMI), which considers both weight and height. The BMI does have limitations—a performance athlete with a lot of heavy muscle could be defined as overweight despite his low body fat percentage—but for the most part it's a useful measure. You might be obese and not realize it because you think, "Well, I'm a little heavy, but I'm not obese—those people can't fit in an airplane seat." If you're heavy enough for your weight to affect your health, you need to recognize it and own it so that you can start to change it.

Many Americans have resorted to drastic measures to reduce weight: the American Society for Metabolic and Bariatric Surgery estimates that 220,000 people had weight-loss surgery in 2008. And of course we have a multi-billion dollar diet industry in this country that has not had success in changing our overall trend toward greater obesity. Ageless Boomer nutrition is not a diet—it's a way of life.

As I'll explain in detail in the nutrition section of this book, as you replace non-nutritious food with nutrient-rich food, you'll radically change the shape of your body. Our nutrition problem in this country is not quantity—it's quality.

BONE AND JOINT DETERIORATION

Kenneth and Tyler Cooper point out in *Start Strong, Finish Strong* that after age 25, you will lose 2 percent of your bone mass every year unless you actively work to prevent that loss. You'll lose 1 percent of your muscle mass each year as well. (If you do strength training you won't.) These trends, along with stress on tendons, ligaments, and cartilage over time, add up to joint pain and loss of mobility. More and more older adults are getting joint replacements to combat pain and lost mobility. The American Academy of Orthopedic Surgeons reports that every year they perform around half a million knee replacements and more than 175,000 hip replacements. In the next 20 years, they expect to perform far more: 174 percent more hip replacements and 673 percent more knee replacements. Do the math—that's around three million knee replacements per year by 2034.

No one wants to live with pain in their knees and hips, but there are alternatives to surgery. Jim and Phil Wharton of the Wharton Clinic in New York City have been helping "everyday athletes" rehabilitate their bodies so that they don't have to go through surgery to get relief from pain and to strengthen their joints. I went to the Wharton Clinic myself when I had a shoulder injury. They helped me rehabilitate my shoulder to the point where I had full strength and range of motion, and I never had to go through surgery.

Cancer is the second-highest cause of death for Americans, claiming 574,743 lives in 2011. The most common cancer is lung cancer, causing more than 157,000 deaths annually. But nearly every part of the body is vulnerable to cancer.

Many of you may have experienced cancer already— breast cancer, prostate cancer, testicular cancer, and skin cancer are not uncommon before age 50. However, as the AARP notes, cancer occurs more often in older adults, meaning it's still high on the list of Boomer health worries.

Because cancers are so varied and affect different individuals and different parts of the body in inconsistent ways, it can be hard to make generalizations about prevention. Still, mounting research shows how much we can control cancer's expression through healthy choices.

"As 10,000 baby boomers reach 65 each day, the incidence of cancer is increasing, estimated to increase by 67 percent between 2010 and 2030, bringing attention to the nation's response to cancer care. Cancer is diagnosed at a higher rate ... and results in more deaths than in younger patients."

— Science Daily

DEMENTIA

One of the biggest sources of stress for Baby Boomers is being the "sandwich" generation— caught between caring for children and caring for aging parents. Among the most difficult challenges we face in caring for parents is dealing with age-related mental decline, especially Alzheimer's disease. Not only do we experience the strain and grief of providing care for suffering parents, but we also have an ongoing reminder that the same disease could strike us as we age.

One in eight Americans over age 60 are already starting to experience symptoms of dementia, according to a 2013 CDC report. Only 35 percent of those people, however, report these symptoms to their doctors.

In fact, one in eight Americans over age 60 are already starting to experience symptoms of dementia, according to a 2013 CDC report. Only 35 percent of those people, however, report these symptoms to their doctors.

A 2013 study by the Rush Institute for Healthy Aging predicted that the number of people living with Alzheimer's will triple by 2050 as Boomers age. The Alzheimer's Association reports that one in eight Baby Boomers will develop this debilitating disease after they turn 65, and that by the time they turn 85, one in two Boomers will have it.

Alzheimer's disease is a complicated medical condition and many factors play a role in its development. However, research is revealing that exercise and plant-based eating slashes your Alzheimer's risk.

REJUVENATION: AGELESS BOOMER BENEFITS

Let's bring some bright sunshine into this gloomy health picture. It's inspiring to know that all of these serious health problems can be prevented by lifestyle choices. Heart disease, for example, can be virtually eliminated by the adoption of a whole-food plant-based (WFPB) diet. Just ask Caldwell Esselstyn's patients.

Esselstyn is a cardiologist who, in 1985, recruited 18 of his patients into a study of the effect of diet on heart disease events. These 18 patients had had 49 coronary episodes between them before they started the diet. After, only one patient had one episode, and that patient had gone off the diet.

"A half-century of research, both mine and that of many others, has convinced me [that] what you eat every day is a far more powerful determinant of your health than your DNA or most of the nasty chemicals lurking in your environment."

— T. Colin Campbell,
Whole

Is heart health the only benefit of Ageless Boomer practices? Hardly. T. Colin Campbell, author of *The China Study* and *Whole*, lists dozens of positive health effects from a WFPB diet. Jordan Metzl, in *The Exercise Cure*, describes the effects of exercise as if it were a miracle drug: "What if I told you this drug treats *everything*? And what if I told you this drug treats every illness you *might* get, including certain types of cancer?" In *Healthy at 100*, John Robbins describes octogenarians so spry that they climb up and down mountains while leaving younger people in the dust.

Let's look at just a few.

STRENGTH

Building and maintaining strength is a core goal for Ageless Boomers. I don't mean muscle bulk, although men in particular will find themselves gaining visible muscle with this approach. (Men and women both gain strength with muscle building but the physical evidence tends to look different.) I mean strength everywhere in your body—strong bones, strong heart and lungs, strong joints, and strong cells. The nutrition I'll discuss will strengthen all your body processes, and you'll phase out dysnutrition that harms you.

Ageless Boomer exercises will bring even more dramatic results. Aerobic training will strengthen your heart, lungs, and even your brain cells. Strength training will augment and improve your aerobic training. As the Mayo Clinic explains, "Strength training ... helps you develop strong bones...control your weight, [and] boost your stamina ... Building muscle also contributes to better balance, which can help you maintain independence as you age."

In addition, strength training can help you stave off dementia. In 2012 researchers at the University of British Colombia found that an exercise plan for seniors that included strength training increased mental skills like selective attention, conflict resolution, and associative memory. I describe meditation as "push-ups for your brain"; it turns out that push-ups are also push-ups for your brain!

In this book I'll be discussing very simple, very accessible, low-impact practices for both aerobic exercise and strength training. No matter who or where you are, you can start building strength and stamina.

"But you're not destined to grow softer and weaker just because you're getting older. Experts say most muscle loss comes from not using your muscles enough as you age, rather than aging itself. Using your muscles regularly will help them stay strong and firm, regardless of age, an important reason for older adults to strength train."

— AARP

STAMINA

"I just don't have as much energy as I used to." It's the refrain we've all heard, and you may be using it yourself these days. If you don't do anything to intervene, age will sap your stamina, but there are so many things you can do.

Nutrition plays a huge factor in your energy levels—food is our fuel, and what we eat affects our ability to use our bodies. Throwing your blood sugar into peaks and valleys with refined carbohydrates is a surefire way to leave yourself feeling drained. A WFPB diet, on the other hand, will give you long-lasting energy that doesn't drop off suddenly when you need it most.

You also have to keep your body in tune by exercising it. Steadily increasing your aerobic exercise will build your stamina in every aspect of life. As I noted earlier, strength training also helps increase your stamina. Doing aerobic and strength training together multiplies the positive effect. Even conditioning your mind with meditation will help your stamina; as you control and manage your stress, you will be able to respond to challenges with a better attitude and a better opportunity for success.

The best way for me to tell you about the benefits of the Ageless Boomer lifestyle for mobility is sharing a story from Robbins' *Healthy at 100*:

> One day, [researcher Alexander Leaf] accompanied [Abkhasian] Markhti Tarkhil on his morning plunge and was astonished by the vitality and physical agility of the 104-year-old. It was a steep and rugged half-mile climb down from the road to the river, but Markhti moved with confident speed and agility … Leaf, a physician coming from a society where elders have thin and fragile bones, was concerned that the old man might fall, and thought he should accompany Markhti down the hill and see to it that he didn't slip. But he was unable to do so, because he couldn't keep up with the pace of the far older man, who as it turned out never lost his footing.

For many Baby Boomers, the idea of climbing down a steep slope like this 104-year-old man did would be an unthinkable risk. But this kind of mobility is exactly what I intend to have when I'm 104 and older, and it's the kind of mobility I hope I can help you achieve with Ageless Boomer practices.

If you already feel confident about your joints and bones, these practices will help you maintain their health, increase their strength, and increase their flexibility with the right kind of range of motion exercises. If you have joint problems or other mobility problems now, Ageless Boomer practices will help you address many related problems such as weight, strength,

If you have joint problems or other mobility problems now, Ageless Boomer practices will help you address many related problems such as weight, strength, and stamina. With appropriate rehabilitation, they may be able to help you regain mobility and avoid surgery.

and stamina. With appropriate rehabilitation, they may be able to help you regain mobility and avoid surgery.

MENTAL CLARITY

In *AARP The Magazine* (Feb/Mar 2012), Beth Howard pulled together a list of things you can do to "Age-Proof Your Brain." They included these approaches:

- Do aerobic exercise
- Strength train
- Seek out new skills
- Meditate
- Eat leafy greens
- Eat essential fatty acids (flaxseed is my favorite)
- Eat herbs and spices
- Set and follow goals
- Maintain a healthy social life

- Reduce risk from obesity, diabetes, and hypertension

Sound familiar? Ageless Boomer practices cover all of these areas. Another risk area for older adults that we haven't discussed in depth yet is depression. Avoiding loneliness by maintaining social connections is very important to long-term health.

The previous items in this list describe how the nourishment and exercise of the Ageless Boomer lifestyle improve the way you look, feel, and think, but the most profound effects are things you will never see—the health of your organs, systems, and cells.

Three of the authors I have mentioned in this section—Campbell, Robbins, and Metzl—all used a "miracle drug" metaphor to describe an Ageless Boomer practice. These two cures individually help treat and prevent a profound list of diseases: obesity, cancer, osteoporosis, heart disease, stroke, Type 2 diabetes, even colds and flu. Just imagine what they will be able to do together!

I'm only scratching the surface of the benefits the Ageless Boomer lifestyle provides. In the next chapter, I'll start to explain the Ageless Boomer practices in more depth, and you'll start to see how profoundly these choices can change your life.

"The foods you consume can heal you faster and more profoundly than the most expensive prescription drugs, and more dramatically than the most extreme surgical interventions, with only positive side effects."

— T. Colin Campbell,
Whole

23

CHAPTER 3

LIVING YOUNG FOR THE REST OF YOUR LIFE: THE AGELESS BOOMER PRINCIPLES

■ ■ ■

Nourishment + exercise = optimal health. The formula is simple, the ideas are simple, and the practices are simple. The only thing complicated about becoming an Ageless Boomer is challenging the concepts you've been taught for decades.

THE CHOICE IS YOURS

How do you want to live your later years? Do you want to be sick, tired, weak, and frail? Do you want to be healthy, strong, vital, and energetic? Do you want to put a limit on your lifespan, or do you want to extend your vibrant years beyond the age of 100? If you've read this far, you want the latter: you want to be an Ageless Boomer. As I said earlier, the great news is that you can control the outcome by making the right choices now and for the rest of your life.

One of the best things about aging is that you know yourself well. You know how you learn, you know what feels good and what feels bad, and you know how to motivate yourself. You're in a better position to take control of your life than ever. The hardest thing you'll face is your habits, which you've followed without thinking for decades. That's how habits work. We're going to replace unhealthy habits with healthy ones, and that will make your transition much easier.

By now you're wondering exactly what kind of choices I'm talking about. If you want to be an Ageless Boomer, one of the biggest changes you will need to make is to your diet. Nutrition is the key to long-term health, and the best research on diet says that if you want to live without heart disease, cancer, dementia, and diabetes, you need to adopt a whole-foods, plant-based (WFPB) diet.

A WFPB diet is nutrient-rich and wildly varied because our world is populated by massive numbers of delicious edible plants. It takes advantage of the amazing combinations of nutrients available in simple fruits, vegetables, seeds, nuts, and legumes. As the quote from T. Colin Campbell (left) suggests, whole plants are miraculous nutrient bombs, and the whole is greater than the sum of the parts. You'll learn about many foods you should avoid and why, but I want you to stay focused on the huge numbers of foods available to you.

I'll give you lots of reasons why this nutrition plan is rewarding in every sense, but if you need a big dose of confidence, I recommend the documentary *Forks over Knives*. It features extensive interviews with both Campbell and Caldwell Esselstyn as well as many patients who have dramatically changed their lives with nutrition alone. These are people who have seen their Type 2 diabetes disappear. People who had multiple heart attacks and were told they should prepare for death. People who have battled cancer successfully by changing to a WFPB diet.

> "What happens when you eat an apple? The answer is vastly more complex than you can imagine. Every apple contains thousands of antioxidants whose names, beyond a few like vitamin C, are unfamiliar to us, and each of these powerful chemicals has the potential to play an important role in supporting our health…But calculating the specific influence of each of these chemicals isn't nearly sufficient to explain the effect of an apple as a whole."
>
> — T. Colin Campbell, *Whole*

It's a life-changing film that I recommend everyone see.

Nutrition choices may be the biggest changes you make, but becoming an Ageless Boomer means making other smart choices about your nourishment and exercise. You'll also need to give your body nourishment in the form of water (a big enough component of nutrition that it deserves its own chapter), sleep, and sun. You need to protect yourself from poor nutrition that harms you. You'll need regular exercise and meditation that keep your body and mind strong.

In this chapter I'll introduce you to the basic nourishment and exercise of the Ageless Boomer lifestyle. I'll explain each one more extensively later in the book. For now you can get an overview of what to expect and what kind of difference it will make for you.

MODERATION VS. PROGRESS

I will never tell you that moderation is good enough. "Everything in moderation" sounds nice, but most of the time people use moderation as an excuse to compromise the good work they've been doing elsewhere in their lives. If you fall back on "it's OK, I'm just going to have a little," you won't be able to commit to long-term change.

As Campbell says, "Health is more than a few superficial expressions like 'eat a good diet' or 'use the stairs, not the elevator.' Of course there is merit in these statements, but for the most part they dismiss the possibility of real change. They are politically correct statements lacking specificity and substance." If you want great health in your extended third trimester of life, you have to commit to real change.

Progress is a different thing. Making significant lifestyle changes is a transition process—I'll discuss that transition in detail later on. I fully believe you should celebrate the milestones you reach in making good health choices (just celebrate with an apple, not champagne). If your path to good health starts by not eating red meat, celebrate it, especially if you've been eating cheeseburgers for lunch every day for ten years. *But don't stop there!* Don't say, "That's good enough." Set your next goal right away, make a plan to achieve it, and put that plan into action.

Setbacks are part of this process too. Don't let them discourage you. Use it as a lesson—what triggered the setback? Figure out how you can avoid that trigger in the future. In *Forks over Knives*, San'Dera Nation, one of Esselstyn's patients, shared her mantra: "Win the war. Do not let one lost battle end the war. If you do break down and give in to temptation, do not

"Not eating the right foods can cause nutritional stress: Not eating enough natural, unprocessed foods rich in vitamins, minerals, enzymes, high-quality protein, fiber, essential fatty acids, antioxidants, and good bacteria (probiotics) is a major source of stress on our bodies."

— Brendan Brazier, endurance athlete and author of Thrive

27

quit. Just get right back on track. Not tomorrow, but right now."

What's true for nourishment is true for exercise. I don't advise that you do only aerobic exercise and not strength training, or that you only do physical exercise and neglect meditation. Moderation, in these areas, is not positive. But progress is positive. All of the exercise plans I lay out in this book will let you develop at a pace that's safe and comfortable for your body. And if you go backward, "just get right back on track."

NOURISHMENT: GREAT FOOD FOR GREAT HEALTH

Every bite of food you eat is a net positive or a net negative for your body. With each bite you get to decide which way you'll go. When you opt for whole plant foods, you get a net positive. What creates a net negative? Animal products, including dairy. Refined sugar. Refined grains. Added oil and salt. Alcohol and caffeine. The nutrition plan I'm giving you will eliminate all those negatives.

"The ideal human diet looks like this: Consume plant-based foods in forms as close to their natural state as possible ('whole' foods). Eat a variety of vegetables, fruits, raw nuts and seeds, beans and legumes, and whole grains. Avoid heavily processed foods and animal products. Stay away from added salt, oil, and sugar."

— Campbell,

Whole

That list may shock you. Don't stop reading because you think you can't give up those foods. If you're eating a standard American diet, cutting out those foods represents a huge change. Never doubt that it is a worthwhile change. In exchange for giving up unhealthy nourishment, your results will amaze you: energy, health, and strength that you can sustain into your 80s, 90s, 100s, and beyond.

When you look beyond the bad foods to avoid, you'll start to see the vast possibilities of the good foods. Nature's infinite bounty provides nourishment, pleasure, and variety. You'll be able to reawaken your taste buds and discover the flavors that salt, sugar, and fat have masked.

PLANT-BASED EATING

Campbell spells out the basics of the WFPB diet in *Whole*: "The ideal human diet looks like this: Consume plant-based foods in forms as close to their natural state as possible ("whole" foods). Eat a variety of vegetables, fruits, raw nuts and seeds, beans and legumes, and whole grains. Avoid heavily processed foods and animal products. Stay away from added salt, oil, and sugar. Aim to get 80 percent of your calories from carbohydrates, 10 percent from fat, and 10 percent from protein."

I actually believe that it's healthy to get a larger percentage of calories from fat—anywhere from 10 to 40 percent, depending on your weight and physical activity—but keep in mind those fats come from nuts, avocados, and other whole plants. It's not from added oil, even so-called "healthy" oils like olive oil. Any oil concentrates fats but eliminates the other essential nutrients from the whole food, including fiber and protein.

Nutrient density is a key concept in a WFPB diet. That's one reason I follow Campbell in avoiding the terms "vegan" or "vegetarian"— these diets only involve eliminating animal products. You can be a vegan and eat french fries and white bread. A search for "vegan desserts" on Amazon yields no less than a dozen different titles for desserts like cupcakes, pies, and brownies that don't use animal products. But that doesn't make those desserts healthy.

The "V" diets do have one thing in common with WFPB nutrition: eliminating animal products. You could say that if you're eating a WFPB diet you're eating a vegan diet, but you can't say that if you're eating a vegan diet you're eating a WFPB diet.

Why is eliminating animal products so important? Because the most comprehensive nutritional study ever conducted demonstrates that animal protein triggers or worsens every age-related disease: cardiovascular disease, cancer, dementia, diabetes, and more. We know this from Campbell's tour de force study, which he explains in *The China Study*, the layman's book about the academic study he and his colleagues produced.

Spurred by the findings of a massive atlas of cancer rates in China, Campbell and his colleagues studied 65 rural countries in China to compare lifestyle factors, especially nutrition, with health outcomes. They found a consistent correlation between high consumption of animal protein and high rates of cancer, high blood pressure, high cholesterol, heart disease, diabetes, stroke, and more.

On the clinical front, doctors including Caldwell Esselstyn and Joel Fuhrman have consistently demonstrated that when their patients switched from a standard American diet

Experts who support WFPB nutrition:

Neal Barnard, M.D.

Brendan Brazier, triathlete

T. Colin Campbell, Ph.D

Caldwell Esselstyn, M.D.

Ruth Heidrich, Ph.D. and triathlete

Doug Lisle, Ph.D.

John McDougall, M.D.

Lindsay Nixon

Dean Ornish, M.D.

Pam Popper, N.D.

of processed foods and animal products to a WFPB diet, their serious health conditions improved and in most cases disappeared entirely. These are conditions such as heart disease and diabetes.

As we've seen, Boomers have huge risks for developing these diseases. Too many already have them! So it's time to change. Let nutrition be your medicine. Let whole, plant-based foods be your fuel in the amazing machine that is your body. Take charge of your choices so that you can tap its full potential for the rest of your life.

MY CHOICE: RAW PLANTS

My diet emphasizes raw WFPB foods, to the point that at times my diet is 100 percent raw. At other times it's 80 percent raw, and the other 20 percent comes from legumes and lightly steamed vegetables. Eating whole plants raw rather than cooked keeps them closer to their original state, keeps more nutrients intact, and avoids the introduction of toxins through browning or blackening (see Brazier's explanation at left). However, I understand that going 100 percent raw might be hard for you, especially at first.

If you're interested in a raw WFPB diet but you fear you won't be able to sustain it, consider a 50 to 90 percent raw diet. In my journey to 100 percent, there was a period when I was high raw (65 to 80 percent), and I felt great, certainly better than when I ate animal-based foods. Eating a high raw plant-based diet versus a 100 percent raw diet is the difference between feeling like a 9 and a 10 (on a scale of 1 to 10).

"Food cooked at a high temperature can also cause inflammation in the body. As well as destroying enzymes and converting essential fatty acids into trans fats…high-temperature cooking creates advanced glycation end products, or AGEs. The body perceives AGEs as invaders so its immune cells try to break down the AGEs by secreting large amounts of inflammatory agents."

— Brazier,
Thrive

There are a few important points to keep in mind should you want to pursue a high raw diet.

- Consistency is the most important thing: stick to whatever goal you set for yourself. If incorporating some cooked foods, such as legumes and grains, into your diet is the difference between long-term success and failure, by all means consider going with a high-raw diet. You have to find a solution that works for you over time, and consistency trumps purity in this case.
- If you decide to go high raw, make sure that your cooked foods are whole, plant-based foods, like legumes and lightly steamed vegetables. It doesn't do as much good to go 80 percent raw if the other 20 percent of what you consume is cheeseburgers. Following the diet I recommend in the book even 60 percent of the time is still much better than the standard American diet.
- Lentils and legumes (beans) are the next tier of the healthiest foods you can eat after raw fruits, vegetables, nuts, and seeds. They are packed with fiber (both soluble and insoluble), low in fat, and high in nutrients, including protein and

antioxidants. They help regulate your blood sugar, and recent studies indicate that they may help prevent colon cancer. Legumes also keep you full for long periods, making them a great weight loss food. Another bonus? There are a wide range to choose from. Whole grains are also high in fiber and nutrients, though they should comprise the smallest percentage of your WFPB diet.

- When you cook food, try to do so at the lowest possible temperature in order to preserve as many of the nutrients as possible. Lentils and beans, in particular, do not need to be cooked above boiling. Steam vegetables lightly and make sure that they retain their crunch. The higher the temperature at which you cook your food, the more nutrients you will lose and the more toxins you will introduce.

- Plan to eat the cooked portion of your meal after your raw food. A typical day for a high raw foodist might be breakfast that consists of a blended salad (including leafy greens and fruit), a juice containing leafy greens and other vegetables, or a fruit meal, and a lunch of a big multi-vegetable and leafy green salad with ground flax seeds. Dinner might start with a raw salad and end with legumes. However you do it, just remember to eat the raw portion of your meal first.

"Hundreds of population studies show that raw vegetable consumption offers strong protection against cancer ... If consumed in large enough quantities, vegetables and fruits protect against all types of cancers, and raw vegetables have the most powerful anticancer properties of all foods."

— Joel Fuhrman, M.D.,
Eat for Health

- Leafy greens are the most important part of any diet. So if you plan to go high raw, make sure you consume plenty of leafy greens, which will ensure that you are absorbing plenty of fiber, some omega 3s, enzymes, chlorophyll, antioxidants, and other nutrients. Sprinkle some hemp seed and/or freshly ground flax seeds on your salad and you'll be set. Blend flax seed, hemp seed, and other seeds and nuts with tomatoes and onions and use it as a dressing for your salad.

Don't dismiss the raw diet altogether if you don't think you can handle going all the way. High raw is an excellent and viable alternative if you don't think 100 percent raw is for you, and you can still enjoy extensive health benefits.

Modern humans consume many, many substances that interfere with physical and mental function. They prevent us from achieving optimal health and accelerate age-related decline.

ANIMAL PRODUCTS

All our lives Boomers were told to eat our meat and drink our milk. John Wayne made us feel like eating beef was a patriotic duty. But as Campbell, Esselstyn, and others have shown, animal protein is just not good for our bodies.

It's not just about animal fat, although the saturated fat in animal products is particularly dangerous. It doesn't matter if we're talking about lean, cage-free, farm-raised chicken, wild-caught salmon, or fat-free, hormone-free milk from grass-fed cows. Animal protein and good health do not go together.

Brendan Brazier has won a huge following by showing athletes that avoiding meat and dairy and eating nutritious plant-based food is the path to great athletic performance. But he notes that it's not just athletes who benefit: "This diet was no longer just for high-level athletes—it was suitable for all people, no matter their activity level: By helping reduce nutritional stress, and thereby overall stress, the Thrive Diet (a WFPB diet) is beneficial for everyone."

"During my laboratory work with aflatoxin, one line of research showed that even when we had genetically predisposed a mouse or rat to develop liver cancer ... the cancer would develop only in the presence of a high-animal-protein diet. In other words, nutrition trumped environment, even when the environment was particularly nasty."

— Campbell,
Whole

Eliminating animal products from your diet is not as difficult as it might seem. When you replace animal products with nutrient-rich plant foods, you'll find that you're sated, rested, and energized, and you won't miss the meat and dairy at all.

REFINED SUGAR

When Boomers were growing up, our parents told us not to eat sugar because it would give us cavities or a stomach ache. Today, though, we know that the effects of refined sugar go far beyond teeth and stomachs: obesity, diabetes, high cholesterol, and heart disease are all results of too much refined sugar.

In a new documentary, *Fed Up*, executive producer Katie Couric exposes shocking truths about American sugar intake and its effects. For example, in 2012, Americans consumed an average of 765 grams of sugar every 5 days, or 130 pounds each year. The organization Kick the Can, which encourages people to stop consuming sugary beverages, explains that "Sugar-sweetened beverages are the single largest source of added sugars in the American diet, with the average American drinking nearly 45 gallons of sweetened beverages a year, the equivalent of 39 pounds of extra sugar every year."

If you're not sick yet, refined sugar will make you sick. If you are sick, it can kill you.

The WFPB diet offers a delicious alternative: fruit. Nature is packed with sweet options that are healthy too: cherries, figs, apples, bananas, mangoes, papayas, peaches, pineapple—that's just scratching the surface of the natural sweets available to us. When you sate your sweet tooth with nutrient-rich fruit, you won't miss cakes and sodas.

FATS AND OILS

As most Americans know by now, trans fats are about the worst form of fat you could consume. They're like heart-attack time bombs, helping create plaques that will pop, block arteries, and give you a heart attack or stroke.

Unfortunately, many Americans then think that any non-trans-fat is fine, especially if it's an unsaturated fat. We need to understand that the sheer caloric density of processed fats and oils throws off the body's ability to track satiation, leading us to overeat.

Forks over Knives uses a simple graphic to explain the way different foods signal receptors in the stomach that we're full. Five hundred calories of nutrition-dense foods from plants fill the stomach, but five hundred calories of fat (about five ounces) fills only a small portion of the stomach. Therefore people overeat just to feel full.

PROCESSED FOODS

We've talked about sugar and fat—what's left to say about processed foods? Plenty.

Processed foods, by which I mean any food that has been fried, condensed, powdered, enriched, bleached, or any of the many changes that companies make to whole foods to make them more "appealing," are primary sources of added fat and refined sugar. They are also sources of excess salt, preservatives, and refined grains.

No one should eat refined grains, which take whole plant foods and crush out the fiber, bleach out the nutrients, and bake out any remaining nutritional value. Refined grains affect the body in the same way as refined sugar, creating a burst of energy that opens the door for inflammation and fat accumulation. If you eat grains, make sure they are whole grains or grain-like seeds.

Salt is necessary for human life, but plant foods are already full of salt. We can get all the salt we need from plants, and anything more contributes to an imbalance that can trigger high blood pressure.

Preservatives have been linked to breathing problems and increased hyperactivity in children, but processed foods are packed with so many different preservatives in so many different combinations that we can't assume we've uncovered all the possible effects. If you're eating a WFPB diet, you don't have to worry about it— the only preserving device you'll need is your refrigerator.

CAFFEINE

Fifty years ago, caffeine was synonymous with coffee. Coffee was, and is, America's favorite stimulant. But today coffee competes with sodas, energy drinks, energy "shots," and other sources to keep America hopped up.

These days, drinks like coffee and tea are being touted for their health benefits. In *Super*

Immunity, Dr. Joel Fuhrman discusses the strange phenomenon of coffee reducing the risk of diabetes. He explains the sad truth of this benefit: "It is most likely that the standard American diet is so nutrient-poor that a significant portion of people's phytochemical intake comes from their morning coffee! ...It is doubtful that coffee would offer any additional protection on top of a nutrient-dense diet."

Caffeine, first and foremost, is an artificial stimulant. It's a drug that silences important messages from your body—fatigue, lack of focus, and sleepiness. If you think you need caffeine to function, that's because you're consistently ignoring your body's cries for help in the form of better sleep and nutrition.

On top of that, long-term caffeine consumption creates strain on the adrenal glands, the organs that produce the stress hormone cortisol. The adrenal glands are responsible for our critical fight or flight response, but caffeine, like chronic stress, stimulates the release of cortisol that we don't need and in fact damages our bodies in many ways. High blood pressure, high blood sugar, and adrenal damage are all long-term effects of caffeine use.

"The fact that coffee is shown to have some phytochemical benefits offering a degree of protection against one disease or another does not make coffee a health food. Caffeine is still a drug. It is a stimulant—it gives you a false sense of increased energy, allowing you to get by with an inadequate amount of sleep...Inadequate sleep promotes disease and premature aging, and can fuel overeating behaviors."

— Joel Fuhrman, MD,
    Super Immunity

As an Ageless Boomer, you won't need caffeine. When you switch to a WFPB diet and you start giving your body adequate nourishment, you'll find that you have energy and focus without artificial stimulants.

"Alcohol does all kinds of things in the body, and we're not fully aware of all its effects. It's a pretty complicated little molecule."

— James C. Garbutt, MD,
    professor of psychiatry at the University of North Carolina at Chapel Hill School of Medicine

ALCOHOL

By this time in your life, you know someone, maybe many people, who have suffered serious addictions to alcohol. You may be a recovering alcoholic yourself. You know that alcohol can be dangerously addictive.

The National Institutes of Health report that nearly 85,000 people die every year from alcohol-related causes. "In 2009," they state, "liver cirrhosis was the twelfth-leading cause of death in the United States, with a total of 31,522 deaths—664 more than in 2008." Even though we know how dangerous alcohol can be, Americans still drink huge amounts of alcohol every year.

"Alcohol does all kinds of things in the body, and we're not fully aware of all its effects," says James C. Garbutt, MD, professor of psychiatry at the University of North Carolina at Chapel Hill School of Medicine and a researcher at the university's Bowles Center for Alcohol Studies (in an interview with WebMD). "It's a pretty complicated little molecule." WebMD identifies twelve health risks linked to chronic heavy drinking: anemia, cancer, cardiovascular disease, cirrhosis, dementia, depression, seizures, gout, high blood pressure, infectious disease, nerve damage, and pancreatitis.

Like coffee, red wine has been touted as a health food because it contains the powerful antioxidant reservatrol. But like coffee, it's most likely only a "health food" because the standard American diet is so nutrient-poor. If you eat lots of red fruits like grapes, berries, and cherries, you are going to get all the health benefits of reservatrol with none of the risks of alcohol.

"Seaweeds are rich in iodine, vitamins, and other protective substances. Iodine not only protects the thyroid from radioactive carcinogens, it supports the adrenal glands, helps with digestion, and improves immunity. Common edible seaweeds include nori, wakame, dombhu, arame, dulse, hijiki, kelp, and agar agar."

— Stephen Sinatra, MD

RADIATION

Older Baby Boomers like me grew up with the fears of the Cold War and nuclear bombs. Since then, we've all learned to be afraid of "radiation." Scientifically, the term radiation refers any kind of electromagnetic wave, but when we talk about radiation as a health concern, we're interested in ionizing radiation, the kind that can do damage to our cells.

According to the United Nations Scientific Committee on the Effects of Atomic Radiation, globally about 80 percent of the ionizing radiation in our environment is natural—it comes from outside the earth in the form of cosmic radiation and from the earth itself in the form of naturally occurring radioactive substances. The other 20 percent comes from man-made sources, in particular from medical imaging (e.g., x-rays, CT scans).

The best defense against radiation is—you guessed it—nutrition. Radiation is one of many stressors that increase cancer-causing free radicals in the body. Antioxidant-rich fruits and vegetables neutralize those free radicals, protecting your cells from damage. You can also limit your exposure by not having unnecessary imaging done to your body. Taking the Ageless Boomer approach to optimal health will help reduce the need for medical care that requires radiation imaging.

It's worth noting that the biggest source of radiation—not ionizing radiation—in our lives is the sun. We've all heard the warnings about UV radiation and skin cancer, and research has certainly demonstrated a link there. However, sunscreen and sun avoidance are not the only ways to reduce skin cancer risk, and both of those approaches cut you off from the benefits of sunlight. I'll talk more about this debate later in this chapter.

TOBACCO

If you want to be an Ageless Boomer but you're using any kind of tobacco, quitting tobacco needs to be your number one priority. I want you to embrace all of these other changes as well, but if you don't quit smoking (or chewing), then you won't see the benefits from better nourishment and exercise. You're putting poison into your system—you can't thrive until you stop.

Food is one of several critical sources of nourishment your body needs. It requires a lot of discussion because our environment is so full of poor nutrition choices that it can be difficult to navigate our way to good choices. The other sources—water, sleep, and sunlight—are vitally important, but for the most part you know how to get these things. We can, however, find ways to get this nourishment in higher quality or greater amounts.

WATER

Drink plenty of clean, pure, filtered water. As I explain in more detail in the "Water" chapter, water enables our body to work more efficiently in a variety of ways, one of which is our ability to burn fat. If you don't drink enough water, you can't eliminate waste as effectively, and the liver then gets called in to cleanse you of those toxins. But what the liver really should be doing is metabolizing fat so you don't store it. By drinking enough water and eating water-rich foods, the liver can focus on its real job, which means less fat stored on your body. Also, you may actually be thirsty when you think you're hungry, so have a glass of water before reaching for that snack.

SLEEP

Most of us underestimate the importance of sleep. Thanks to electricity, we have become accustomed to pursuing many activities after dark, and the modern age is full of diversions and distractions that lure us out around the clock. We have in-home entertainment centers, news 24/7, and work encroaching on us at all hours. We rely on caffeine and various other stimulants to fight our natural fatigue, and the modern age encourages us to go-go-go all the time. We've lost all respect for our natural circadian rhythms.

> "The cells of a hydrated body swell, causing an anabolic response (growth of muscle tissue), speeding up cellular renewal. As well, hydrated cells remain alkaline. A catabolic response (breakdown of muscle tissue) will occur if the cells become dehydrated, advancing degeneration."
>
> — Brazier,
> Thrive

Instead of taking fatigue as a sign that our body needs to rest and recuperate, we fight it all the way—with bright lights, loud music, stimulants such as coffee and energy drinks, and more. But pushing our body beyond its natural limits diminishes our mental and physical capacities in the short term and takes an inevitable toll on our health in the long run.

SUNLIGHT

As I mentioned in the discussion of radiation, sunlight is the largest source of radiation in our lives, but it's not ionizing radiation. The debate about how to balance the risks and benefits of sun exposure is raging strong in the medical community.

One thing we know is that sunlight is our best source for vitamin D, a critical nutrient. Supplements containing vitamin D, including fortified milk, which you should avoid anyway, aren't absorbed by our bodies as well as naturally produced vitamin D from sun exposure. A 2005 study by Ashraf Zadshir and colleagues found that a large number of Americans, especially minority Americans, didn't have enough vitamin D in their diets.

For my part, I try to spend plenty of time in the sun and I use antioxidant-rich foods to protect myself from sunburn. If you or your family members have a history of skin cancer, you have to decide for yourself how to handle sun exposure. But even ten minutes of sun exposure a day can help you create all the vitamin D you need.

EXERCISE:
THE ACTIVE BODY AT ANY AGE

One of the worst excuses people make for not exercising is "I don't have time." No, you don't have time to NOT exercise. If you don't engage in regular physical activity, you're shortening your life. You might save minutes but lose years. And the years you keep will be far less healthy.

So let's get moving, and let's remember the most important thing about it—it should be enjoyable and interesting! Enjoy your body and its many abilities; the more you do, the more you will be able to do.

WALKING: CARDIO FOR EVERYONE

Could any form of exercise be more natural than walking? Walking is accessible to everyone, and no matter what your fitness level, you can start walking now and increase your health over time. Many Boomers worry about stress on their joints from exercise, but walking is low-impact and can be a great cardiovascular exercise. You won't hurt yourself walking.

In addition, I'm going to introduce you to the idea of walking with "Nordic sticks" or poles. Not only do these ples increase the overall aerobic value of walking by incorporating your upper body, they also give you additional supports to make walking on uneven terrain safer.

"Walking is one of our most natural and fundamental physical activities. Natural because our bodies have evolved to do it easily, efficiently, and comfortably. Fundamental because it's at the root of how we move around every day."

— Mark Fenton,
    The Complete Guide to Walking

And I hope you'll take your walking out into wilder natural spaces. Walking itself is beneficial for the body wherever you do it, but putting yourself in a natural, plant-filled, quiet setting is beneficial for your mind and soul.

REBOUNDING: SPRING IN YOUR STEP

Remember how much you loved to bounce on your bed as a kid? One of my favorite exercises is rebounding, which involves bouncing on a mini-trampoline. This simple bouncing motion does the body a world of good and helps to strengthen cells. The process of acceleration and deceleration with gravity also helps flush out the lymphatic system, aids with digestion and elimination, improves balance and coordination, circulates more oxygen to your tissues, and keeps bones strong. And all these benefits come from a low-impact exercise that doesn't stress your joints.

It's also a wonderful form of relaxation. In fact, it's so meditative that I often incorporate gentle rebounding (feet don't leave the mat) into my pre-sleep ritual. Last but not least, it's fun!

BODY-WEIGHT EXERCISE: STRENGTH TRAINING FOR ANY TIME, PLACE, OR BODY

You don't need a gym or any kind of fancy equipment to get a strong body. You just need to know how to use your own body weight and resistance to build your strength. I'll describe two kinds of body-weight exercises: slow-motion resistance (SMR) and calisthenics. They're both good and work together well.

SMR is the simplest, most effective, most portable method of strength training I have ever found, and I think I've tried just about every kind of strength training out there. It's portable because there aren't any machines or weights involved—you're just using one muscle to oppose another. It's simple—a handful of exercises will work all of the areas of your body. And it's effective—by doing these exercises consistently, you will increase your lean muscle and increase your strength-to-weight ratio, the most important measure of strength.

All of these exercises give you the opportunity to start slow and work up to more difficult levels. And as your body grows in strength, you'll be able to apply more resistance, so these exercises will increase in challenge as you increase in strength.

I'll also discuss calisthenics like push-ups, which you can scale to your level of strength. If you don't have enough strength to do one push up, you can start by doing push-ups against the wall. When you have enough strength, you can start doing them against a counter or table. Eventually you can start doing them on the floor military-style.

Don't be put off by the word "meditation" if it conjures up images of New Age crystal shops and patchouli incense. If you don't want to think of this mental work as meditation, don't. Meditation is part of a larger process to increase health by reducing stress.

While mindful meditation has been practiced around the world for millennia, medical practitioners are increasingly embracing various forms of "mindfulness" therapies to help people experiencing depression, dementia, and other conditions. It's important to remember that mindfulness is not restricted to sitting cross-legged in a quiet space, although that approach works for many people. Mindful walking and exercising (like tai chi or yoga) help some people more than sitting.

I'll guide you through some of my favorite techniques later in the book. I encourage you to try them and explore your own preferences to find the stress-reducing mindful meditation that works best for you.

"Stress is like fire: When controlled and used for a purpose, it serves us well. Left unbridled, it can consume us. In amounts that our body is capable of adapting to, certain stresses are beneficial. Exercise, for example, is a stress. Exercise and then rest, and your body will grow stronger. However, stress has become, now more than ever, a real threat to our health and livelihood, often overwhelming us and, in some cases, even controlling us."

—Brazier,
  Thrive

John Donne wrote, "No man is an island,/Entire of itself,/Every man is a piece of the continent,/A part of the main." Human beings are social creatures, and our health is directly impacted by our social connections. A 1988 article in *Science* reported that social connections might have a greater influence on health than obesity, smoking, and high blood pressure.

As important as they are, social connections are not always easy. You have to work on relationships the same way you work on exercise or meditation. You may have wonderful relationships with your family members, or you might have terrible relationships with them. Or, like many people, your relationships may be somewhere in between, a source of both happiness and stress.

Whether you're friends with your family or you've made friends who have become your family, it is vital to your health that you maintain and strengthen those relationships. If you don't have many connections, look for ways to build more. These connections will help you stave off dementia, depression, and many other diseases exacerbated by stress and loneliness.

And there you have it—the overview of what it takes to become an Ageless Boomer. All these benefits are within your reach because none of these approaches are difficult. They may seem strange now, but as you try them and you begin to see the results, you'll be thrilled to discover that these new ideas become the new normal, and you won't look back.

PART 2

CHAPTER 4

NOURISHMENT: THE BUILDING BLOCKS OF LONG-TERM HEALTH

■ ■ ■

The substances you put into your body have a profound impact on your health and longevity. You've heard this a hundred times, but have you taken action yet? Reward your body with the food, water, sleep, and sunlight that will keep it strong and healthy. Stop starving yourself of the nourishment you need.

CHOOSE NOURISHMENT AND GAIN HEALTH

You are what you eat, the old saying goes. I would add that you are what you eat, drink, and do. Your body is the result of all the good and bad choices you make about what you consume, what you spend your day doing, and even what you think about (especially if you dwell on things that make you angry or anxious).

The Four Essential Sources of Nourishment:

Food

Water

Sleep

Sunshine

Part II of this book is called "Nourishment," inspired by Hippocrates' quote, "If we could give every individual the right amount of nourishment and exercise, not too little and not too much, we would have found the safest way to health." Nourishment is mostly about food, but also about a few other things you need to keep your body and your mind healthy.

FOUR SOURCES OF NOURISHMENT

Food and water, sleep and sunshine. Your body's most basic needs are as simple and ancient as the human race itself. Even older, in fact—almost every animal needs these basic things to survive and thrive.

These sources of nourishment don't exist in isolation from one another. They interact at every level: without water we couldn't digest our food; sunlight gives you vitamin D so that you can absorb the calcium in your food; sleep allows our metabolism to recharge and convert our food into energy; sunlight helps our brains regulate our sleep hormones so that we sleep better.

To be an Ageless Boomer, you need to get high-quality nourishment and enough of it. When you have balanced amounts of good nourishment, the result is a leaner, stronger, healthier, and more vital body and mind.

FOOD: LEAVE OUT THE BAD, PUT IN THE GOOD

As I explained in Chapter 3, you can make huge improvements in your body's health, strength, and energy by changing the foods you eat. Many of my recommendations will seem familiar: you already know that you should eat a wide variety of fruits and vegetables. You may even know that these foods supply essential micronutrients, including vitamins, minerals, antioxidants, enzymes, and more. What you may not know is that fruits, vegetables, seeds, and nuts contain all the macronutrients you need to thrive: fat, protein, and carbohydrates. I'll break down some of the biggest myths about these nutrients and explain how you can get everything you need in a plant-strong diet.

"Plant-strong" is a phrase used by authors such as Rip Esselstyn, author of *The Engine 2 Diet* and *My Beef with Meat*. I want you to think of whole-food, plant-based (WFPB) eating as plant-strong: not only is WFPB eating strong in plants, it also strengthens your body and your health. When you look at vegetables you're buying at the market or store, see them for the strong building blocks they are.

Q: WHY SHOULD I EAT A PLANT-STRONG DIET?

A: In a nutshell, studies have linked the consumption of animal products to all kinds of diseases—cancer, heart disease, diabetes, etc. Other studies have shown that if you want to protect yourself against obesity, gout, arthritis, kidney stones, and all manner of other ailments, you'll go 100 percent plant-based, preferably high raw. Plant-based eating is good for your own health, for the environment, and for the treatment of animals.

I asked my friend Jon Hinds, founder of the Monkey Bar gym, trainer to professional athletes, and gold medalist in jiu-jitsu, what book he would choose if he could recommend only one book on healthy nutrition. While John is good friends with T. Colin Campbell and greatly admires *The China Study*, he recommended *Your Healthy Journey* by Fred Bisci. (I hope that *Ageless Boomers* will become one of his favorites, as well.) Bisci is thriving in his eighties, still doing long-distance runs and enjoying a vibrant life. Bisci's slim book is filled with great nuggets of advice, but the primary lesson comes down to two things:

- What you leave out
- What you put in

I've used those phrases in the titles of chapters 5 and 6 because I am inspired by the concept. Healthier nutrition comes from leaving out unhealthy foods and adding in healthy foods. It makes sense: if you eat more healthy foods, you won't have room for the unhealthy foods.

Bisci emphasizes that what you leave out makes a bigger difference than what you leave in, so if you're not sure about how to begin, start by avoiding the foods that hurt your body: animal products, processed foods, and foods cooked at high temperatures. I'll explain more about all these foods in Chapter 5.

Of course, once you take those foods out of your diet, you'll need to fill in those calories with other foods. That's where "what you put in" becomes important. In Chapter 6 I'll give you some more details about these terrific foods and some advice on how to incorporate them into your eating plan.

WATER: YOUR MOST BASIC NEED

Water is life, but many of us exist in a state of low-grade dehydration because we don't drink enough water. The simple step of drinking enough pure water (and consuming it through foods and juices) can give you a huge bump in your health and energy. In Chapter 6 I'll discuss some of your body's cues that it needs water and how to ensure that you're getting enough.

SLEEP: REPLENISH YOUR BODY AND MIND

Sleep is one of the greatest victims of our modern lifestyle. As wonderful as electricity is, our wired society has eroded the quality of our sleep. Televisions, bright lights, tablets, mobile phones, and other sources of light, sound, and stimulation throw off our natural rhythms, making it difficult to fall asleep and stay asleep. What's more, we undervalue sleep, so when we have a lot to accomplish, we sacrifice sleep; when we sacrifice sleep, we sacrifice our health in the short term and the long term.

"Many things that we take for granted are affected by sleep. If you sleep better, you can certainly live better. It's pretty clear."

— Raymonde Jean, MD, director of sleep medicine and associate director of critical care, St. Luke's-Roosevelt Hospital Center, New York City, in Health magazine

Chapter 7 will discuss the value of sleep as well as simple changes you can make to get more high-quality sleep (yes, you need quality as well as quantity when it comes to sleep!). When you put these changes into practice you'll notice immediate benefits, and you'll build the foundation of long-term health.

SUNSHINE: LIGHT UP YOUR LIFE

Sunshine has gotten a bad reputation in the past few decades as dermatologists proclaim that even a tiny amount of sunlight each day puts us at risk for skin cancer. What we don't hear about is the benefits of sunlight, from regulating sleep and reducing depression to providing us with the essential nutrient vitamin D. In fact, sunlight is the safest and most effective source of vitamin D. In Chapter 8 we'll take a look at these benefits and the much-discussed risks so that you can make an informed choice about your sun exposure.

START YOUR TRANSITION TODAY

You don't have to wait to start feeling better. You can start today. If you love sweets, you can start feeling better immediately by cutting down your intake of refined sugar and replacing it with fiber-rich whole fruit. You will feel the difference within hours as your blood sugar maintains an even level instead of spiking and crashing.

Other benefits will take more time, but they will come. It can take weeks to see a major drop in blood pressure or cholesterol, but it will happen (some people do see a dramatic change almost immediately). The increase in your overall energy level happens slowly as your body gets used to easier digestion and increased amounts of bioavailable nutrients. If you're looking to lose weight, that change will happen steadily if you choose a WFPB diet (if you go cold turkey, you will almost certainly loose a good amount right away; more on that later in this chapter). Transitions can be difficult and stressful—especially life transitions that have the potential to effect great change, such the transition to a whole-food plant-based (WFPB) diet. This change will make you reframe your thoughts about yourself, about your priorities, about your relationships with food and exercise, and about your world. As Brendan Brazier points out in *Thrive*, making lots of big changes at once can put your body under a lot of stress, and stress is not healthy.

Know that *you* are in control of this change. You can make the transition easier with preparation and some simple tools:

- Choose the right approach for you
- Learn about your food options
- Pay attention to your body

Remember that setbacks are okay, as long as you acknowledge them and keep moving forward with your eyes on the main objective: becoming the Ageless version of yourself.

Take three steps to start your transition:

Choose the right approach for you

Learn about your food options

Pay attention to your body

"Know thyself" is an ancient Greek saying that holds true today. And one advantage of being a little older is that you know yourself better. You have the benefit of experience and you know how you will deal with change.

Do you commit 100 percent to a change and stick with it, no matter the obstacles? Do you commit to a change and then find yourself discouraged, at which point you abandon that change? Are you a person who likes to try new things, or are you a person who avoids change? At this point in your life, you know the answers to these questions, so choose your path accordingly.

I've outlined two approaches to adopting a WFPB diet: "cold turkey" and "easing in." Read about them and decide what approach you think will be most successful for you. I would love to see everybody on a WFPB diet as quickly as possible, but I would rather see you get there slowly than not get there at all.

APPROACH 1: COLD TURKEY

When I switched to a vegan diet, I didn't go cold turkey: I allowed myself "cheat days" to eat other foods. If I had to do it again, though, I would commit to a fully WFPB diet at once because I would have felt so much better, so much faster. When you go cold turkey, the benefits hit you between the eyes. It can be hard to make the big change all at once, but if you do, you'll feel like a different person within a day or two.

Joel Fuhrman, author of bestsellers *Super Immunity* and *Eat to Live*, recommends a fairly rapid shift to a plant-based diet in both books. Fuhrman wrote *Eat to Live* for everyone, but especially for people with heart disease, diabetes, and other chronic diseases who needed to change their diets to save their lives. Cardiologist Caldwell Esselstyn, who helped put the nutrition-based cure for heart disease on the map, insists that his patients go cold turkey. He points out that after a few weeks, they're rewarded by decreased chest pain, increased mobility, and weight loss. But you don't need to be suffering from a chronic disease to see dramatic results.

"A phytochemically deficient diet is largely responsible for a weak immune system. Populations with a much higher intake of vegetables have much lower rates of cancer, and the longest-living populations throughout history have been those with the highest intake of vegetables in the diet."

—Joel Fuhrman, MD,
Super Immunity

Most of the experts on WFPB eating suggest that you commit to an all plant-based diet sooner rather than later. If you're feeling gun shy, they suggest you keep to it for set span of time, usually three weeks to a month. Caldwell Esselstyn's son Rip is a world-class triathlete and former firefighter who has authored two books on WFPB eating, including *The Engine 2 Diet: The Texas Firefighters' 28-Day Save-Your-Life Plan that Lowers Cholesterol and Burns Away the Pounds.*

His diet plan differs from mine in a few areas, but the gist is the same: give your body one month on a WFPB diet and you will not believe how much better you'll feel.

For many years after I switched to a vegan diet, I let myself eat whatever I wanted one day each week. That one day, I would go crazy, eating out at restaurants, indulging in pizza or steak, cake or candy. But over time I realized I wasn't enjoying those days as much as I once had and always paid the price the next day or two. I noticed that my body reacted strongly to those heavy, cooked, processed foods, basically rejecting them. My body was sending me a powerful message.

Gradually, I came to associate those foods not with good times, but instead with lethargy. And I found myself starting to skip my one day of indulgence each week. I simply didn't need or want it anymore.

I actually crave the foods in my diet now. I can go off to the best steakhouse in the world (Peter Lugers in Brooklyn, New York, in case you want to know) with friends, and I don't even crave the steaks and home fries that my friends order. I bring my own salad and some seeds and nuts or a trail mix, and I am utterly content. My taste buds have adapted, and they're not leading me down the path to temptation.

It took me several years to go 100 percent raw (WFPB with no cooked foods), which I continue for sometimes months at a time before I go back to eating WFPB cooked foods like lentils,

legumes, and lightly steamed vegetables. But had I known then what I know now, I wouldn't have made so many mistakes and it wouldn't have taken me as long to get here.

If you go cold turkey, you'll have more energy and probably find that you need less sleep. You may even find that you won't need that cup of coffee in the morning that you once did. You will gradually find that you are getting hooked on feeling good. It will get progressively easier to resist temptation, as you'll find that you're not craving the unhealthy food that makes you feel lousy.

Please note that the cold turkey approach does not have to happen in one day—the transition process may still take you a few weeks. You can even use the approach I describe next, just at a faster pace. If you want to feel the fullest benefits of the change to WFPB eating, aim to achieve a fully WFPB diet within about three weeks.

APPROACH 2: EASE INTO THIS NEW LIFESTYLE

Fuhrman also wrote a book called *Eat for Health* that explains how you can gradually introduce more and more WFPB eating (Fuhrman's term is "nutritarian") into your diet over the course of many months. There are a number of ways you can ease into this new lifestyle. Take the transition to a plant-based diet in stages to give your body a chance to adjust and

"This is the biggest obstacle to the adoption of a plant-based diet: most people who hear about it don't seriously consider it, despite the truly impressive health benefits.

"If you are one of these people ... then I know that no amount of talk will ever convince you to change your mind.

"You have to try it."

— T. Colin Campbell,
The China Study

detoxify gradually. Start with only one meal a day and work up from there.

Ease in Step By Step

Step 1. Replace your heavy breakfast with a green breakfast juice or blended salad.

Step 2. Replace your morning snack with fresh fruits.

Step 3. Replace your lunch with a big salad.

Step 4. Replace your afternoon snack with fruit.

Step 5. Replace your dinner with a WFPB meal, which can be a salad, vegetable soup, cooked whole grains and legumes, etc.

If you choose the gradual method, breakfast is the best meal to start with. I highly recommend vegetable juice as a way to jumpstart your day. You'll immediately begin to enjoy the benefits of renewed vigor and vitality, and that will encourage you to stay the course. If you're not quite ready for 100 percent green juice (which is my personal favorite), start with a sweeter mixture, such as half carrot, half leafy greens, with celery or cucumber. It's very palatable for a beginner and has a sweet, mellow flavor, thanks to the carrots. Be sure not to eat any other food for at least half an hour after your vegetable juice (I usually wait an hour or two because I exercise after my vegetable juice). The idea is to have your first meal quickly absorbed into the bloodstream without digestive stress and not to have it slowed down by anything else.

Whatever you do, it's a mistake to start with a heavy breakfast (by heavy I mean dairy, grains, and meat). Your body has to stop the elimination cycle to digest a heavy breakfast. And since it has had to stop working on eliminating waste from the previous day, you'll end up with an accumulation of toxic waste. Starting the day off on the standard American diet basically throws everything off course. So start out strong, with vegetable juice or even just some of your favorite organic, ripe, in-season raw fruit, and then progressively add in denser foods over the course of the day. It won't take long for you to start feeling more energetic than you've felt in years.

After you've gotten used to having your morning vegetable juice, try to eat only fruit until one hour before lunch. Fruit is ideal, because it's high in fiber that works like a broom, sweeping the waste right out of your body.

Once you've gotten your morning routine set, plan on having a big salad for lunch. For a high-energy day, snack on fruit until dinner. You can go from melons to citrus to apples to bananas in the afternoon (moving from the least dense to the densest fruits).

At each stage of this transition, you should be eating less and less processed food and animal food. Refined sugar, white flour, refined grains, meats, and dairy should start to give way to whole, plant-strong foods.

By this point, you're almost there! Now you can start changing your dinners. Try to have just WFPB fare at dinner (lentils, beans, quinoa, or buckwheat) along with raw or lightly steamed vegetables (so they maintain a slight crunch). Once you adjust to that routine, you can try to have one raw dinner each week, i.e., a large salad with a seed or nut dressing. I like blending tomatoes with scallions and seeds and/or nuts.

The idea is to eat the highest water-content foods early in the day, which will give you lots of energy. Toward the end of the day, you can consume some foods that are denser because you won't need quite as much energy before bedtime.

I follow this daily model of increasingly dense foods even on my exclusively plant-based diet: I drink my vegetable juice first, then fruits during the day, and save the seeds, nuts, or avocado salad or cooked grains and legumes for the last meal of the day.

Right now you may be thinking that this diet is limiting, but if you take the time to learn about the astonishing variety of fruits, vegetables, seeds, and nuts out there, you'll find no end of satisfying foods. Spend extra time in the produce aisle. Read WFPB books and websites. Try newly ripe, in-season organic fruits and vegetables you've never tasted before. Experiment with different combinations. In short, take the time to educate yourself. Your efforts will open up a whole new world for you and eliminate any sense of deprivation.

RECIPES VS. MEAL CREATION

You won't find a lot of recipes in this book because I don't cook from recipes. To me, recipes just add confusion to the process of meal planning. However, I recognize that for a lot of people in our generation, following a recipe is the preferred way to put a meal together.

A recipe is just a set of instructions. Certain types of food (not the types I'm recommending, mind you) need a lot of careful instructions to make them turn out the right way. These foods involve a lot of chemical processes—combining acids and alkalines, emulsifying fats, heating ingredients, and so on—and without instructions, you can do things wrong.

WFPB eating is so much simpler than traditional cooking. The only cooking you'll do is gently steam vegetables or simmer beans. It's extremely basic; you just need to know how to heat water.

Instead of putting your time and energy into complicated recipes, you can put it into beautiful presentation. Plant foods are beautiful—their intense colors, interesting shapes, and diverse textures make meal preparation an enjoyable and creative experience. You can play with different flavor combinations to create a meal you've never had before. (When you're starting out, I recommend following the food combining rules in Chapter 10. Once you're used to WFPB eating, you can combine your foods much more freely. You should pay attention to how your body feels after you finish a particular combination and discover what works well for you and what doesn't.)

ENJOY THE UNBELIEVABLE VARIETY

You might worry that you're limiting yourself by excluding animal products from your diet, but consider this: I can count on my fingers the number of animal foods in a typical American's diet. It's chicken, beef, pork, fish, turkey, eggs, and milk products. That's not a lot of variety.

Vegetables and fruits, however, come in a staggering array of species, and different varieties within those species! For a small sampling, take a look at my food pyramid in Chapter 6. Try new things: apples, oranges, and bananas are great, but don't forget about pineapples, berries, melons, pomegranates, kiwis, pears, and many other fruits. Keep the carrots, celery, tomatoes, and cucumbers, but try the bok choy, artichokes, kale, watercress, beets, radishes, and all the other wonderful veggies available to you. Herbs like cilantro, parsley, rosemary, and basil are delicious, nutrient-rich herbs you can add to your meals.

Another thing to experiment with is alternative flavorings. For instance, I use dulse (a kind of seaweed) on my salads instead of salt. The dulse is packed with nutrients and doesn't have any of the negative side effects that come with salt (for example, dehydration, high blood pressure, and high acidity). I also use avocado as a salad dressing instead of oil and vinegar. If you mash it to a smooth paste, it works well as an alternative to traditional dressing, but you're still consuming a whole food rather than an extracted oil. You can also try combining avocado and an acid fruit, such as tomatoes or raspberries. Try using lemon instead of vinegar. If you'd like a smoother dressing, you can throw your dressing ingredients in the blender.

Try this terrific dressing: use tomatoes as a base (as many as you need depending on their size) and add hemp seed, flax seed, walnuts, almonds, and a whole bunch of scallions (green onions). Put it all in a blender and blend until smooth. It's the best dressing I've ever had in my life! It also delivers all your omega 3 fatty acids in one go.

Q: WHAT ABOUT SALT?

A: Humans do need salt to live, but most Americans are eating far more salt than they need, and much more than is healthy. I say throw away the salt shaker.

Humans also need iodine to live, and iodized salt has become our primary source of that mineral. Brenda Davies, author of *Becoming Vegan* and *Becoming Raw*, writes, "Several studies suggest that vegans who avoid iodized salt may be at risk for iodine deficiency. Vegetarian diets that are rich in foods containing natural goitrogens, such as soybeans, cruciferous vegetables, sweet potatoes, millet, and raw flaxseed may reduce iodine uptake. However, these foods only appear problematic when iodine intake is inadequate. The adult RDA for iodine is 150 mcg, and can easily be met with one-half teaspoon of iodized salt daily." So a tiny amount of table salt covers that need.

If you're following my suggestions, though, you do need a source of iodine, and luckily sea vegetables are great sources. "Seaweeds are ... rich iodine sources and are an excellent choice for those wishing to limit sodium consumption. Only one-tenth of a teaspoon of kelp powder per day is necessary to provide the RDA of 150 mcg iodine," Davies explains. Don't go overboard, though: "The upper limit for iodine is 1100 mcg, which can be exceeded with large intakes of seaweed."

RAW, HIGH-RAW, AND COOKED

In my diet, I prioritize raw foods over cooked foods. There are times when I eat a 100 percent raw diet, but other times I eat what's called a high-raw diet, where 60-80 percent of your food is raw and 20-40 percent is cooked. I recommend a high-raw diet because you get so many wonderful micronutrients from raw food. However, whole foods that are gently cooked (no hotter than boiling) are just fine, and in some cases are beneficial. For example, beans are wonderfully nutritious, but without cooking, most beans are inedible.

Likewise, most grains require cooking or sprouting. Personally, I don't eat very much grain—I prefer to eat foods more densely packed with micronutrients, so I stick to vegetables, fruits, seeds, nuts, and cooked legumes. I do occasionally eat some grain-like seeds such as quinoa, buckwheat, and amaranth. These seeds are commonly mistaken for grains because their texture when cooked is similar to grain.

But whole grains are a staple in the diets of some of the longest-lived people in the world, as John Robbins explains in his book *Healthy at 100*. Robbins looks at the lifestyles of four groups of people, scattered around the globe, who routinely live healthy, vital lives in their eighties, nineties, and beyond. It's a wonderful book, and I highly recommend it.

All of the people he researched eat large amounts of fresh fruits and vegetables as well as whole grains. They eat little to no animal products. The elders of Okinawa, Japan, eat 32 percent of their diet in grains, while Americans eat only 11 percent of their diet in grains. And those grains aren't equal—the elders of Okinawa eat almost exclusively whole grains while Americans eat almost exclusively refined grains.

Whole grains can be somewhat nutritious, but refined grains cannot. Refined grains strip away all the fiber and micronutrients in the germ and bran, leaving only the starchy interior. Those starches, uncoupled from fiber, will spike your blood sugar and cause inflammation and weight gain just as surely as white sugar.

I also recommend grain-like seeds. Quinoa is often mistakenly regarded as a grain, and it substitutes well for rice in many dishes, so it's an excellent choice as you start out. Buckwheat, which is also a seed and has no relation to wheat at all, is also acceptable.

Quinoa (pronounced KEEN-wah): A seed that, when cooked, has a very grain-like texture. It's delicious, easily digested, and protein-packed.

Raw diet: A WFPB diet with no cooked foods.

High-raw diet: A WFPB diet with 60-80 percent raw foods and 20-40 percent cooked foods.

Legumes (beans and lentils) are terrific foods that require some cooking. Lentils, which don't require presoaking, and black or pinto beans are among the best. Black beans and quinoa is a delicious dish for WFPB eating; if you mix in a little avocado too, it tastes great.

High-raw (60-80 percent raw) is an excellent goal. If you eat cooked foods, it's not so much what you're eating, but what you're not eating that is important. Grains and legumes are much better than the processed and refined foods that make up the standard American diet.

Q. IS RICE SAFE? I'VE HEARD IT CONTAINS ARSENIC.

A. In 2012 *Consumer Reports* published test results that indicated a concerning amount of arsenic in rice products in the U.S. The FDA and the rice-growers' association insist that it's safe, but *Consumer Reports* and others disagreed.

Consumer Reports published further results in 2015 that give some helpful guidelines for safe rice choices. The highest levels, they found, appeared in rice grown in Texas, Arkansas, and Louisiana. Rice grown in California, India, and Pakistan had lower levels.

They found that brown rice has higher levels of arsenic than white rice because the arsenic is most concentrated in the outer layers. However, that doesn't mean you should eat white rice instead of brown rice! Look for safer sources like California-grown brown rice.

Even with safer rice choices, you should mix in some different grains. Amaranth, buckwheat, and millet all had lower levels of arsenic than rice.

Q. SHOULD I TAKE A FISH-OIL SUPPLEMENT FOR MY OMEGA-3 FATTY ACIDS?

A. No! You may already know that fish products can contain dangerous amounts of mercury and heavy metals, but even if you have a brand that says it's mercury-free, it's a bad choice. Fish oil is packed with cholesterol, which is not healthy. Finally, the strong and distinctive odor of the added citrus can mask the smell of rancid fish oil.

Instead, consume hemp seed, flax seed, and walnuts. If you eat them daily, you'll get all you need for omega-3s and other essential fatty acids.

LESSEN CRAVINGS WITH TRANSITION FOODS

It can be hard to give up foods you love—remember, those foods don't love you back. It can help to substitute some vegan options to make the transition easier.

If you need a sweetener while you're in transition, honey is an option, but keep in mind that it is a transition food. I recommend manuka honey, which comes from the rain forests in New Zealand and is not as sweet as most other honeys. Use up to a teaspoon, eating it with a high-fiber fatty food, such as nuts, to slow the release of sugars. However, as soon as you can, transition from honey to consuming raisins, fresh and dried dates, dried figs, or other sweet fruit.

Fresh, right from the tree Medjool dates are amazing.

Be careful with dried fruit, however. Normally fruit fills you up quickly because it's full of water, but that doesn't happen with dried fruit. It's also naturally high in sugar, so if you go overboard you can give yourself an unwanted sugar spike. Finally, those sticky sugars can wreck your teeth (see sidebar), so you must brush your teeth and floss right after you eat dried fruit. For all these reasons, eat dried fruit in extreme moderation if at all.

Are you worried about missing chocolate? Go for the source of chocolate: cacao beans. Cacao nibs are broken up pieces of the beans used to make chocolate. They're delicious on

Protect Your Teeth!

Your permanent teeth have to last you for the rest of your life, and if you're living an Ageless Boomer lifestyle, it's going to be a long one. Proper care of your teeth is absolutely essential. Brush and floss daily and visit the dentist once or twice a year.

In addition, when you eat dried fruit you must brush your teeth and floss right after. Dried fruit is full of sugar and is as sticky as candy, so you have to protect your teeth by getting that sugar off the surface right away.

their own, but they aren't nearly as sweet as processed chocolate because they don't have added sugar. If you need to get yourself used to the taste of cacao, you can start by blending the nibs into blended salads with bananas or another sweet fruit. (Just make sure you blend fruits—

never juice them. Juicing removes the fiber from the fruit, creating a sugar spike.) Cacao is a great source of magnesium, which has a very calming effect. Mix it with some nuts and it's delicious. However, use cacao in moderation—in some people it causes insomnia and anxiety.

PREPARE TO OVERCOME TEMPTATION

A diet that is very different from the standard American diet can be inconvenient, but I have found many ways to stick to my eating plan despite those difficulties. In the beginning, try to anticipate and prepare for situations that will tempt you to go off your healthy diet. For instance, don't go to restaurants hungry. Eat an apple or two beforehand. I always bring my own food to restaurants, but if you're not ready for that, at least plan what you want to order ahead of time. (See the box on the following page.)

Sometimes, you won't feel like explaining your new diet to colleagues or acquaintances, especially when you've done it dozens of times already. In that case, I don't see the harm in a little white lie. I can't tell you how many times I've told people that I'm participating in a study and am on a special diet. No one has ever batted an eye.

When I'm invited to someone's home, I explain to them that this is my diet. Would they mind terribly if I brought my own food? Some people may not understand, which again means a little white lie might help. I sometimes say I've volunteered to be part of a study and can't break my pledge. I therefore have to bring my own food. You can also tell them you have severe allergies or that you're following a doctor's orders. You can even volunteer to make the salad. (The only danger is that the host or hostess may not like the other guests' enthusiastic reaction to the beauty and taste of your WFPB salad with a seed-, nut-, or avocado-based dressing.) If the person pauses or hesitates, just remind them that the reason you want to be there is because you're looking forward to all being together. Just be charming about it. You'll feel energized after your meal, and you'll be the life of the party.

The social contact of dining out or going to a party is much more important than what you eat. There are lots of ways to enjoy going out, socializing with friends, and participating in gatherings of all kinds without consuming food that you don't want to eat. If you find yourself at a restaurant or a big social function and without your own food, you can always take a bit of food and move it around on the plate. Just be sure to eat beforehand so you're not hungry. And remember the main purpose of the party is to socialize with friends. The food is incidental.

"Food bullies generally have a strong need to control and dominate. If a food bully's intended target exhibits a 'defeated attitude' in response to their pushiness, then the bullying is likely to continue. If you are a people-pleaser, you may be tempted to give-in to food bullies and compromise your own health goals by eating disease-promoting foods. Recognize where you are vulnerable and be prepared with strategies to stand your ground."

—Fuhrman,

"Is Pleasing Grandma Ruining Your Health?"

TRICKY SITUATION: BUSINESS LUNCH

If I need to meet a client at a restaurant for business, I'll go 20 minutes early, ask to see the chef, give him my own food, and ask him to please serve it in a very delightful way. I've never yet been refused. I always let the waiter know my plan and tip well in advance (if it's a small party). When the waiter takes my order, I just say, "The chef knows what I like."

I used to go to the best restaurants in New York City and ask the waiter to make me a vegan meal. My clients would always want to try, and invariably someone would say "take my meal away and bring me that!" Because the chefs loved a challenge. Give the chef 24-hours notice and they'll have all the ingredients on hand. A couple of times I went back and I noticed a vegetarian option, and it was the meal they had newly created just for me.

When I travel, I do my homework in advance and call the hotel to find out if any health food supermarkets or stores are in the neighborhood where I'll be staying. Before I go to the airport, I just put trail mix in a plastic bag in my pocket. I have found that trail mix is the easiest and most compact snack to carry along. However, I won't eat it if it has gone through the X-ray machine.

I highly recommend that you keep a diary when you start the transition to a WFPB diet. Note what you're eating and when, and describe how you felt after the meal and the next day. Write down your workout, your sleep routine, how much time you spent in the sunlight that day and the time of day, and any outside stresses that might influence your energy levels. Also note how you're feeling over the course of the day. After keeping track of all this for a few weeks, look back over your diary and see if you can identify patterns. Was there one thing that consistently left you feeling tired? What meal and exercise left you with the highest energy and easiest recovery? Have you noticed a change over time in your mood, energy levels, or training regimen? Note your setbacks—see if you can identify a situation or craving that triggered each one. If you've been eating a lot of processed foods, you won't be able to trust your cravings at first. As I'll tell you in the next chapter, the multi-billion-dollar processed food industry banks on creating foods that will make you crave more. Foods with lots of fat, sugar, and salt trick your body into thinking it needs more when it really needs zero junk food. Keeping a diary will help your weather these tricky cravings.

"Over time, the body will begin to crave high net-gain foods and lose interest in processed foods. Also, by making high net-gain foods a large part of the diet, there will simply be no room for others. The body will get all the nutrition it needs from the new diet and then turn off its hunger mechanism."

— Brazier,

Thrive

After a while, you won't need a diary—much of this mental work will become intuitive. Over time, you will find yourself less and less tempted by the foods you once used to eat, and your body will begin to crave the things that are good for it, so you can just listen to your body.

As you start to adopt this lifestyle, take the time to tune into your body's cravings and energy levels. There's no need for you to ever feel hungry on this diet, but listen to your body and eat when it's telling you it's hungry, not just because it's a prescribed mealtime. And in fact, don't deprive your body if it's hungry—that defeats the whole purpose. If you reach for an apple, orange, veggie, or salad, you can eat any time.

Also, as you increase your intake of fruits and vegetables, you'll start to taste them more intensely, too. By eliminating all the sauces and additives and condiments that you need for animal and processed foods, you'll get to the essence of the flavor of your food. You'll suddenly find that you are better able to distinguish between different varieties of blueberries, dates, and apples.

DETOXIFICATION:
GETTING THE SLUDGE OUT OF YOUR SYSTEM

As you make the transition to a plant-based diet, you need to learn about the process of detoxification and what your options are for the best ways to help your body through this phase. Every body is different, and there is no single detox approach that works for everyone.

To begin, a WFPB diet is tremendously good at detoxification. Not only are you replacing bad foods with good foods, but also the fiber-rich plant foods do an excellent job of sweeping out your digestive system. Once you adopt a plant-strong diet, you're already beginning the process. Eventually you will detoxify just by eating the diet—how long depends on your body. It could take a week, a month, or six months. If you want to help the process along, additional methods are available.

Most of us have been eating foods that our body has had difficulty digesting for the better part of our lives: high-temperature cooked foods, meat, dairy, and, processed foods. Since we were never really meant to eat that way, our bodies are not very efficient at digesting those foods, which means that we don't flush all the waste out of our systems whenever we eat those foods. The result is a slow but massive buildup of waste and toxicity in our large intestine and colon, which,

"Common detoxification symptoms include headache, bloating, diarrhea, nausea, fatigue, and sleep disturbances. It's important to remember that detoxification involves cleansing symptoms. Severe symptoms, however, are an indication that you should reduce the rate at which you are implementing the change. Keep in mind, though, that the worse you feel initially, the more there is to be gained."

— Brazier,

Thrive

over time, affects every single part of our body—every gland and every cell.

As a result of our overtaxed colons, it is also more difficult for us to absorb the nutrients we are consuming. As veteran nutritionist Norman Walker said in his book *Colon Health*, "The very best of diets can be no better than the very worst if the sewage system of the colon is clogged with a collection of waste and corruption." This backlog also creates extra weight that we're dragging around all the time. Remember: waste = weight. So, the first step toward good health is not only a change in diet but the process of cleansing and flushing out the colon. Colon purification is essential to a successful transition.

Unfortunately, the process of removing decades of buildup is not entirely pleasant. As you begin to work on flushing out the waste, those released toxins can get into your bloodstream and make you feel pretty lousy. The loosened-up toxins will try to escape any way they can, and you may feel any of a wide range of symptoms: headaches, skin breakouts, bad breath, foul-smelling elimination, fatigue, and sluggishness. The good news, and the thing to keep in mind at all times, is that detoxification is temporary, and you will feel extraordinary benefits once you reach the other side. You will feel like an entirely new person:

lighter, more energized, with glowing skin and brighter eyes. You'll experience enhanced memory and mental clarity, better physical and mental balance, lots of energy, and a general sense of well-being that you probably haven't felt in years.

In Chapter 10, I'll discuss several detoxification processes that may help you, including food combining and fasting. These processes can help you anytime, but they can be especially helpful during transition. Another very helpful practice is rebounding, which I've covered in Chapter 15. You can "jump" ahead to that chapter and find out just how energizing and beneficial rebounding can be—it can really help you through this change.

DIET VS. NUTRITION: STOP THE YO-YO

How many diets have you tried in your life? One? Five? Ten? If you're reading this book, chances are they didn't work and you're looking for another solution. It's important that you understand WFPB eating is not a diet—it's a lifestyle change. It can help you lose weight, but weight-loss is a side effect of healthy eating and exercise; the goal is health and longevity. You will find, for example, that exercise changes your size and shape (it redistributes your weight away from your middle), but may not change the number on the scale. Muscle is heavier and denser than fat, so as you lose fat and gain muscle, you may not see a huge dip in your weight. You will see and feel the difference in your clothes, though! When you make this change, you'll feel the benefits in every part of your life.

Despite the thousands of diet books flooding the market, they seem to be doing us precious little good. People try one diet, decide it doesn't work, give up, try another, lose some weight, gain it all back, try another, and finally give up.

Americans continue to pile on the weight in ever-more-alarming quantities.

Why are there so many diet books on the shelves? Because they don't work. Ineffective diets are intensely frustrating, but we're now learning that yo-yo dieting, or weight cycling, is also taking a huge toll on our health. A 2012 study examined a group of postmenopausal women who lost significant weight on a five-month diet. The women who gained weight after the diet ended had higher cholesterol and insulin levels than they had before they started the diet, even if they didn't gain back all the weight they lost. In other words, that yo-yo diet hurt their health.

It's time to get our facts straight about diets and why they don't work once and for all. When you understand the way our bodies react to crash diets, you will see why they will never, ever, ever be a long-term weight solution. And you will realize you must find another more effective way to reach your healthy weight and ideal body shape.

Let's look at what happens when we go on a crash diet. The human body was designed to withstand starvation, which means that it quickly kicks into emergency mode when it detects that it's not getting enough food. The first thing the body does when it senses deprivation is to slow its metabolism down, wanting to stretch any food it gets as far as it can go. This means that it will slow down the calorie-burn rate. This approach worked well for our ancestors who needed to survive unpredictable food shortages, but it's bad news for us when we're trying to drop a few pounds.

"Instead of 'dieting,' we must change our lifestyle to include a diet that promotes health. People who adopt a WFPB diet find that most of their health problems were caused or significantly worsened by their old diets and resolve naturally and quickly once the body starts getting the proper fuel."

— Campbell,

Whole

The instant you go on a diet, your body reacts by slowing down your metabolism. Plus, your body starts storing fat rather than burning it, and you lose half fat and half muscle, especially if you're not strength-training, in order to hold on to your body's now-precious fat reserves. So, yes, in the beginning, if you deprive yourself of calories, you may lose a few pounds, half of which are from fat and half of which are from muscle.

The problem comes once you return to your normal eating habits after your diet. Even though you're consuming more calories, your metabolism continues to operate at a reduced rate. And it may take up to a year to restore your metabolism to its pre-diet rate, providing you don't crash diet during this time. This means that you are eating the same as before, but your body is not burning calories as effectively. So you are adding weight back on, but it doesn't return as half-muscle, half-fat, but instead is all fat (unless you are strength-training). So you're worse off than when you started—with more fat, less muscle, and a slower metabolism.

Once you've put on a few pounds, you may decide it's time to try another crash diet, and the cycle repeats itself. Over time, you've wreaked havoc with your metabolism, reduced your muscle mass (your single most effective calorie burner), increased fat, and probably gotten terribly demoralized in the process. Eventually you give up. As a result, you may find yourself resorting to increasingly ridiculous and unhealthy diets to compensate (high protein! low carb! instant miracle!). But none of them is any more effective than the last. It's a self-defeating, downward spiral—one in which all too many Americans are stuck.

So how can you stop this unhealthy cycle and lose that weight once and for all? Well, in addition to building muscle mass, increasing your functional strength (the kind of strength that enables you to accomplish daily physical tasks), and increasing the calorie-burning efficiency of your metabolism, there are several other steps you can take to reach your ideal weight.

The first and most important step is to establish long-term changes, not short-term fixes. The goal of this book is to help you with those long-term changes so that you will have long-term success. Don't look at these solutions as something to try until you reach a goal weight—look at them as your new normal.

The second step is to replace high-calorie, low-nutrient food with high-nutrient food, period. I'll explain the basics of this diet in the next chapter. Some of these foods, like avocados and nuts, are high in calories, but they're rich in micro- and macronutrients. Other foods, like kale and spinach, are nutrient-rich but have minimal calories. You'll learn how to make the most of them.

The third step is to eat smaller meals more frequently—about three meals and two snacks spread roughly three hours apart throughout the day. This accomplishes three things. One, eating nutritious food satiates hunger, which reduces your sense of deprivation and temptation. Two, it sends the message to your body that you are in the "land of plenty" and it can reliably expect to be fed on a regular basis, so it will actually release the fat reserves that it has stored for emergencies. If you eat a large meal, however, you experience a bigger insulin boost, which sends the message to the body to store fat. Besides, if you eat too much at one meal, it will take a long time to digest that food. Even good fruits and vegetables will putrefy if you eat too many of them at one time. Three, your metabolic rate goes up when you eat, so small meals help give it a little extra boost. Bottom line: eat modest amounts at a reliable frequency. Remember, though, these should be small meals; we'll look at appropriate meal sizes in later chapters. Eventually you'll eat only 2-3 meals a day—it's really all you need because you've satisfied your body with nutrient-rich foods.

Keep in mind that it takes about 20 minutes for your body to feel full and register that you are satisfied. If you eat too quickly, your body won't have the chance to send the signal that you've had enough. You'll have overeaten before your body transmits the signals to your brain. So slow down, take your time, and chew your food well. Break the cell walls of your food as thoroughly as you can to make it easier on your body to digest and assimilate the food. Chat with your family, put your fork down, and stop while you're still just shy of complete satiation.

Combined with the other core essentials of a health promoting lifestyle, balanced activity or exercise and adequate sleep, you'll not only lose weight rapidly and healthfully, but you will eventually look and feel the best you've ever felt. Any other option just places you at needless risk.

The fourth step is to drink plenty of clean, pure, filtered water and eat water-rich vegetables and fruits. As I explain in more detail in chapter 6, water enables our body to work more efficiently in a variety of ways, from our ability to burn fat to the efficient delivery of nutrients to the body. Water flushes toxins from your organs so that the liver can process them; it carries nutrients to your cells to give you energy, fuel growth, and repair damage; it keeps your digestive system moist so that you can digest foods effectively. It can even help the liver burn fat by reducing the burden of toxins on the liver. Water is so important that it can trigger hunger: you may actually be thirsty when you think you're hungry, so have a glass of water before reaching for that snack.

The fifth step is to find a form of exercise you love. As you'll see, I highly recommend body-weight training as presented in Part III. It's the most effective way to reach your ideal weight and continually build muscle while giving you a great short-burst cardiovascular workout as well. But it's vital that you find a form of exercise you love because that's the only way you'll incorporate it into your life over the long term. If you really don't like exercise, you need to build in a reward system for yourself. Variety can help: focus on upper body exercises one day and lower body exercises the next. The important thing is to incorporate intervals into your training regimen, as a steady cardio workout, such as long-distance running, is not an effective muscle-builder over the long term (in fact, you lose muscle by doing long, slow, distance workouts). What you need in your workout—whatever you choose—is a pattern of intense bursts followed by active rest because this approach builds muscle and increases your metabolic rate. If you're running, jog to rest, if you're walking fast, walk slower, and so on.

Finally, don't aim to lose too much weight too fast. The human body perceives rapid weight loss as starvation, so is will use all its resources to hold on to its energy reserves—i.e., fat. A good goal is to aim to lose half a pound a week or two pounds a month. This slow rate of loss won't trigger any starvation reflex in your body and will allow you to find your optimal weight. It may sound slow, but that's 24 pounds a year! Think of it as a change in lifestyle, not a temporary weight loss plan. If you go cold turkey, you will lose weight very fast at first, then you will level off and lose it slowly but steadily until you reach your optimal weight.

CHANGE YOUR THINKING

If you decide to go on this plant-based diet permanently, you will find your optimal weight without even thinking about it. The human body developed to eat balanced, plant-based, nutrient-rich foods, so it becomes exceptionally proficient at regulating itself and will find its natural weight all on its own. In fact, I eat as many fruits and vegetables as I want and I have hardly any fat on me.

That's because the body weight to strength ratio is so important—for both men and women. Women sometimes avoid strength-building because they think muscle isn't feminine, but everyone needs muscle. Research shows that postmenopausal women especially need strength-building exercise for everything from bone health to heart health to mental health. No matter who you are, your strength should be directly proportional to your body weight. High-nutrition foods combined with strength-building will naturally, gradually, and consistently build a lean, strong body. I haven't been on a scale in years. As an added bonus, in addition to losing weight, you'll feel like a kid again.

So throw out the crash diet books (your first muscle-building activity) and focus on changing your thinking. You'll be extremely gratified by the results.

CALORIE RESTRICTION DONE RIGHT

Here's one of the most widely proven, least-talked-about truths of longevity: eating fewer calories leads to longer, healthier lives. As early as 1934 researchers discovered that rats who ate fewer calories than a control group lived up to twice as long as the controls. Roy Walford and Richard Weindruch expanded on these findings during the 1980s, finding that mice who ate a low-calorie, high-nutrient diet lived longer, looked younger, acted younger, and stayed healthy longer. Since then additional studies in non-human primates have confirmed the results of all these studies. As Dr. Gabriel Cousens puts it in his book *Rainbow Green Live Food Cuisine*, "Calorie restriction is the only thing we know that is able to consistently slow aging in all varieties of animals, including the mammalian species." What's more, he points out, Walford and Weindruch's research showed significant anti-aging benefits even on middle-aged mice—so no matter when you start, you can benefit from a calorie-restricted diet. And it's quick—anti-aging effects appear in the body within one month of adopting a healthy calorie-restricted diet.

But remember, not all calorie sources (foods) are the same. And restricting yourself to the wrong foods will not add years to your life or life to your years.

The nutrition approach I've outlined in this book offers a healthy, filling way to restrict calories, and I'll give you all the details in the next few chapters. In the meantime, remember the following guidelines:

Avoid animal protein. Yes, even "healthy" foods like low-fat dairy, fish, egg whites, and grilled chicken. As Joel Fuhrman, M.D., explains in several of his books, including *The End of Dieting* and *Super Immunity*, animal protein triggers the increase of the hormone insulin-like growth factor 1, or IGF-1. IGF-1 triggers the aging process in the body, and it's like fertilizer for cancer cells, promoting their proliferation and growth. Less IGF-1, by contrast, is linked to lower oxidative stress, reduced inflammation, and increased lifespan. Reducing your calories but increasing your animal protein intake, therefore, just pumps up your levels of IGF-1, and you undo any benefit you gained by reducing calories. (In fact, Fuhrman argues that caloric restriction works because the restriction of animal proteins leads to reduced IGF-1 levels.)

Eat nutrient-rich foods. If you want to reap the benefits of calorie restriction, you can't skimp on nutrients, and whole plant foods give you major nutritional punch. As you'll see in the next few chapters, plant foods are not only capable of supplying all the macronutrients (carbs, fats, and proteins) you need, they're also the best source of micronutrients (vitamins, minerals, enzymes, and more).

Don't starve yourself. While eating fewer calories is highly beneficial to your health, letting yourself get hungry can undermine healthy choices. So how do you eat fewer calories without starving yourself? You can avoid hunger by making sure your calories are nutritionally dense and full of fiber and water. Fiber and fluid fill your stomach, making you feel full even though they're not calorie-packed. Don't stuff yourself—if you leave a little room in your stomach it's easier to digest your food; 80 percent full is a good goal.

The beauty of WFPB eating is that it naturally restricts calories. Raw vegetables, which are the foundation of this way of eating, are low in calories but high in nutrients, and their fiber and water content fills you up so that you don't feel hungry. Fruits, while slightly higher in calories because of their natural sugars, are still nutrient-rich and high in fiber and water. You have to be a little careful with calorie-dense foods like nuts and avocadoes, but they will be an important part of your diet. By eating a WFPB diet, you gain the life-extending benefits of calorie restriction without feeling hungry or deprived.

CHAPTER 5

KILLER FOODS: WHAT TO LEAVE OUT

■■■

The evidence is piling up: cardiovascular disease, dementia, even cancer are not genetically determined fates, they are heavily—some say exclusively—determined by lifestyle. Can I promise that if you become an Ageless Boomer you'll never get cancer? No. But I would bet on it. I have enough faith in the power of nutrition over cancer that I became an Ageless Boomer despite my family history. And if I hadn't, I believe I may not have been alive to write this book.

DON'T LET FOOD
COMPROMISE YOUR HEALTH

When you're ready to improve your health by eating better, you need to look first at what to not eat, then look at what you should eat. That's because certain foods are actively damaging your health. You need to stop hurting yourself before you can really benefit from healthy foods. (Of course, the great thing about WFPB eating is that you can do both!)

PROCESSED FOODS FATTEN YOU UP
AND STARVE YOU FOR NUTRITION

In *Your Healthy Journey*, Fred Bisci compares half a dozen different diets and comes up with one common denominator: they all recommend that you cut out processed foods. "In the short term," he writes, "exclusion rather than inclusion is the key, and many diets will at first make you feel and look better because they succeed with the part of the equation that is **what you leave out** (emphasis in original)."

This quote tells us a couple of things. First, many nutritionists and experts have concluded that avoiding processed foods will improve your health, even if they disagree on nearly everything

Which foods are actively damaging your health?

- Processed foods, including refined sugar
- Animal foods
- Foods cooked at high temperatures

Start taking these foods out of your diet so that they can't continue to cause harm.

else. Second, enough people have told us this lesson that we all know that we should avoid these foods.

And yet people still eat them. Why?

"A good rule is to avoid anything that is 'white,' such as sugar, white flour, white pasta, white potato, or white rice. Remember this rhyme: 'The whiter the bread, the sooner you're dead.'"

—Joel Fuhrman, MD,
Super Immunity

PROCESSED FOODS ARE NUTRITIONALLY BANKRUPT

Let's start with a definition. What are processed foods?

Bisci gives this one: "A processed food is something that you can't see in nature. The more highly processed it is, the less it looks like something you could theoretically grow in your

66

garden." In The China Study, T. Colin Campbell explains that most of the refined foods we're eating are carbohydrates, "found in foods like white bread, processed snack items including crackers and chips made with white flour, sweets including pastries and candy bars and sugar-laden soft drinks."

Michael Moss sums it up in the title of his book: *Salt, Sugar, Fat*. I'm going to follow Bisci and add two more big categories: alcohol and coffee.

Americans eat massive quantities of processed foods, even though we know they're unhealthy. The people who manufacture and sell processed foods are not interested in your health. They are interested in your money. Food companies have spent decades carefully manipulating their food, its packaging, and its advertising to get you addicted to their products.

Addicted is not an exaggeration here. Food companies want you to crave their products so that you will buy and consume more of them. They know their foods are unhealthy, but they make them worse anyway. If you want to dig into the dirty details of the food industry's efforts to get you eating their products, take a look at Moss's book, which is subtitled "How the Food Industry Got Us Hooked."

SUGAR WITHOUT FIBER IS A RECIPE FOR OBESITY AND DIABETES

I'm talking about refined sugar here: white sugar, brown sugar, raw sugar, corn syrup, and others. Natural sugars in whole foods are fine because they occur with fiber, and fiber slows the absorption of sugar into the blood. Refined sugar is completely separated from any fiber in its source food. (Some WFPB proponents are comfortable with honey and maple syrup. I don't recommend them because they don't have fiber, so they can still create that sugar rush and insulin spike.)

In *Healthy at 100*, John Robbins notes that almost one-third of the calories in American's diets come from refined sugar and corn syrup. He explains, "Food manufacturers put such massive amounts of refined sugars in foods for a simple reason—to stimulate appetite ... People eating highly refined and processed foods typically consume 25 percent more calories than those on a more natural diet."

All those refined sugars are terrible for the body. They create blood sugar and insulin spikes that, over time, lead to insulin resistance, metabolic syndrome (pre-diabetes), and then finally type 2 diabetes. They also lead to added weight: sugars can give us a quick burst of energy, but if they don't get used right away, the body stores them as fat. If you drink a 200-calorie soda, you'd have to go for a 15-

> "When you take fruit, for instance, and you cook it and put it in a can and add sugar to it, even though it tastes good, it in no way compares to when you're eating a piece of fresh fruit."
>
> — Fred Bisci,
> Your Healthy Journey

minute run to burn off those calories. And that's not happening for most Americans, so the sugars turn into fat and added pounds.

It's important to note that nearly every processed food, from candy to crackers to spaghetti sauce, contains added sugar. It's the food industry's leading weapon for creating cravings, so it ends up in nearly everything they make.

By the way, artificial sweeteners are not a good alternative. Studies have linked diet sodas (a favorite source of artificial sweeteners) with weight gain, even though the drinks themselves have no calories. The reason for the weight gain is unclear—researchers speculate that the body compensates for the lack of sugar in the artificially sweet drink by causing cravings for other sources of sugar. The bottom line is that you can't fool Mother Nature, so get your sweets from whole, ripe, organic fruits.

> "When you next go into your local supermarket, you may wonder if there's anything in the store that you can eat. The regrettable truth is that most of the shelves are filled with processed, unnatural products that do not qualify as healthy foods. When you clean out your mind, body and spirit, and your vision becomes clear, you will walk into a supermarket and instead of seeing a cornucopia of foods, you will see rows of inert products that have little or no vital force left in them."
>
> — Fred Bisci,
> Your Healthy Journey

REFINED GRAINS ARE NEITHER WHOLE NOR WHOLESOME

In a very telling chart in *Healthy at 100*, Robbins shows 18 important nutrients that are diminished or deleted when whole wheat flour is refined into white flour. Fiber and Vitamin E are both reduced by 95 percent, calcium by 56 percent, potassium by 74 percent, and so on. And that's just for 18 well-known nutrients ... plant foods have many more, and we don't know how many of those are lost through refining.

Robbins writes, "In the United States, 98 percent of the wheat eaten today is eaten in the form of white flour." That flour appears in pasta, bread, cookies, crackers, and many other foods. Other whole grains get stripped as well—white rice is probably the second most common refined grain in American diets (not counting corn in the form of corn syrup; wheat is the first). But our reliance on white flour is a major problem.

Refined grains act in a similar way to refined sugars. "White flour, white rice, and other refined grain products are absorbed rapidly into the bloodstream, causing rapid fluctuations in blood sugar levels," Robbins writes. In fact, almost any flour, including whole wheat flour, will give you a blood sugar spike.

> "Do you know why they call it Wonder Bread? Because if you eat it, it's a wonder you're still alive."
>
> — John Robbins,
> Healthy at 100

I'll discuss the pros and cons of fat later in this chapter, but when it comes to processed foods, you can bank on that fat being bad for you. Food manufacturers are experts in altering and manipulating fats. The deadly trans fats that we all avoid now were the creation of the food industry, which created "hydrogenated" fats in order to make fats more shelf-stable. Trans fats have since been linked to high amounts of bad cholesterol, which, in turn, leads to increased risk of heart attack and stroke.

As Moss explains in *Salt, Sugar, Fat,* the food industry is still playing with fat. The labels may say "No Trans Fat," but that doesn't mean the fat in those foods is good for you. Just stay away.

MORE SALT THAN YOU CAN EVEN TASTE

Adding salt to your food is a great way to cause dehydration, retain water (a result of dehydration), and increase your blood pressure. Processed foods are packed with salt because not only does it "enhance" flavor, it also helps preserve foods, giving them a longer shelf-life. I put quotes around "enhance" because in reality, added salt tends to dull your taste buds, requiring you to add more and more salt to perceive a "salty" taste. Stop adding salt to your food and you will find, over time, that you can taste much more, and what you taste is delicious.

LEGAL DRUGS: ALCOHOL AND COFFEE

Alcohol and coffee are drugs. Alcohol is a depressant, coffee is a stimulant, and although both drugs are legal, that doesn't mean you should consume them. Both of these drugs have a powerful effect on the body, both create dependence, and both have substantial negative effects.

It's best to avoid these drugs, but if you're already using them, you may need to taper back their use to avoid painful side effects. If you are drinking heavily (several alcoholic beverages a day, or binging on alcohol at any time), you many need to consult a professional to help treat your addiction.

ANIMAL FOODS AND
THE PROTEIN MYTH

Protein is without a doubt the most misunderstood of the three essential macronutrients (fat and carbohydrates being the others). If we want to start taking better care of ourselves, it's essential that we get our facts straight and change the way we think about our protein intake. Unfortunately, this involves scrapping most of what you think you know about this vital nutrient and learning a whole new way of incorporating it into your life. For one thing, we need a lot less protein than we've been led to believe. For another, protein sourced from vegetables and nuts is far healthier than the protein found in meat and dairy. (Shocking, right?) You can dramatically change your outlook for lifelong health when you incorporate protein into your diet in a new way.

Let's begin by explaining protein's role in the body. Protein is composed of strings of amino acids, and different foods contain different combinations of amino acids. You may have heard people talk about "complete proteins" or refer to "high-quality proteins" versus "low-quality proteins." They're talking about the completeness of a chain of amino acids in a given food. Some foods contain most or all of the essential amino acids needed to form a "complete" protein, while some foods need to be combined with others so that the different amino acids can link together to create complete proteins. If you eat a good variety of vegetables, fruits, seeds, nuts, and legumes, you really don't need to worry about getting all the essential amino acids.

And what exactly does this macronutrient do for us? Protein is essential for growth and repair of body tissue. For example, it's especially vital that you get sufficient protein when you exercise because you break down your muscles during exercise, and protein helps build muscle back even stronger than before. As muscle mass and strength increase, those muscles will work more efficiently. Babies and children also need extra protein in order to grow. (It's an interesting fact that breast milk contains only six percent protein, and that's enough to help babies double their weight in their first few months of life.) Every adult needs protein to help maintain healthy muscles. The bottom line is that we all need protein. But what you'll find out next may surprise you.

> "It is most likely that the standard American diet is so nutrient-poor that a significant portion of people's phytochemical intake comes from their morning coffee!"
>
> — Joel Fuhrman on studies that found a reduction in diabetes risk among coffee-drinkers, in Super Immunity

Q: CAN YOU REALLY LIVE EXCLUSIVELY ON VEGETABLES, FRUITS, SEEDS, NUTS, WHOLE GRAINS, LENTILS, AND BEANS? WHAT ABOUT THE FOUR FOOD GROUPS?

A: Every nutrient that your body needs can be found in fruits, vegetables, seeds , and nuts. Fruits and vegetables supply water, minerals, vitamins, phytonutrients, antioxidants, enzymes, and fiber. You'll get all the protein you need from leafy greens, seeds, nuts, and beans. Even fruit has some protein. Fruits provide simple carbohydrates, and you'll get good-quality fats from avocadoes, seeds, and nuts. Variety is key. You need to draw from vegetables, fruits, seeds, and nuts to be healthy.

THE DANGERS OF ANIMAL PROTEIN

Ask Americans about the best sources of protein, and you'll hear plenty about meat and milk, cheese and eggs. Even kindergarteners seem to know that they should eat their meat at dinner because it has protein and will help them grow. The standard American diet is built around protein because meat is one of the densest (read: most efficient) ways for us to get what is called "high-quality" protein. If you compare 100 calories of meat and 100 calories of spinach, the spinach has far more protein. However, you can eat the meat in about two bites, compared to an entire bunch of greens. Since meat is the most compact way to consume protein, we mistakenly think of it as the "best" source of protein. But it turns out this is a big mistake.

T. Colin Campbell grew up on a dairy farm. He believed that milk was a perfect food and that eating meat was vital to human health. He started his research career with those ideas in his mind, but he discovered, over decades, that everything he believed about the value of animal foods was wrong.

Campbell has explained his findings in his books, *The China Study* and *Whole*, both of which are excellent. While investigating the relationship between protein and cancer, he and his team found that animal protein was a leading trigger of cancer growth. Experiments with multiple types of cancer in different species and at different points in their life cycles all showed the same results: Animal protein sped up the rate of cancer growth; without animal protein, cancer growth stopped or never occurred.

"A pattern [in our research findings] was beginning to emerge: nutrients from animal-based foods increased tumor development while nutrients from plant-based foods decreased tumor development."

— T. Colin Campbell,
The China Study

In *The China Study*, he compares cancer growth to the growth of a lawn. You have three phases: seeding, growth, and overgrowth into your sidewalk or flower beds. Cancer works in a similar way—carcinogens "seed" our cells, but cancer cells won't grow unless they have the right conditions. Those conditions include a lack of antioxidants, but more importantly, the presence of animal protein. Once the cancer growth reaches a certain point, "overgrowth" appears in the form of tumors and metastasized sites.

Campbell explains that most of the time, we can't stop the seeding process. Carcinogens get into our systems despite our best efforts. A healthy immune system can help prevent some seeding, but it's likely to happen. The growth process, however, we **can** control—his experiments showed that they could "turn on" and "turn off" tumor growth in rats simply by changing the amount of animal protein.

"But what about humans?" you ask. That's where *The China Study* comes in. In a massive study carried out in cooperation with a Chinese research team, Campbell and his colleagues studied diet and health variables among 6,500 Chinese in 65 counties. They found a consistent trend. In regions where people ate large amounts of animal foods, cancer rates rose in proportion. In regions where animal food consumption was low, cancer rates were low as well.

"In America, 15-16 percent of our total calories comes from protein and upwards of 80 percent of this amount comes from animal-based foods. But in rural China, only 9-10 percent of total calories comes from protein and only 10 percent of the protein comes from animal-based foods."

— *T. Colin Campbell,*
The China Study

Campbell's findings have been largely ignored by many in the medical community and the federal government. He delves into the reasons why in *Whole*, but the bottom line is you probably haven't heard this very important information from your doctor or your local health agency. Nevertheless, a growing number of nutritionists, physicians, and health-conscious individuals like me are heeding his warnings.

My doctor was one of those people. When I went to see him at the age of forty, he told me to go on a WFPB diet if I didn't want to die of cancer the way my parents had.

HOW MUCH PROTEIN DO WE REALLY NEED?

You'll get a wide range of answers depending on whom you ask. I've heard some people say that you should eat 2 grams of protein for every pound you weigh. If a person weighs 150 pounds, that means they'd have to consume 300 grams every single day. That's 10.6 ounces of protein— a staggering amount! I remember working out in high school and college and being told over and over again that I needed to consume more protein. So I took a vile-tasting protein supplement and gulped it down, as did all my teammates. We thought it would help us build muscles fast and improve our athletic performance. (What builds muscle is exercise—period. But we'll get to that later.) I'm convinced to this day that greatest accomplishment of that protein supplement was to line the pockets of its manufacturer.

Everyone seems to be talking about getting enough protein. The standard American diet centers on protein; most parents plan meals around a protein source (typically meat); and many people consume protein supplements just to be sure they're getting enough. In fact, the single most common question I get when people hear I'm on a plant-based diet is: "But where do you get your protein?" They've been led to believe that an abundance of protein is essential for their health, and they worry unnecessarily about how they'll get enough and where it will come from. I think it may also be one of the main reasons people have trouble making the switch to this diet.

But have you ever heard of anyone having a protein deficiency? Except for cases of starvation, you won't. That's because there's increasing evidence that we need a whole lot less than we thought. In *The China Study*, Campbell points out that those consuming what was thought to be a much-too-low protein diet in rural China—no more than 10 percent protein—had a much lower rate of cancer, heart disease, and many other afflictions. He makes the case that the typical Western diet, which is astoundingly high in protein by comparison, is the culprit here.

It may be hard to get used to the idea that your meals don't have to revolve around meat, but it gives you a lot more flexibility. Once you eliminate the meat and the need for a sauce or accompaniment to give the meat some flavor, you'll discover an astonishing variety of plant-based foods that meet all your nutritional needs.

Here's another way to look at how much protein we really need. Breast milk is considered to be the perfect food for a growing baby, enabling an infant to double its weight in six months. But breast milk contains only 6 percent protein! That's a fraction of what we've been led to believe we need, and most of us are certainly not aiming to double in size.

So how much should we be getting? Based on my studies and experience, if you consume seeds, nuts, legumes, and plenty of leafy greens and other fresh raw vegetables, you don't have to worry about your protein intake. Calorie for calorie, leafy greens have more protein than meat. Let me emphasize this: *all plants have protein!* Some, like seeds, nuts, lentils, beans, and grain-like seeds, are excellent sources of protein.

The "paleo" diet—which is really a hodgepodge of different diets promoted by different people—says that we should eat like humans did in the Paleolithic period because our bodies haven't evolved since that time. While one thing is true—human bodies haven't evolved much since the Paleolithic era—most of the other claims of paleo promoters are confused or outright wrong. You could write a book on the problems with the paleo diet, but I'll just touch on a few major issues:

There is no single "paleo" diet. Our ancestors ate a lot of different types of diets depending on what part of the world they lived in and what types of food were available at that time. We have no idea what kind of health outcomes they experienced based on diet, so we can't say one paleo diet is better than another just because ancient humans ate it.

Many indigenous peoples have health problems when they eat meat. Some paleo proponents argue that we should look to indigenous peoples who are eating diets similar to the diets of their ancestors. For one thing, indigenous peoples have varied diets, just like our ancestors did (see above). For another, high amounts of animal foods can be bad for anyone, even indigenous peoples. As Esselstyn points out in My Beef with Meat, "There are two populations today that still eat large amounts of meat. First, the Maasai tribe of East Africa, who basically live on blood, milk, and meat. Although many people think these people are free of heart disease, it's not so … Harvard's George Mann conducted fifty autopsies on the Maasai in the 1970s and found their bodies were loaded with heart disease—but unlike the arteries of Americans who eat a great deal of meat, the Maasai arteries were also dilated, allowing for more blood flow, due to their high degree of physical activity." In other words, if you live a life where you're constantly in motion, like Paleolithic man and the Maasai, you can live longer with heart disease, but you'll still have heart disease if you eat nothing but meat.

Esselstyn goes on to explain that the other indigenous population that eats a great deal of meat, the Inuit people who live in northern Alaska and Canada, have very negative health outcomes as well. Medical examinations of Inuits past and present reveal heart disease and bone loss. He quotes pathologist Arthur Aufderheide as saying, "the spines of many [Inuit] women who died 8,000 years ago, nearly all before age 40, look like the hunched backs of 85-year-old American women today."

Humans evolved to eat plants. If you want to look backward to see the right way to eat, you can look all the way back at our closest animal relatives, chimpanzees and bonobos. These apes eat a plant-based diet (with a few insects thrown in) and they are healthy and amazingly strong.

My Beef with Meat tackles the myth that humans evolved to eat meat by comparing our teeth and digestive systems with those of carnivores. Carnivores, Esselstyn explains, have sharp teeth for tearing flesh and no grinding teeth. They have highly acidic stomachs and short, relatively straight intestines which process animal flesh quickly. Herbivores have grinding teeth to break down fiber, less-acidic stomachs, and long, slow-moving intestines, all of which work best to pull nutrients out of plant foods. Can you guess which group the human digestive system fits in? Yep, the herbivores. We have evolved to eat plants.

The positive of paleo. Despite the problems, I can point to a couple good pieces of advice from paleo promoters. One, eat lots of fresh vegetables, fruits, seeds, and nuts. Two, avoid processed foods, including refined sugar, refined grains, and added salt and oil.

Basically, instead of looking at the dubious science supporting paleo, look at the solid science supporting WFPB eating. Your body will thank you today, tomorrow, and for many years to come.

As Rip Esselstyn explains in *My Beef with Meat*, "the World Health Organization recommends the following formula to calculate your daily protein requirements: (0.8 grams) x (your ideal body weight in kilograms) = protein in grams. So, for a 175-pound guy like me using the above formula I should be getting 64 grams of protein per day." If you're a little smaller (or want to be), say 150 pounds, the amount is closer to 54 grams.

Q: WHAT ABOUT CALCIUM? WILL I HAVE ENOUGH CALCIUM IF I DON'T DRINK MILK?

A: Milk is not the excellent source of calcium we've all been led to believe. Dairy, like meat, creates an acidic state, which means you have to draw alkaline calcium from the bones to balance the body's acidity, thereby weakening the bones in the long run.

Gabriel Cousens, M.D., author of several books including *There Is a Cure for Diabetes*, cites research that suggests even less protein is fine. More importantly, he argues that too much protein, particularly animal protein, contributes to numerous degenerative diseases and premature aging in general.

Some argue that a low-protein or plant-based protein diet will diminish their energy, but that simply isn't true. Protein is not an energy source. Fat and carbs deliver energy to your body, protein doesn't. I eat a lower protein diet and people actually admire my overabundance of energy. For other examples, consider Bill Pearl, a former Mr. Universe, who became famous as the "Vegetarian Bodybuilder." As he says, "They think that to have big muscles you have to eat meat—it's a persistent and recurring myth. But take it from me, there's nothing magic about eating meat that's going to make you a champion bodybuilder. Anything you can find in a piece of meat, you can find in other foods as well."

Since I've spent most of this section debunking long-held myths, let me explain some of the easy ways to get healthy protein into your system. Let's start with the fact that all fruits and vegetables have some protein. Leafy greens top the list, but broccoli is another good choice.

Even fruits, which are not protein powerhouses, provide you with a good amount of protein. In *My Beef with Meat*, Rip Esselstyn includes the following list of fruits and how much of your daily protein needs (according to the USDA) they supply:

1. Oranges (1 navel): 7.4 percent
2. Strawberries (1 cup, whole): 8.3 percent
3. Kiwi (1 whole fruit or 1 cup sliced): 7.5 percent
4. Apple (1 medium): 2 percent
5. Pineapple (1 cup, chunks): 4.3 percent
6. Peach (1 medium): 9.3 percent
7. Banana (1 medium): 4.9 percent

I often throw a few leaves of romaine in a blended salad. I hardly notice it's there, but it's an easy way to get the added protein boost. A huge salad with guacamole dressing will give you plenty of protein.

Beans are packed with protein (as well as fiber, good carbs, and micronutrients). Enjoy the huge variety of beans of every flavor and texture.

Seeds and nuts are excellent sources of protein as well. One ounce of almonds, for example, contains about 6 grams of protein. You have to be a bit careful though, since nuts tend to be high in fat (although a much better type of fat than you get in meat). Just remember that a little bit goes a long way. Hemp seed is a protein-packed miracle food (10 grams of protein in a one-ounce [30 gram] serving), so if you're still worrying about your protein intake, throw a bit in your blended salad.

If you're exercising a lot, eat more beans, leafy greens, and a higher amount of nuts and seeds because you'll need the extra for optimal recovery. Let me emphasize that **athletes do not need to eat meat!** Plants are much better for you. From endurance athletes like Esselstyn and Brazier to football stars like Herschel Walker, Arian Foster, and Ricky Williams, athletes are demonstrating that plant-strong diets translate into optimal results. My own experience taught me the same thing decades ago.

Remember, supplements are not the answer. We need to consume protein as part of a whole food or in the form of a juice or blended salad in order for that protein to be bioavailable to us. Save yourself a lot of money and forget about protein supplements.

> "I provide nutritional counseling to world-class and professional athletes to maximize their performance and to increase their resistance to infection. One key feature of the eating style I recommend to them is that most of their protein and fat needs are met by consuming seeds, nuts, legumes, and avocadoes instead of more animal products."
>
> —Joel Fuhrman, MD,
> Eat for Health

The message is simple: don't worry about your protein intake. If you eat a natural diet with a good variety of fruits and vegetables, enhanced with a small amount of seeds and nuts, lentils, beans, and grains, you will get all the protein your body needs. Balance and variety are the keys to a healthy diet. It's not necessary to fret too much over the specific quantities. One of the best things about this diet is that you don't really need to think about protein at all. It may take some getting used to, but enjoy being untethered from the demands of the protein myth and the renewed energy and good health that go along with it!

"[Athletes are] often afraid of changing their diets because they think that change might hurt their performance. So they get stuck in the old status quo: Meat is good. Plants are bad. Phooey! The truth is that plants are the dope. In fact, plants are nature's legal performance-enhancing drug."

— Rip Esselstyn,
My Beef with Meat

THE STRAIGHT SCOOP ON FAT

After protein, fat is probably the second-most misunderstood macronutrient. (Although low-carb diets have done a good job making carbs misunderstood as well!) On one hand fat has been demonized beyond recognition, on the other it has been praised as the (counterintuitive) path to weight loss (such as the Atkins' Diet). It's time to get our facts straightened out about fat.

Let's begin with what fat accomplishes in our body. Fat is our most efficient source of energy, containing more than twice as much caloric energy per gram as carbohydrates. In addition to creating energy reserves, it also carries certain fat-soluble vitamins (A, D, E, and K) to our various organs, provides cushioning for our organs, and creates a layer of insulation for our bodies. It lubricates joints, helps our brains function better, and gives our skin elasticity. Finally, fat curbs hunger. It takes longer for us to digest it, so we remain full longer and experience fewer cravings. So a certain amount of fat is crucial to our well-being. If you don't get enough of it for a prolonged period, you'll subject your body to a whole range of problems. Fat should be about 20-40 percent of your diet (by calories).

Now, before you reach for the olive oil, remember that every gram of fat packs a wallop in terms of calories, and not all fats are equal. Read on to learn what fats to eat and how much of them to consume.

There seems to be a good deal of confusion about the right amount and right types of fat. Start by throwing out everything you've ever heard about going on a low-fat or high-fat (Atkins' type) diet. Instead, you need to pay attention to the type of fats you consume and consume them in moderation. When you eat unprocessed plants, you always consume the right kinds of fats. You just need to exercise a small amount of restraint in the amounts you consume.

Seeds and nuts are terrific sources of healthy fat. Keep in mind that it's important to eat a variety of seeds and nuts because they contain different nutrients.

I have very little body fat. When people look at me, they're surprised to hear that I eat as much fat as I do. But that's because I eat the right types of fats. So where do I get it on this plant-based diet? Mostly from seeds and nuts, which are both very high in fat. Seeds and nuts are a fabulous source of fat and protein, and our body digests them slowly, so they'll keep you from craving a lot of other food. They also contain plenty of other vital nutrients. Brazil nuts, for instance, are an excellent source of selenium; pumpkin seeds are great for zinc; hemp and flax seeds are full of omega-3 essential fatty acids. As I mentioned earlier, be sure you consume only raw unsalted seeds and nuts because roasting seeds and nuts introduces carcinogens and damages the nutrients. Blend seeds and nuts with tomatoes for a healthy, delicious dressing.

I love avocadoes, which are high in monounsaturated fat. I also use them on occasion as dressing for my salads.

Don't overdo it with fat, though. Fat is vital, but it is also tasty and easy to overindulge. One to six ounces of seeds and nuts a day is a good amount. (In the next chapter I'll explain how much is best depending on your physical needs.) Listen to your body and adjust as you see how your body responds to different foods. Each person is different, and each day is different. If you're eating too much fat, you'll know because you'll feel sluggish and gain weight. Many WFPB eaters get carried away with nuts, and many raw food restaurants use very rich, heavy nut bases, but this can lead to weight gain, lethargy, and digestive stress. Pay attention to your body's reactions, and when in doubt, have less.

ESSENTIAL FATTY ACIDS—EMPHASIS ON ESSENTIAL

One of the biggest reasons you need a sufficient amount of fat in your diet is essential fatty acids—those omega 3s and omega 6s that have gotten a lot of press lately. They're called essential for the simple reason that our body cannot produce them—we must get them from outside sources in order to survive. They're key for most of our internal systems, including our cardiovascular, nervous, and immune systems. They help with cell repair and regeneration. They have anti-inflammatory powers, give skin elasticity, help lubricate joints, improve brain function, contribute to longevity and general health, and on and on. But the main point is that you want to get a good and balanced dose of them on a regular basis.

Soak chia seeds before you eat them: I soak about 24 grams of chia in about 6 ounces of water for at least 10 minutes.

The best sources of essential fatty acids are seeds and nuts. Hemp seeds, flax seeds, chia seeds, and walnuts are all excellent sources of omega-3 essential fatty acids. I grind the flax seeds into a fine meal, then add them to blended salads or sprinkle them on salads to add taste and texture. They have a nice, nutty flavor and they are easy to incorporate into any meal. With chia, I soak about 24 grams of chia in about 6 ounces of water for at least 10 minutes. Then I add them to my blended salad dressing.

UNHEALTHY FATS: ANOTHER REASON TO AVOID ANIMAL FOODS

But not all fat is created equal. The foods I described above are all healthy sources of fat. Consumed in moderation, this kind of fat is vital to good health. These monounsaturated fats, consumed in small amounts, would not interfere with blood flow or heart health. What you want to avoid at all costs are saturated fats, which come mostly from meat and dairy products. Meat is relatively high in saturated fats. So while you're getting your protein from your meat, you're also getting a high percentage of saturated fat. Some meats are over 90 percent saturated fat, and these are very hard for the body to digest. This means you're directing energy to your digestion, and therefore reducing the amount of energy you have for other tasks. In addition to making you lethargic, this type of fat clogs arteries and restricts blood flow. Reduced blood flow means less oxygen is reaching your muscles, including your heart, which is especially crucial for those in training who are determined to reach their peak athletic performance.

This is also true of dairy products, whether you're consuming milk, eggs, or cheese. Animal fat is going to clog your arteries and reduce blood flow. At best, your body will be less efficient at everything; at worst, you'll suffer heart attacks, strokes, and cancer.

Cardiovascular disease is the number one killer of Americans. Don't increase your risk with animal fats.

> "High-fat plant foods are high in the essential fatty acids that your body needs. Nuts and seeds and avocado are some of nature's ideal foods for humans and the best source of healthy fats. They can satiate true hunger better than oils because they are rich in critical nutrients and fibers and have one quarter the calories of an equal amount of oil."
>
> — Joel Fuhrman, M.D.,
> Eat for Health

A. In late 2014 we started to hear a lot of buzz about high-fat diets being better than high-carb diets. Soon a throng of people were claiming that steak and butter were healthy foods because they were high in fat. Some people even claimed that bacon was healthy because it contains niacin (vitamin B3). (Eating bacon to get your niacin instead of, say, mushrooms or sweet potatoes is not a good idea.)

To make things worse, some of the people who promote a steak- and butter-filled diet are denouncing WFPB diets as unhealthy because they are "high-carb" and "low-fat." They'd have you believe that bacon and eggs are a better choice than oatmeal and blueberries.

This debate will probably continue to rage for years, and I can't refute every argument here. In the meantime, consider the following guideposts as you make your choices:

Whole-food carbs and refined carbs are not equal. One of the biggest problems about the high-carb/low-carb war of words is that the anti-carb believers don't separate good carbs, like whole fruits and vegetables, from bad carbs, like refined sugar and white bread. *Every* WFPB proponent will tell you not to eat refined carbs because they will create blood sugar spikes and lead you down the road to insulin resistance and eventually diabetes. You **must** eat carbs with fiber, in whole foods like ripe fruit.

Animal protein is a troublemaker in your body. As I explained a few pages ago, animal protein is not good for your body. T. Colin Campbell's studies show a strong link between animal protein and cancer. In addition, as Dr. Gabriel Cousens points out, animal protein contributes to the metabolic imbalances that promote diabetes. You should avoid animal products.

Fat is essential—just don't go overboard. Plant foods can provide you with the healthy fats your body needs. Eat **whole** plant foods like nuts and seeds, but don't add oil. Oil packs anywhere from 100 to 120 calories per ounce, so adding oil can add pounds you don't want or need.

Don't be afraid of fruits and vegetables. If you're eating a variety of whole fruits and vegetables, you don't need to worry about them hurting you. Fruit can have a lot of sugar, but as long as you eat it in its whole form with its fiber, and as long as you eat vegetables as well as fruit, you will be fine.

THE RAW AND
THE COOKED

I strongly recommend that you avoid eating foods cooked at high temperatures, specifically temperatures above 212 degrees Fahrenheit, the boiling point of water. In *Becoming Raw*, nutritionist Brenda Davies explains why cooking can be trouble: "When foods are subjected to heat, especially at high temperatures, several byproducts can form that are very damaging to human health. Among the most notorious are acrylamide, advanced glycoxidation end products (AGEs), heterocyclic amines (HCAs), and polyacrylic aromatic hydrocarbons (PAHs)."

That's a lot of long words and acronyms to handle, but the simple explanation is this: heat creates strong chemical reactions. When you heat food, you can create dangerous chemicals that weren't present before.

Research on these chemicals and the dangers they pose to us is still in early stages, but the results so far are disturbing. HCAs, which occur when animal foods are grilled or fried, are known to damage DNA. PAHs, which occur when fats are heated to very high temperatures, may be linked to several types of cancer.

"The body perceives [advanced glycoxidation end products (AGEs)] as invaders and so its immune cells try to break down the AGEs by secreting large amounts of inflammatory agents. If this natural process is called on too often, the result will likely be diseases commonly associated with old age but which actually have more to do with toxins created by high-temperature cooking. Less elastic skin, arthritis, poorer memory, joint pain, and even heart conditions are often attributable to inflamed tissue."

— Brazier,

Thrive

While animal foods produce the most dangerous chemicals, high-heat cooking of plant foods can be dangerous as well. Browning foods and roasting them creates potentially dangerous amounts of AGEs. Davies explains, "There is evidence that AGEs impair immune-system function, accelerate aging, and contribute to the progression of Alzheimer's disease, cardiovascular disease, diabetes, eye diseases, kidney disease, nerve diseases, and stroke."

Although browning or roasting nuts or vegetables may appeal to you, the potential dangers are significant. In addition to introducing dangerous compounds, you're damaging the nutritious micronutrients in otherwise-healthy plant-based foods. You don't have to heat these healthy foods to enjoy their delicious flavor.

Low-temperature cooking of lentils, beans, grains, and grain-like seeds, such as quinoa and buckwheat, does not form dangerous amounts of these compounds. (All cooking can produce some AGEs, but lower concentrations do not seem to be dangerous.) If you're at all worried, go high to all raw.

THE GREAT DEBATE:
WHOLE FOODS VERSUS SUPPLEMENTS

Dietary supplement manufacturers—a thriving, $20+ billion per year industry—want to keep this information under wraps, but the secret is finally out: many nutritional supplements aren't doing you much good, if any at all, and may in fact do you harm. They've been gouging us out of our money for years, including thousands of my own hard-earned dollars, by claiming to promote longevity, lifelong health, general well-being, superior energy, stronger bones, better immunity, and more. But many of their claims, their studies, and their promises are crumbling before our eyes. New studies (ones not funded by the supplement companies) have revealed that consuming a specific vitamin or mineral in pill form does not produce the same effect in our bodies as that vitamin or mineral when it is consumed as part of a whole natural food. All this time, we should have been focusing not simply on what we put in our mouths but on what gets absorbed by the body.

For instance, those who take calcium pills—which we've been told to take for years to strengthen our bones in old age—don't fare any better in terms of fractures than those who don't take the pills. The pills may be composed of 100 percent calcium, but the body can't absorb the calcium in pill form and it simply gets excreted.

"Nobody chooses their diet based on databases and RDIs. But quantifying foods this way reinforces the impression that this is the best way to understand nutrition, and the fear engendered by those reductionist tools leads many people to worry about not getting their daily allowances. Hence Americans spend $25-30 billion or so each year (as of 2007) on nutrient supplements."

— T. Colin Campbell,
Whole

To get calcium into your bloodstream, you need to eat leafy green vegetables. In fact, it's been shown that some supplements can have a harmful effect. According to the National Institutes of Health Medline Plus site, "There is growing concern that taking high doses of antioxidant supplements such as beta-carotene might do more harm than good. Some research shows that taking high doses of beta-carotene supplements might increase the chance of death from all causes, increase the risk of certain cancers, and possibly other serious side effects. In addition, there is also concern that taking large amounts of a multivitamin plus a separate beta-carotene supplement increases the chance of developing advanced prostate cancer in men."

Nutrients change when they are fractured and delivered to the body in pill form. People thought and continue to think that if, for example, the beta-carotene in carrots helps prevent lung cancer, then a greater and more condensed quantity of beta-carotene delivered to the body in pill form would be a great way for people to reduce their risk of getting lung cancer.

But for a long time no one paid attention to whether these nutrients were actually getting absorbed into the bloodstream in the same way as when they were consumed as part of a whole natural food. And it turns out that this difference is critical: our bodies do not absorb fractured, isolated nutrients as well as they do nutrients in their original form. Popping a Vitamin C pill is not the same as eating an orange, and taking a calcium pill every morning is not going to prevent osteoporosis.

It's not all that surprising when you think about it. Our bodies were not designed to absorb intensely formulated and isolated nutrients developed in a chemist's lab. Supplements deliver too much of a given nutrient too quickly, and it taxes our system to try to extract the goodness from a high-density pill. When our bodies can't absorb a substance effectively, they just excrete it; in other words, you're flushing a whole lot of money down the toilet.

On the other hand, sometimes you **don't** excrete it, and that's another problem. As Brendan Brazier explains in *Thrive*, "While [the body will excrete] water-soluble vitamins (vitamins B and C) and minerals such as potassium, chloride, and sodium, fat-soluble vitamins and certain minerals, such as iron, are not so readily excreted … An excess of synthetic fat-soluble vitamins (A, D, E, and K) in the system can have a considerably more negative effect than those that are water-soluble." Instead of excreting these substances, the body builds them up, often with very negative effects. That's

"Are you sitting down? Because I need to explain something that almost no one acknowledges about nutrition: there is almost no direct relationship between the amount of a nutrient consumed at a meal and the amount that actually reaches its main site of action in the body — what is called its bioavailability."

— Campbell, Whole

why these supplements come with warnings about consuming too much. But why bother with supplements when you can get these nutrients by consuming whole plant foods? Vitamins and minerals from whole foods don't build up in dangerous amounts.

You practically can't overdose on a nutrient in food form. Because fruits and vegetables are naturally full of fiber and therefore filling, you're unlikely to eat 20 carrots at one sitting (big carrots, that is, not "baby" carrots). Your body is designed to naturally deter you from overdoing it.

The supplement approach ignores another crucial fact: nutrients function synergistically. For instance, oranges don't contain only vitamin C. They contain a wonderful myriad of other nutrients—more than we have discovered—and all of those nutrients aid in making that vitamin C available and absorbed. As Campbell explains, "**The process of nutrition is profoundly wholistic**, in that the way the body uses a particular nutrient depends on what other nutrients are ingested along with it. **If we just take an isolated vitamin C pill, we miss out on the cast of 'supporting characters' that may give vitamin C its potency.** Even if we add many of those characters to the pill too, which some manufacturers have done with bioflavinoids, we are still assuming that whatever is in the apple and not the pill is somehow unimportant."

Athletes in particular have been told for years that they should increase their intake of certain nutrients—notably protein—in order to achieve peak athletic performance. But all those horrible-tasting protein powders are not and never have been the answer. I'd even venture to say that all those supplements may have actually detracted from those athletes' abilities, because their bodies had to devote extra energy to try to assimilate those fractured nutrients and then excreting what they couldn't absorb, thereby depleting their overall energy level. What they should have done to enhance their athletic performance was adopt a nutritionally dense whole food diet, thereby increasing the number of nutrients in bioavailable form.

What all of this really means to you and me is that whole foods—fruits, vegetables, seeds, and nuts—are the way to go. Nature intended for us to get our nutrients from real food, not pills, and it's still the very best, most effective, most efficient, most delicious, and most satisfying way to get the appropriate balance of vital nutrients. Very simply, our body knows what to do when an orange is ingested. It has evolved over millions of years to extract precisely what it needs from different kinds of food without stressing any of our organs. And less dietary stress means more energy for other things.

If you're not persuaded and want to hang on to those pill bottles as a precaution, at the minimum purchase supplements made from

"The healthiest way to meet nutritional needs is to simply eat a diet rich in whole foods. Food-sourced vitamins and minerals are superior to their laboratory-created counterparts. . . .Many calcium supplements are derived from non-food sources— oyster shells, bovine bone meal, or dolomite—none of which the body is able to use efficiently. Again, the more work the body must do to assimilate nutrients, the less usable energy it will be left with."

— Brazier,

Thrive

whole foods. These nutrients at least started out as natural, whole foods and stand a better chance of being absorbed than anything developed synthetically in a chemistry lab. The only exceptions I would consider are Vitamin B12 and Vitamin D supplements. For those who live in northern climates who don't have regular access to sunshine, Vitamin D supplements are a viable alternative. And Vitamin B12 supplements can be good as an insurance policy. If you go this route, remember to always purchase the best quality supplements you can.

Finally, consider that dietary supplements lack the formal regulation of drug testing, so companies have a lot of leeway in terms of what they can put out on the market, the claims they make, and the doses they suggest. Although persuasive to the consumer looking for a quick and easy health boost, most of the common marketing terms used to trumpet the virtues of supplements ("All natural!") are virtually meaningless. Many of these supplements have not been tested on humans at all, and few have been subjected to rigorous or long-term studies. When ingested at high levels, some of these nutrients function as drugs in our bodies, with all manner of side effects and long-term consequences—from overstressed organs to lack of energy.

I hope that the myth of supplements will continue to crumble and that the vast aisles of supplements in health food stores will be replaced by a bigger produce section, which is really a more colorful, healthy, and tasty way to get your nutrients in the first place.

THE REAL TELL-TALE SIGN OF AGING: TELOMERES

If you want to know how youthful a person is, don't look at wrinkles, look at telomeres—although you'll need a microscope to see them. Telomeres are the caps at the ends of our chromosomes, and they help our genes replicate properly (into healthy cells rather than cancer cells, for example). In the past decade, research into telomeres has revealed that telomere length correlates to lifespan, with longer telomeres correlated to longer lifespan and shorter telomeres to shorter lifespan.

The great news is that healthy choices can keep telomeres long. Research shows that a plant-based diet high in vegetables and fruit, moderate daily exercise, and stress reduction techniques such as conscious breathing and meditation greatly reduce the rate of telomere shortening, as Michael Greger, author of *How Not to Die*, explains. And longer telomeres mean you're young, no matter your chronological age.

CHAPTER 6

FULL-SPECTRUM NUTRITION: WHAT TO PUT IN

■ ■ ■

You know fruits and vegetables are good for you. You know that you should "eat the rainbow" because all those color-saturated plants are filled with vitamins, minerals, and antioxidants that will improve your health. But did you know that you can get all the protein you need from plants? Did you know that you can get all the fat you need from plants? Plants give us full-spectrum nutrition, and it's about time we gave them more real estate on our dinner plates.

WHAT TO EAT—
PUT IN THE GOOD STUFF

During the past several decades, our knowledge of human health and diet has exploded—we've had an explosion of new knowledge, and we've seen many of our long-held assumptions exploded by what we've learned. We've relearned what the ancient physician Hippocrates told us: "Let food by thy medicine, and medicine be thy food." We've also learned that plants are by far the healthiest food choices available.

"Some people think the 'plant-based, whole foods diet' is extreme. Half a million people a year will have their chests opened up and a vein taken from their leg and sewn onto their coronary artery. Some people would call that extreme."

— Caldwell Esselstyn, MD,
Forks over Knives

As I mentioned in Chapter 4, I eat a high-raw plant-based diet, meaning I eat raw fruits, vegetables, seeds, and nuts. Occasionally, the remainder of my diet comes from cooked legumes, grain-like seeds, and lightly steamed vegetables. Some of you might be intimidated by the idea of adopting this kind of a diet; others might think it's extreme.

In *Forks over Knives*, Caldwell Esselstyn offers another definition of "extreme": "Some people think the 'plant-based, whole-foods diet' is extreme. Half a million people a year will have their chests opened up and a vein taken from their leg and sewn onto their coronary artery. Some people would call that extreme." For you, it might take an extreme change to go from your current diet to a WFPB diet, but I believe it's a small change in the face of the extreme risk posed by the standard American diet.

I have been eating a plant-based diet for almost three decades now. I can attest that plants have everything you need for a healthy body and mind. You don't need animal foods for protein. You don't need them for fat. You can get the protein and fat your body needs from plants, and they won't hurt your body the way animal proteins and fats will. And of course, animal foods can't give you any of the incredibly beneficial micronutrients that plants can.

ROD'S WFPB PYRAMID

This food pyramid is my guide for balanced nutrition. I recommend eating the most of the bottom level, a little less of the next level, and so on, keeping the top level to a small but high-impact portion of your diet.

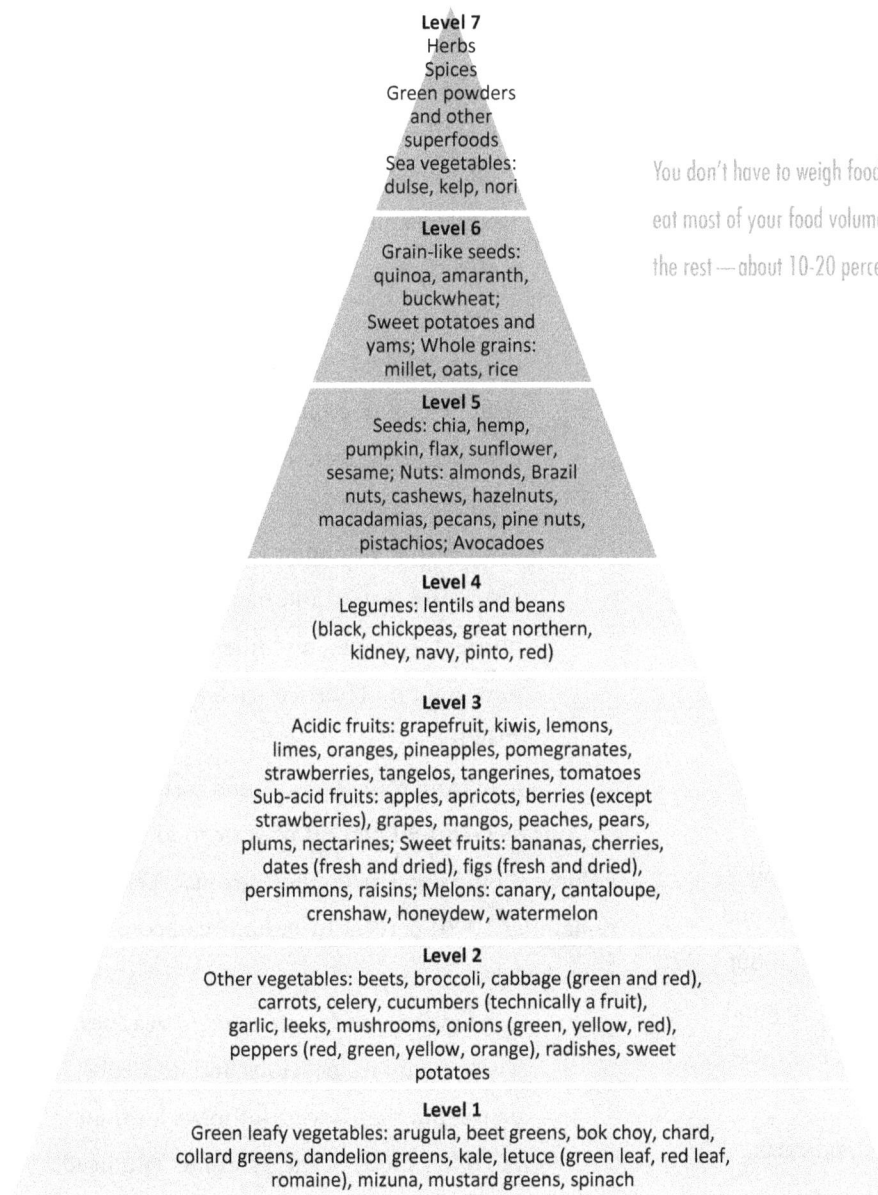

Level 7
Herbs
Spices
Green powders
and other
superfoods
Sea vegetables:
dulse, kelp, nori

Level 6
Grain-like seeds:
quinoa, amaranth,
buckwheat;
Sweet potatoes and
yams; Whole grains:
millet, oats, rice

Level 5
Seeds: chia, hemp,
pumpkin, flax, sunflower,
sesame; Nuts: almonds, Brazil
nuts, cashews, hazelnuts,
macadamias, pecans, pine nuts,
pistachios; Avocadoes

Level 4
Legumes: lentils and beans
(black, chickpeas, great northern,
kidney, navy, pinto, red)

Level 3
Acidic fruits: grapefruit, kiwis, lemons,
limes, oranges, pineapples, pomegranates,
strawberries, tangelos, tangerines, tomatoes
Sub-acid fruits: apples, apricots, berries (except
strawberries), grapes, mangos, peaches, pears,
plums, nectarines; Sweet fruits: bananas, cherries,
dates (fresh and dried), figs (fresh and dried),
persimmons, raisins; Melons: canary, cantaloupe,
crenshaw, honeydew, watermelon

Level 2
Other vegetables: beets, broccoli, cabbage (green and red),
carrots, celery, cucumbers (technically a fruit),
garlic, leeks, mushrooms, onions (green, yellow, red),
peppers (red, green, yellow, orange), radishes, sweet
potatoes

Level 1
Green leafy vegetables: arugula, beet greens, bok choy, chard,
collard greens, dandelion greens, kale, letuce (green leaf, red leaf,
romaine), mizuna, mustard greens, spinach

You don't have to weigh foods and count calories to follow this plan. Just eat most of your food volume — 80-90 percent — from levels 1-4, and the rest — about 10-20 percent — from levels 5-7.

Let me give you a little more detail about each of these levels, starting from the bottom.

Level 1: Green leafy vegetables. You want the greatest bulk of your food to come from this category. These veggies (except spinach) are all cruciferous vegetables, which are the most micronutrient-packed foods available to us. They're low in calories, high in fiber, and full of vitamins and minerals, so you get a nutritional punch that fills you up while consuming very few calories.

Level 2: Other vegetables. This group includes a huge range of vegetables, including some of the fruits we call vegetables (namely cucumbers and peppers) and some fungus (mushrooms). (Note that I haven't listed every veggie in the pyramid—there's no way they would all fit!) In the next section I'll talk about why this vast range of veggies is so good for you. Eat a generous amount of these as well.

As Joel Fuhrman's quote, above, indicates, you should aim to eat **one pound** of raw vegetables (Levels 1 and 2) each day. That doesn't include cooked veggies. If you think there's no way you could eat that much, pick up a few different veggies at your supermarket and put them in the scale until they weigh a little more than a pound (because you'll discard some parts of almost any veggie). It should be a generous plateful. As Dr. Fuhrman says, if you split that up between two meals, it's not that hard to do. And if you want to be 100 percent raw, just eat from levels 1, 2, 3, 5, and 7.

Level 3: Fruit. I have broken this group up into three categories—acid, sub-acid, and melons—based on the food-combining rules I explain in chapter 10. For the purposes of the pyramid, just remember that you should be eating several servings of whole fruits every day (not fruit juice). All fruits are packed with helpful micronutrients, but each fruit delivers a different combination, so eat a wide variety.

Level 4: Legumes. Legumes include beans and lentils, and they are full of nutrients, protein, and fiber. They're an important and nutrient-rich part of a WFPB diet.

These bottom four levels should be the bulk of your diet—80-90 percent of your food by volume should come from these groups. The remaining 10-20 percent by volume can come from Levels 5-7.

Level 5: Seeds, nuts, and avocadoes. These foods are delicious and nutrient-dense, but they have a lot more fat than the other foods in the pyramid. You need to have them in your diet—the fatty acids and micronutrients they supply are essential for good health—but if you overdo it, they can contribute to weight gain. I'll give you some guidelines for this category later in this chapter.

Level 6: Grain-like seeds, sweet potatoes, yams, and whole grains. These foods are nutritious; sweet potatoes, for example, can give you niacin that's hard to find in other veggies. However, all these foods are calorie-packed compared to other plants, so they don't offer you as many micronutrients per calorie as vegetables or legumes. In particular, you should eat fewer whole grains than veggies or legumes. Grain-like seeds, including quinoa, amaranth, and buckwheat, have more protein and less fat than other seeds, so you don't have to be as careful with your quantities as you do with other seeds.

Level 7: Herbs, spices, green powders and superfoods, and sea vegetables. Most of the foods in this category you won't want to eat in huge amounts—you probably want to eat a teaspoon of turmeric rather than half a cup. These foods have a ton of flavor and nutrition in a tiny package, so you only need a little.

When it comes to the pyramid, keep it simple and don't get caught up trying to figure exact percentages. This graphic should be a helpful guide, not a source of stress. Just remember to eat about 80 percent of your food from the bottom four levels (fruits, veggies, legumes, and whole grains) and the remainder from the top two levels (seeds, nuts, avocadoes, spices, herbs, superfoods, sea vegetables).

EAT THE RAINBOW OF FRUITS AND VEGGIES

We've been hearing we should eat our fruits and vegetables since we were in diapers. And we know that's because they're full of nutrients, which keep us healthy and strong. But few of us know much beyond that. This chapter sings the praises of fruits and vegetables and explains in more detail why they're Mother Nature's perfect food and what variables we should consider when we're buying them.

So what is it exactly that makes fruits and vegetables so magical? Well, for one thing,

they're the most nutrient-dense foods on the planet. They've got all the macronutrients (protein, carbohydrates, and fat) in abundance, but also a dizzying number of micronutrients, which are equally important for our long-term health. They've got antioxidants, fiber, carotenoids, and much more. We can't get all of these vitamins and minerals as effectively in any other form. Also, they're low in calories.

Another thing about raw fruits and vegetables is the fact that they are a complete package, containing within them everything we need to help us digest them effectively. Think about it. Many of them have an enticing flavor—carrots are sweet, tomatoes slightly salty, oranges refreshingly acidic (although they produce an alkaline balance in our bodies). Many of them satisfy our innate sweet tooth. Finally, they contain plenty of fiber, which lowers the time it takes for your body to discard any waste. The fiber also slows the rate of absorption so that your body doesn't absorb any single nutrient too quickly. For instance, the fiber in an apple ensures that you get a nice steady release of glucose, not a quick spike, which would create a correspondingly high spike in insulin as a response. Not only do fruits and vegetables supply nutrients, but they also supply compounds that help our bodies extract the maximum benefit from those nutrients. It is all rather elegant when you think about it.

"Since [raw vegetables] have a negative calorie effect, the more you eat, the more weight you will lose. A negative calorie effect means that the food contributes so few calories and is so bulky that it displaces space in the stomach, leading to a full feeling, which has the effect of limiting other, more calorie-rich options."

— Fuhrman,
Eat for Health

Fruits and vegetables are perfectly designed for us: consider the way in which the various nutrients in a given food complement and enhance one another. When we look at an orange, we think vitamin C. But it turns out that we can't absorb vitamin C without the help of bioflavonoids. And guess which foods have an abundance of bioflavonoids? Citrus fruits. So the orange isn't just supplying us with the vitamin C but with the helpers to absorb it. In fact, supplement companies are now introducing citrus extracts into their vitamin C supplements in an effort to replicate the natural synergy that already exists in the orange. Nature provides the nutrients in a synergistic way. There are hundreds of other examples just like this and many more that we don't even know about yet. We have only identified a small fraction of the nutrients in an orange and all other fruits and vegetables. Instead of popping a few supplements, keep in mind that there's far more going on than meets the eye when it comes to fruits and vegetables; eat the real thing instead.

It's one thing to know we should eat more fruits and vegetables and another to embrace that knowledge wholeheartedly and make it happen. Here are some tips on how to successfully incorporate more fruits and vegetables into your diet and start to reap the health benefits. Note that vegetables are highest in minerals, while fruits are highest in vitamins, so you want a good mix of both to get the maximum variety of nutrients.

For starters, consider the staggering variety of fruits and vegetables available to us. While there are only a handful of flesh types that people regularly consume (beef, chicken, lamb, and pork), there are hundreds of different varieties of plants. And that is not only good for our taste buds but for our bodies as well. You see, that variety is vital to our health. Because different fruits and vegetables have different amounts of various nutrients, we need to incorporate an abundance of them into our diet if we are to extract the maximum benefit from them. In fact, it turns out that variety is an important element of cancer prevention.

It can help to think about the food we consume in terms of a rainbow. Our objective should be to select from all the different colors. In fact, those colors are more than just about making them pretty. Those colors represent nutrients—and the deeper the color, the more nutrient-dense they tend to be. For instance, red and purple vegetables and fruits (red cabbage, cherries, blueberries, and so on) are particularly high in the cancer-fighting flavonoid anthocyanin. Green vegetables are full of chlorophyll. Oranges are packed with Vitamin C. So you want to always be sure you're including a mix of berries, leafy greens, oranges, peppers, etc. But don't neglect your white-fleshed foods. New research shows that white-fleshed fruits and vegetables (apples, pears, cauliflower, and so on) play an important role in reducing stroke risk. So, it may help to think of eating the rainbow—and the clouds.

BUILD YOUR BODY'S DEFENSES

As I explained earlier in the book, changing your diet can prevent and even reverse the course of many chronic diseases. This may fly in the face of everything you've been led to believe about heart disease and cancer. But the science is becoming increasingly clear on the matter: we do have the power to prevent, and even reverse, a plethora of chronic diseases that we have long thought to be determined only by genetics.

It certainly worked for Norman Walker, who lived to almost 100 years of age thanks to his juicing and consumption of fruits and vegetables. This was a man who was born in the nineteenth century, an era where the life expectancy was about 40 years. Walker ate a diet of raw fruits and vegetables, and in his eighties he wrote, "I still feel my best years are ahead of me. I never think of birthdays, nor do I celebrate them.

Today I can truthfully say that I am enjoying vibrant health, I don't mind telling people how old I am: I AM AGELESS!" Walker invented the Norwalk juicer, which is still the gold standard.

Not only does a plant-based diet help prevent chronic disease, it also helps prevent colds and flu. I've been eating this plant-based diet for close to 30 years and during that time I have been ill only once. Once! And here's why: after several weeks of working 20-hour days, I had compromised myself with too little sleep and not enough attention to my diet and exercise. I had gone into the UCLA medical center for a checkup (as I explained in chapter 1) and come away with a glowing bill of health. The next week, however, I came down with pneumonia, which I most likely picked up at the hospital. If I had stayed diligent about maintaining my health practices, I would have stayed healthy despite my contact with the pneumonia bacteria.

When you eat a WFPB diet you will not only look healthier and feel more energetic, you will also rarely, if ever, get sick. And if you do get sick, you will recover in a fraction of the time you would if you were on another kind of diet. I never took a sick day in all my years as chairman and CEO of my company (which was just about the time I adopted the WFPB diet). My colleagues were always coming in with colds, but I was entirely immune to all the germs floating around the office and never got sick during my tenure. The reason is simple. I was consuming such a huge quantity of antioxidants, vitamins, minerals, and micronutrients that my body had built a protective shield against germs. Bacteria thrive in a weak immune system but couldn't gain a foothold in mine.

Now getting a cold may not sound like the end of the world. But think of it as the canary in the coal mine. If your body can't fight off a mild cold, then how do you expect it to resist all the

"The best and most effective way to prevent illness is with comprehensive nutritional adequacy maintained all year ... An improved diet is more effective than any ... specific cold [remedy]."

— Fuhrman,

Super Immunity

bigger diseases, such as cancer and heart disease? That cold is telling you that your immune system isn't able to do its job properly, and that you'd better start supplying it with a better arsenal with which to fight off the bigger invaders.

In this day and age, people rely much too heavily on pharmaceuticals. They tend to think of them as a simple cure-all, but the fact is that pharmaceuticals often can only suppress symptoms. They often cannot address the main cause of the problem. Pharmaceuticals are a dangerous and toxic crutch, for they do nothing to keep people from getting sick in the first place.

This is all the more frustrating because the solution is so simple: you are what you eat. If you eat better, you will get sick less, if at all. If you follow this diet, you will significantly lessen your chances of contracting a fatal disease. The body is exceptionally good at repairing itself and warding off disease if given the proper tools to do so. Build an impenetrable immune system as a protective shield, and you can plan to enjoy many healthy years ahead.

FIGHT OFF FREE RADICALS

There's lots of talk about free radicals these days, but what are they exactly? Free radicals are molecules that have lost an electron, which renders them unstable. In order to re-stabilize themselves, they have to steal an electron from a

stable molecule, thereby turning it into a free radical. Oxidizing processes, many of which are necessary for survival, create free radicals, but an overabundance of free radicals can set off dangerous, cell-damaging chain reactions. The cell damage from these reactions can have many detrimental consequences for our bodies. Although some effects are mild (fatigue, increased signs of aging), other consequences of letting free radicals go unchecked are much more damaging. Cancer is the most notorious effect, but stroke, lung disease, liver trouble, glaucoma, and cataracts are other adverse effects of free radicals.

The bad news is that a certain amount of exposure to free radicals is inevitable. Free radical damage comes from sunburns, toxins in the environment, cigarette smoke, pesticides in our food, stress, even an extra-hard workout session. It's part of modern life.

FRUITS AND VEGETABLES COUNTERACT FREE RADICALS

The good news is that you can build an army to stop these free radicals in their tracks. The conquering army in this case consists of a group of nutrients called antioxidants, and they're found in abundance in fruits and vegetables. You're undoubtedly already familiar with some of them—Vitamins A, C, and E are antioxidants,

"Since neither processed foods nor animal products contain a significant load of antioxidant nutrients or any phytochemicals, the modern diet is dramatically disease-promoting. In other words, we are eating ourselves to sickness."

— Fuhrman,
   Super Immunity

as are certain phytochemicals. Unlike free radicals, which are missing an electron, antioxidants have one or more extra electrons to donate. Antioxidants release electrons to the free radicals without becoming unstable themselves, effectively neutralizing the free radicals and stopping them from causing any kind of chain reaction.

You have far more control over your long-term health than you have been led to believe. The science is clear: proper nutrition is very powerful. And this is due in large part to the protective shield created by an abundance of antioxidants.

ANOTHER REASON TO CHOOSE ORGANIC

Many of us already know that organic food is preferable to conventional, since it was not grown with harmful pesticides. We obviously should not be eating food that contains toxins. What you may not know is that organic food actually contains a higher nutrient content than conventionally grown foods. Here is why: when plants are grown without pesticides, they have to deal with insects, which is stressful. This stress causes the plant to produce a greater number of antioxidant compounds so that they can defend themselves. They are stronger (more nutritious) as a result. The organic plants therefore are more packed with phytonutrients; when we eat them, those phytonutrients in turn help us fight disease. You'll also find they taste better. So if disease prevention is a priority for you (and it should be), then it is worth making the switch to more nutrient-dense and disease-resistant organic food.

PLANTS ARE RICH SOURCES OF ANTIOXIDANTS

It's hardly surprising that antioxidants have become a buzzword in the health and beauty supply world. Beauty creams tout antioxidants as a way to fight free radical damage to the skin. Vitamin supplement companies have also jumped on the bandwagon, claiming that increasing your dose of antioxidants will ward off all sorts of disease. But as you've probably guessed by now, the best way to get your fill of antioxidants is from an organic WFPB diet.

Colorful fruits and vegetables are, without any doubt, the best possible sources of antioxidants. Carrots, kale, peaches, and cantaloupe for beta-carotene, which is then converted to Vitamin A; citrus fruits and green leafy vegetables for Vitamin C; seeds and nuts and leafy greens for Vitamin E; Brazil nuts for selenium; purple grapes, cranberries, and pomegranates for flavonoids; flax seeds for lignans; tomatoes, pink grapefruit, and watermelon for lycopene, and so on. All of these are different varieties of antioxidants, and they are incredibly easy to come by when you're on a plant-based diet. (You can look up the ORAC scores on the Internet for a list of foods highest in antioxidants.)

"Low in calories and high in life-extending nutrients, green foods are your secret weapon to achieve incredible health."

— Fuhrman,

Eat for Health

RADIATION

Radiation fears spike every few years when it makes the news: people started paying close attention to radiation after several of Japan's nuclear reactors were damaged by the earthquake and tsunami in March 2011. Everyone wanted to know about the potential dangers of the leaking radiation.

The bad news is that radiation is all around us, all the time. However, the kind we have to worry about is ionizing radiation, which can create large numbers of cancer-causing free radicals. Since radiation is cumulative, the biggest threat to our health comes from the low levels of radiation that we all experience: electromagnetic fields, airport and medical X-rays, cell phones, microwave towers, UV radiation, and so on. We all are accumulating these low levels of radiation all the time.

Now for the good news. Just about all of the recommendations in this book help protect against radiation, especially eating sea vegetables, including dulse. As Dr. Gabriel Cousens explains, sea vegetables contain multiple compounds, including iodine and sodium alginate, that work to neutralize radioactive materials in your body. If you adopt this diet, you will, in fact, be adopting an anti-radiation diet at the same time. The anti-radiation diet is high in minerals, many of which are cancer-inhibiting. The iodine, calcium, zinc, iron, selenium, and potassium you're getting from raw vegetables can improve your body's ability to repair the negative effects of radiation. Think leafy greens, such as spinach, chard, and kale, as well as citrus fruits, watermelon, and pineapple. A diet high in antioxidants neutralizes free radicals. When you switch to a plant-based diet, you will be consuming many, many more cancer-fighting substances than you did before, and your protection against free radicals will be better than ever.

So despite all the bad news out there, you can take control and keep radiation at bay through nutrition. Fortunately, it's the exact same diet that we already recommend for a variety of other reasons. So this is just one more reason to start making the transition today.

One group of plants that is considered particularly effective in the fight against cancer (especially estrogen-triggered cancers such as breast cancer) are the cruciferous vegetables. Named after the cross-shaped flowers that grow on these plants, these consist primarily of leafy greens (kale, arugula, bok choy, cabbage, collards, and mustard greens), but also include broccoli, cauliflower, turnips, radishes, and rutabagas, among others. These vegetables are packed with phytonutrients, which create a strong protective shield against harmful carcinogens. In particular, they contain isothiocyanates (ITCs), which are credited with helping us break down toxins. Note that you must consume these vegetables raw in order to enjoy the benefits of these phytonutrients. If you cook them, their health-enhancing properties will be compromised. To derive the maximum benefit from them, you should chew, juice, or blend them. These

"Cruciferous vegetables in particular, broccoli, Brussels sprouts, cabbage, kale, bok choy, collards, watercress, and arugula, to name a few, are loaded with disease-protecting micronutrients and powerful compounds that promote detoxification and prevent cancer."

— Fuhrman,

Eat for Health

techniques break down the cell walls and make the phytonutrients more bioavailable. If you eat them whole, be sure to chew them for a long time. Also, lightly steaming broccoli, cauliflower, cabbage, and so on is just fine. If I steam them, I only do it for about two minutes (less time than most cookbooks recommend). I like to pour the extra water from steaming on my food to add flavor and moisture.

Remember, supplements are not the way to increase your nutrient intake. Nutrient-dense foods have tremendous health benefits. Those nutrients taken in fragmented form do not. In fact, they can even have adverse effects. For instance, folic acid (the synthetic form of folate) in pill form has been linked to triggering certain cancers, while folate in leafy greens helps in preventing them. The answer is simple: eat your vegetables (especially cruciferous leafy green vegetables).

GO NUTS (AND SEEDS)

Nuts and seeds are a terrific source of micronutrients as well as healthy fat. As Joel Fuhrman states in his terrific book *Eat for Health*, "Believing fat is the villain is wrong. Eating a bread, potato, and pasta-based diet is not as healthful as a diet higher in fat, where the extra calories come from seeds and nuts." He also encourages us to eat avocadoes, which are rich in micronutrients, fiber, and healthy fat.

"Well-controlled trials that looked to see if eating nuts and seeds resulted in weight gain found the opposite; eating raw nuts and seeds promoted weight loss, not weight gain."

— *Fuhrman*
Eat for Health

VEGGIES VS. PHARMACEUTICALS

Drugs that treat erectile dysfunction (ED) have launched a multi-billion-dollar industry and created a cultural phenomenon among aging men. What most men don't know is how completely unnecessary those drugs are.

Doctors know that ED is the canary in the coal mine for cardiovascular disease. Rip Esselstyn explains the issue beautifully in *My Beef with Meat*. "To help you understand why the artery to the penis tends to block up first and foremost, let's take a look at the diameter of two arteries. The coronary artery that flows to the heart is about 5 mm wide, or the size of a normal drinking straw. The artery to the penis is a mere 1 mm wide, or the size of a little coffee stirring straw." That's a pretty clear picture.

If you decide to take a pill to treat ED without changing your diet, you're doing a disservice not only to your sex life, but also to your life in general. Research shows that ED is not something men will absolutely experience with old age. Instead, it's almost always the result of poor diet and lack of exercise that have led to cardiovascular disease. So forget the drugs and eat your veggies!

HOW MUCH IS ENOUGH?

But as I said earlier, we have to be a little careful about seeds, nuts, and avocado because they are so calorie-rich. As Fuhrman says, "Don't sit in front of the TV and eat an entire bag of nuts in an hour. Nuts and seeds contain about 160-175 calories per ounce, and a handful could be a little over an ounce."

Not everyone has the same fat needs. If you're already healthy and moderately active (the way I hope you'll be as you become an Ageless Boomer), you can have 3-4 ounces per day: "Most healthy, normal-weight individuals who exercise moderately and are in good shape can eat 3-4 ounces of seeds and nuts a day. That will bring their fat intake up to about 30 percent of total calories." If you have avocado on a given day, reduce your nut intake by an ounce or so that day.

"One form of omega-3, ALA, which is found in certain nuts and seeds, can be converted in the body to the other forms, making fish consumption unnecessary."

— Campbell,

Whole

If you're overweight, nuts will help you lose weight, but you need to eat less. "If you are significantly overweight and want to maximize your weight loss, you should limit your intake of seeds, nuts, and avocadoes to one (one-ounce) serving a day since they are calorie-rich,"

Fuhrman says. "However, you should not exclude these healthy, high-fat foods completely from your diet …. Studies show including some seeds and nuts in your diet actually aids in appetite suppression and weight loss."

If you're very active, Fuhrman says you can eat more nuts and seeds as well as avocado because you'll be burning up more calories. "A competitive athlete may require 4 to 6 ounces or more of raw seeds and nuts a day, in addition to an avocado." The bottom line is that each of us has different calorie needs, and we should adjust our consumption of calorie-rich foods accordingly. If you're living an Ageless Boomer lifestyle, you can probably have 3-4 ounces a day, and if you're very active athletically, you can have 6 or more ounces plus an avocado.

Incidentally, nuts can be a little hard to digest at times; you can soak seeds and nuts for up to 10 hours to make them easier to digest. (You should always soak chia seeds for about 10 minutes before you use them.) The downside is that most nuts don't taste as good when they're soaked. Soak almonds because they're among the hardest to digest, but don't remove the nutrient-rich skin. I don't soak nuts very often, but I do chew them really well so that they're easier to digest.

NUTS FOR NUTS

Dr. Fuhrman gives the following summary about the benefits of different nut varieties on his web site, drfuhrman.com:

Almonds are rich in antioxidants. In one study, people ate either almonds or a snack with a similar fat profile each day for 4 weeks, and the subjects who ate almonds showed reduced oxidative stress markers.

Walnuts. Diabetics who ate walnuts daily for 8 weeks experienced an enhanced ability of the blood vessels to dilate, indicating better blood pressure regulation. There is also evidence that walnuts may protect against breast cancer. [Walnuts are also high in omega-3 fatty acids.]

Pistachios and **Mediterranean pine nuts** have the highest plant sterol content of all the nuts; plant sterols are structurally similar to cholesterol, and help to lower cholesterol levels. Pistachios reduce inflammation and oxidative stress as well as cholesterol.

Mediterranean pine nuts contain a specific type of fatty acid that has been shown to curb appetite by increasing hormones that produce satiety signals.

Flax, hemp, and **chia seeds** are extremely rich sources of omega-3 fatty acids, and **hemp seeds** are especially high in protein, making them a helpful food for athletes.

Pumpkin seeds are rich in iron, calcium, and phytochemicals, and may help to prevent prostate cancer. [These seeds are high in the essential nutrient zinc.]

Sesame seeds have the greatest amount of calcium of any food in the world, and provide abundant amounts of vitamin E and contain a lignan called sesamin; lignan-rich foods may protect against breast cancer.

(Content above quoted from www.drfuhrman.com. Bracketed text added to quoted material.)

LOVE YOUR LEGUMES

Legumes, which include beans, peas, and lentils, are a healthy, hearty way to round out a vegan diet. As athlete and nutrition expert Brendan Brazier says in his book *Thrive: The Vegan Nutrition Guide,* "High in protein, fiber, and many vitamins and minerals, a variety of legumes are part of my regular diet." Fuhrman calls them "the perfect carbohydrate" because they're much more nutritionally rich than other carbs such as grains (even whole grains).

If you're worried about missing iron and calcium when you stop eating animal foods, legumes are a terrific source of both. Esselstyn shows in *My Beef with Meat* that soybeans, lentils, kidney beans, lima beans, navy beans, black beans, pinto beans, and tofu are among the best plant sources of iron. A cup of boiled soybeans can give you 50 percent of your daily iron needs. And, he writes, "Just 2 cups of black beans contains more than 90 mg of calcium, and a cup of delicious white beans has a whopping 130 mg."

Fuhrman explains how the starches in beans are perfect for weight loss and management: "Beans and other legumes have uniquely high levels of fiber and resistant starch, carbohydrates that are not broken down by our digestive system. Though indigestible, these carbohydrates have a number of valuable health effects. First, because they are indigestible they reduce the total number of calories that can be absorbed from beans. Fiber and resistant starch also limit the glycemic (blood-sugar-raising) effects of beans. Finally, when resistant starch and some fibers reach the colon, they act as food for our healthy gut bacteria, which then ferment it into anti-cancer compounds in the colon." (From "Beans: The Ideal Carbohydrate" on www.drfuhrman.com.) In short, legumes are superfoods.

As with all plant foods, you should eat a variety of different legumes because each type of bean delivers a different combination of nutrients to your body. Brazier sings the praises of yellow peas for the amino acids and B vitamins they supply. Black beans are packed with antioxidants. White beans, as Esselstyn noted, are packed with calcium. And all of these beans combine deliciously with vegetables to make terrific, hearty meals.

Finally, consider this thought from Fuhrman's *Eat for Health*: "[An important longitudinal] study found legumes were associated with long-lived people in various food cultures, such as the Japanese (soy, tofu, and natto), the Swedes (brown beans and peas), and the Mediterranean people (lentils, chickpeas, and white beans). Beans and greens are the foods most closely linked in the scientific literature with protection against cancer, diabetes, heart disease, stroke, and dementia." In other words, if you want to eat like an Ageless Boomer, eat your beans!

MANAGING THE MUSICAL FRUIT

Beans are notorious for giving people gas, but that doesn't mean you need to equate beans with discomfort. If you haven't been eating a lot of beans, you just need to take it slow, as Fuhrman explains: "If beans give you gas or bloating, make sure that you start chewing them very well. It takes some time for your digestive tract to grow the bean-digesting bacteria to digest them better. You may have to start out with a smaller quantity and increase the amount gradually. Don't stop eating beans entirely. It will make things worse when you try to eat them again. Instead, just eat a smaller amount first, gradually increasing over time." (*Eat for Health*) Brazier offers this tip in *Thrive*: "Another way to improve the legumes' digestibility is to add seaweed to the pot when cooking them, to release the gas. A short strip of seaweed is enough for a medium-sized pot."

Another important measure of good long-term health is acidity. Foods are naturally acid-producing or alkaline-producing, and our goal should be to keep our bodies balanced, or even slightly alkaline. If the foods you eat produce too much acid, your body will have to draw calcium from your bones to make the body alkaline, thereby weakening the bones.

Brazier has an excellent explanation of acid- and alkaline-producing foods in *Thrive*: "An acidic environment within the body negatively affects health at the cellular level. It is not possible to be truly healthy when the body is in a

"So if you want to have strong bones and be healthy, here's the trick! Avoid diets rich in animal-based proteins, which will decrease the pH level of our blood, draining that precious calcium from our bones."

— *Esselstyn,*
 My Beef with Meat

constant state of acidosis (characterized by excessively high acid levels)."

Over time, an overly acidic diet can reduce our body's strength and its capacity to fight disease. Brazier points out that because acidity is a stressor, it can raise your levels of cortisol (the stress hormone) and lead to fatigue. An acidic body is like a petri dish for viruses and other chronic diseases. For example, you may experience osteoporosis or increased bone fractures because your body has been diverting calcium, an alkaline mineral, from your bones to

fight the acidity in your system and restore your acid/alkaline balance.

Recent studies have demonstrated a link between high-acid-producing diets and a wide range of diseases and debilitations, including bone loss, joint and muscle pain (due to lactic acid buildup), autoimmune diseases, and more. And the reverse is true: 2004 study of Boomer women (ages 45-54 at that time) showed that women who ate less acid-producing foods had higher bone density and bone mass. Athletes should note that a high-acid-producing diet can cause inflammation and muscle tension, neither of which will help enhance athletic performance.

For optimal health, your goal should be to maintain a balance on the pH scale, even aiming to stay slightly more alkaline than acid. The most acid state is 0 and the most alkaline is 14. Your body has natural systems and buffers that work to keep your pH in the range of 7.3 to 7.4. You don't have to worry about the technical details as long as you follow a WFPB diet because plant-based foods are overwhelmingly alkaline-producing. As Brazier explains, even the acid-producing plant foods like nuts are only slightly

"Fruit is vital to your health and well-being and can contribute to lengthening your life."

— *Fuhrman,*
 Eat for Health

acid-producing (animal foods like milk or meat are highly acid-producing).

It's important to understand that acid-producing foods are not necessarily those that taste acidic to us (citrus fruits, for instance, are not acid-producing but alkaline). That's why I've used the term "acid-producing" rather than "acidic." The measure of a food's capacity to produce an acidic or alkaline state is not based on its taste when we eat it but on the effect it has on our bodies after it has been digested.

For example, meat and dairy, as well as all processed foods, such as white bread and pasta, are highly acid-producing. What foods are high alkaline producers? Vegetables, especially leafy greens. In fact, if you want a simple way to know the difference between acid- and alkaline-forming foods, use this as your litmus test: if it came out of the ground or off a tree, it's highly likely that it's alkaline-forming. If it was processed in any way, it's likely to be acid-forming. Simply by increasing your intake of leafy greens, you can lower your body's stress levels, increase your immunity, and improve your prospects for long-term health.

"H=N/C [Health equals Nutrients divided by Calories] is a concept I call my health equation. It stresses the importance of focusing on the nutrient density of your diet. If your nutrient intake is low and your calories are high, your health will be only a fraction of what it could be if you were consuming a high level of nutrients in each calorie."

— Fuhrman,
The Eat to Live Cookbook

Leafy greens are also a great source of chlorophyll, another wonder nutrient credited with wide-ranging healing powers (but remember that you have to eat those leafy greens in a raw state to enjoy the benefits of chlorophyll). Vegetable juice is a great option, as are salads. Many fruits are also quite alkaline, including kiwi, all citrus, papaya, pineapples, figs, olives, some stone fruits such as cherries, and some berries. Fruits in the middle of the scale include apples, cucumbers, tomatoes, apricots, peaches, blueberries, strawberries, and nectarines. Note that some foods on this plant-based diet are somewhat acid-producing (nuts and some fruits, such as avocadoes), but they are balanced out by the rest of your plant-based diet. (For a detailed, multi-page chart of acid- and alkaline-producing foods, check out Brazier's *Thrive*.) Although we can't tell whether a food is alkaline or acid just by looking at it or tasting it, if you eat a wide variety of fruits and vegetables and avoid animal products, you won't have to spend time thinking about the pH scale.

Finally, pay attention to your fiber intake. Fiber is the all-important broom that sweeps out toxins and other waste. It's vital to your long-term health. Now, if you adopt this whole-food plant-based diet, you'll never have to give fiber another thought. You'll be getting more than enough in all the foods you consume. But I mention it because colon cancer, one of the most common cancers in the country, is associated with toxic buildup in the colon. Fiber flushes that debris out of your colon, radically diminishing your chances of contracting cancer there.

Fiber is also an important element in the fight against heart disease, which kills more people in this country than any other disease. Fiber helps reduce cholesterol, which is responsible for all manner of heart-related problems and a key risk factor for heart attacks. In fact, the plant-based diet developed by Dr. Dean Ornish, founder and president of the nonprofit Preventive Medicine Research Institute, is so successful at combating (both preventing and reversing) heart disease that his clinic is now being covered by insurance companies (who clearly see the bottom line benefit of a diet-based cure over high-priced quadruple bypass surgery).

GARLIC, ONIONS, TURMERIC, AND OTHER SPICES

Whenever anyone asks me what to take to help cure an ailment, I always tell them to eat vegetables, fruits, seeds, and nuts, and to add more raw garlic—no matter what the illness may be. Garlic has an astounding number of health benefits. It has been used to heal people for thousands of years. Greek and Roman warriors are said to have consumed it because they believed it magnified their strength and endurance. As recently as World War II, wounded Russian soldiers consumed garlic to prevent infection; as a result, they dubbed it Russian penicillin. They also used it in poultices applied directly to their wounds.

"Increased consumption of allium vegetables [garlic and onion] is associated with lower risk of cancer at all common sites."

—Fuhrman, Super Immunity

Modern research proves that the ancients were right to use garlic for healing. It reduces risk for heart attack and stroke, has cancer-fighting properties, brings down blood pressure, helps cure infections, boosts the immune system, works as an antibiotic, an antifungal, and an antiviral. The doctor who told me to go vegan, Dan Miller, also recommended garlic to me because research studies showed a strong protective link between garlic consumption and decreased cancers of the stomach and colon

Garlic has both preventive and curative powers, so be sure to add it to your salads and blended salads on a regular basis. Note that you need to peel and mince it, then eat it fairly soon after that. I also love to use garlic when I cook, but there's a trick to it. You have to mince the garlic and then wait ten minutes before you add it to the cooking pot. I learned this trick from Dr. Andrew Weil, who says, "This allows the allicin—the active component of garlic—to form, as it needs air to do so. Once the allicin is formed, it does not deteriorate while cooking." You can buy various preparations of garlic in supplements, but as with all supplements, I would stay away from them and always opt for the real thing.

Although onions have a less pronounced effect than garlic, they have many similar benefits. Green onions are some of the best sources of nutrients, and their mild flavor makes them perfect for everything from blended salads to cooked grain dishes.

I also believe strongly in the curative powers of spices. All kinds of herbs and spices have healing properties. Spices are a great source of antioxidants and are powerful anti-inflammatories. Turmeric, for example, contains curcumin, an anti-inflammatory compound that has been shown to have a preventive effect on Alzheimer's disease and helps with mental focus. Cayenne pepper contains the compound

"Curcumin also has a potential role in the prevention and treatment of [Alzheimer's Disease (AD)]. Curcumin as an antioxidant, anti-inflammatory and lipophilic action improves the cognitive functions in patients with AD."

— Neurology researchers Shrikant Mishra and Kalpana Palanivelu, "The effect of curcumin (turmeric) on Alzheimer's disease: An overview"

capsaicin, which not only gives the pepper its heat but also is great for circulation, heart health, and easing muscle soreness. Ginger has been used for centuries in traditional Asian medicine; it's very good for soothing an upset stomach or providing relief for a sore throat. And sweet, fragrant cinnamon delivers a powerful anti-inflammatory kick that can help lower blood sugar. And, according to *Men's Journal*, "Cinnamon also kills bacteria, so the next time you get a cut, you can actually sprinkle the spice on the wound." (You should check with your doctor about that practice, though.)

So keep a supply of fresh organic spices on hand. Cinnamon, cloves, cumin, pepper, rosemary, thyme, and basil are just a few of the amazing herbs and spices you can add to your foods. Not only will they promote health, they also add a pleasant variety of flavors to your meals.

PASS UP THE SALT, PLEASE

One food that I strongly disapprove of is salt. It does not matter what kind of salt it is (sea salt, rock salt); we were never meant to consume it in the quantities that we do today. Processed foods are packed with salt, and Americans are consuming 600 to 800 percent more salt than they need each day. The effects are catastrophic: high blood pressure, osteoporosis, and more. Although it may take a little while for you to wean yourself off it, you will soon discover that your vegetables have plenty of natural sodium in them (celery and tomatoes have a wonderful natural saltiness). Also, your taste buds will become more responsive and will be better able to detect the natural sodium in the foods.

Many people worry about getting enough iodine if they stop eating iodized salt, and it is an important concern. As Dr. Gabriel Cousens, a doctor and holistic medicine practitioner, explains, iodine is critical for proper thyroid function, protection against radiation, and a host of other functions in the body. In addition, Brazier writes, "High levels of iodine are lost in sweat, making active people's requirements higher than those of less active people." You can get iodine by eating sea vegetables like dulse, kelp, and nori. Half a handful of dulse leaf will take care of your iodine intake and give you lots of other great nutrients.

"Sea vegetables are among the most nutritionally dense foods in the world. Containing about 10 times the calcium of cow's milk and several times more iron than red meat, sea vegetables are easily digestible, chlorophyll-rich, and alkaline-forming."

— Brazier,

Thrive

Sea vegetables are also great for giving your food a salty taste. You can add some sodium to your food by sprinkling kelp or dulse on your salads. You can put kelp in your salt shaker. But I strongly advise that you give up adding any kind of salt to your food altogether.

DIGESTION AND ENERGY

Many of the suggestions I'll give you throughout this part of the book have to do with reducing the work of your digestive system. Most people treat digestion like cleaning—they only notice it if the work doesn't get done. People don't think about their digestive systems until they act up in the form of bloating, gas, constipation, and other symptoms that cause inconvenience, discomfort, or worse.

The digestive system is one of the body's powerhouses, and it's terribly underrated and misunderstood. We really treat it like a black box—food goes in, waste comes out, and in between we get nutrition. I want to help you understand how much you can do to improve that system and reduce the drain on energy caused by digestive stress.

Digestion itself is an energy-intensive process. The energy our bodies use in digestion is called "diet-induced thermogenesis" or the "thermic effect of food." You actually use some of the calories you consume to digest that very food.

I recommend eating foods that minimize the labor of your digestive system. For one thing, your digestive system doesn't need extra stress—it works hard for you all day, every day, so there's no reason to make it work harder. For another, I'd rather have that extra energy available to exercise, play, work, and enjoy life. Once you find out how easy it is to get that extra energy, you'll want it too.

When we get to chapter 10, I'll go into great detail about many ways you can fine-tune your digestive system to optimize your energy use. Until then, remember that by packing your diet full of fiber-rich foods you are actually giving yourself an energy boost.

THE RAW ADVANTAGE

For the past six months (as of this writing), I have eaten a 100 percent raw diet and I intend to continue eating this way for the rest of my life. When I eat an all-raw diet, I feel my very best— my energy is high and my strength is excellent. I've been doing push-ups in sets of fifty, and when you do that many push-ups in a row it's tough to maintain perfect form. However, I asked my son-in-law to watch my form, just to make sure, and he told me that my fiftieth push-up was as good as my first. I'm not alone, either: Dr. Gabriel Cousens recounts his experience in his book Rainbow Green Live Food Cuisine: "In a personal observation of this diet, in my sixtieth year I was able to do 601 consecutive push-ups." This kind of physical performance is the raw advantage.

If I were to give just one reason for eating raw vegetables, fruits, seeds, and nuts, it would be enzymes. (It's not the only reason for eating raw, as I'll explain shortly.) Enzymes are small proteins that help us digest our food. They exist in all live food—fruits, vegetables, seeds, and nuts. But they're fragile little things and die when exposed to heat. So if you're eating a primarily cooked diet, you aren't getting very many of these nutritional powerhouses into your system. If, however, you introduce more raw food into your diet, you'll start to experience the myriad and powerful benefits of these enzymes. So basically, the raw food diet is all about preserving the enzymes and other nutrients in fruits, vegetables, seeds, and nuts.

The role of plant enzymes in human digestion is a matter of debate between raw food proponents and traditional nutrition specialists. Brenda Davis, a registered dietician and nutritionist and author of *Becoming Raw* (among other books), discussed the disconnection between what she learned about plant enzymes in college versus what she learned when she started researching her books. She was taught that plant enzymes don't matter—when they reach our stomachs, they get broken down, so it doesn't matter whether they get cooked. However, she found many researchers who said intact (raw) plant enzymes had a host of positive effects. She went to them and asked them to show her their

> "To help you remember the importance of raw vegetables, put a big sign on your refrigerator that says, 'The Salad is the Main Dish.' … Eating a huge, delicious salad is the secret to successful weight control and a long healthy life."
>
> — Fuhrman,
>   Eat for Health

research; when they did, she came away with a very different view.

Davis learned that plant enzymes perform at least two valuable functions: they "convert certain phytochemicals to their bioactive metabolites," and they "can aid in the digestive process," as she explained in a 2010 lecture at the University of Alberta. She went on to explain how this process works with myrosinase (found in broccoli) and allinase (found in onions and garlic), but I won't hammer you with those details. The point is, as T. Colin Campbell pointed out in *Whole*, that plants are full of complex nutrients that react with each other and with the human body in complex ways, and our research is only scratching the surface of the ways they work.

> "One of the least appreciated yet most important components of our diet, enzymes are vital to achieving optimal health. An absence of enzymes in your diet can result in the same sickness and disease associated with malnutrition, even if your diet is otherwise healthy."
>
> — *Brazier, Thrive*

Our own bodies produce enzymes that perform the important task of breaking down our food into small bits so that the nutrients can enter the bloodstream and be taken to the various organs and cells throughout our body. They're not just an essential part of the digestive process—they *are* the digestive process. Davis compares enzymes to garden shears that cut plants into small pieces; they come in all sizes and so that they can "cut" the molecules of food down into smaller and smaller pieces that the body can use.

Davis explains that during the early part of digestion, while foods are in the upper part of the stomach, plant enzymes can aid digestion because the acidity is low enough for them to survive. In addition to doing the immediate work of aiding digestion, enzymes are responsible for a long list of other health benefits, such as being responsible for breaking down, separating, and eliminating waste. When we provide our body with a big natural enzyme boost, we're enabling it to function at a higher level.

If you've eaten a raw enzyme-rich meal, the reserves aren't drained, which enables you to keep more enzymes in the bank for a rainy day, and the enzymes that you consumed with your fruits and vegetables get to work cleansing your system. A cleaner system means that your body is strong enough to resist germs, regenerates more effectively, and generally runs more efficiently.

Here's an example of just how effective enzymes can be at purification. I visited a colon hydrotherapist a few years ago because I heard that people felt great after cleansing their colon (effectively removing a long buildup of toxins there). When I arrived, the colon hydrotherapist told me that she had clients who had to come in 75 to 100 times before they were completely detoxified (one person came in over 200 times!). But after a single session, she told me I never had to come back again. There was no toxic buildup at all and she pronounced me clean. I credit the fruits and vegetables and the abundance of enzymes I consume for that happy diagnosis.

Enzymes are also a good way to prolong your health (remember all that toxic waste has been eliminated) and slow aging. In fact, I would venture to say that enzymes are the closest thing to the Fountain of Youth. I fully credit enzymes with my sharpness and clarity of mind, my vitality, and the radiance of my skin. Dr. Norman Walker was one of the first people to believe in the benefits of raw food. He became famous for his books on the merits of juicing, and he was perfectly healthy up until the day he died at the ripe old age of around 100. And what did he do? He consumed massive quantities of enzymes through his raw vegetable juices.

LIFE IS THE SOURCE OF LIFE

Whenever people meet me, they inevitably comment on how much energy I have. I attribute most of that to my intensely enzyme-rich diet. They are literally a life force in themselves. And when you think about it, it only makes sense. How can dead food nourish a live person? How can we possibly expect to get energy from something dead? How can we be expected to live a long and healthy life if we consume foods that we were never meant to eat? Life is the source of life. Live foods are the way to harness that vitality we all have within us, but that is all too often suppressed or drawn upon to do extra work it should never have had to do. Give your body the chance to achieve vitality, and it will reward you many times over.

As for how I get all those enzymes, I've found that a leafy green raw vegetable juice first thing in the morning, fruit a couple of hours later, and a vegetable salad with seeds/nuts in the evening is the answer. I generally consume from a pint to a quart (16–32 ounces) of vegetable juice a day. It would be difficult to consume in whole vegetable form all of the vegetables that I put into my juicer, which might include a bunch of spinach leaves or other dark leafy greens (especially cruciferous leafy greens like kale, bok choy, collards, etc.), several stalks of celery, and a bunch of parsley. It actually ends up being a slightly different combination every day. But condensed into juice form, it is a nutritious, hydrating drink that is literally supercharged with enzymes. With so many enzymes and so little fiber, the juice gets readily absorbed into my system, and I'm off and running for the day. I even "chew" my juice a bit (meaning that I let it rest for a moment in my mouth before swallowing) in order to allow it to mix with my saliva (which has lots of enzymes), jumpstarting the digestive process. And I drink it very slowly in order not to overwhelm my system. (You can read more about the benefits of juicing in chapter 10.)

"Not eating enough natural, unprocessed foods rich in vitamins, minerals, enzymes, high-quality protein, fiber, essential fatty acids, antioxidants, and good bacteria (probiotics) is a major source of stress on our bodies."

— Brazier, Thrive

As I explained in chapter 4, you can improve your longevity by eating fewer calories—far fewer than our standard American diet includes. A raw food diet provides an easy, healthy way to reduce your calorie intake naturally. As Dr. Cousens explains in *Rainbow Green Live Food Cuisine*, "On a healthy live-food [raw] regime one automatically gets the anti-aging calorie-restriction effect without having to diet."

Cooking foods, he explains, destroys the nutrients in the food: 50 percent of the protein, 60-70 percent of the vitamins and minerals, and 100 percent of the enzymes. When you eat your foods raw, you don't lose half of your nutrients in the cooking process, so you get more nutrition in each bite. "It becomes rather obvious," Cousens writes, "that by eating live foods, we are able to get complete nutrition with eating 50-80 percent less food."

EAT TO LIVE, DON'T LIVE TO EAT

We can control our prospects for a long and healthy old age. Before you're forty, you can get away with a lot, and you may feel immortal. But after forty, you pay dearly for what you practiced before you were forty. And you'll feel the effects of a poor diet more and more strongly over time.

On the other hand, if you take charge and give your body the tools it needs to stay healthy, you'll feel an increasingly vital and dynamic aging process that can only be described as reversing the clock. I can certainly confirm that's been the case for me.

CHAPTER 7

WATER — THE BODY'S MOST BASIC NEED

■ ■ ■

Water is the lubricant for the human machine and supports every cell in your body. Your body cannot survive without adequate water intake, and even just a 1-2 percent drop in hydration levels can lead to lower cognitive function and a drop in energy levels. Everyone knows how to recognize thirst, but how do we know how much hydration is enough, and how do we hydrate effectively?

Water is the single most important source of nourishment. Our bodies need it more than anything else. Consider the fact that we can last for weeks without food—but only about three days without water.

Take another step in becoming an Ageless Boomer through the long-term benefits of adequate hydration:

Look and feel younger

Boost mental clarity

Control body weight

Reduce the risk of disease

Improve digestion

Relieve back and joint pain

Our bodies consist of a little more than 60 percent water. It is essential to every single one of our organs and bodily functions. It helps build muscle, delivers nutrients to our cells and organs, lubricates joints, removes toxins, flushes out waste, smoothes out our complexions, helps us lose weight, remedies constipation, regulates our hormones, helps with mental health conditions, and on and on the list goes.

Water is absolutely vital to our well-being, and yet we give it remarkably little thought. We know that water is the great revitalizer, a symbol of lushness and fertility, but in terms of our own bodies we know little more than the fact that when we get thirsty, water quenches our thirst. This chapter explains why water is so essential to our health and why we should pay more attention to our consumption of it. It will address how much you need, when to consume it, and benefits of drinking water and eating water-rich plants that you may not even know about.

AVOID DEHYDRATION

Dehydration contributes to a multitude of problems such as constipation, water retention, reduced energy, headaches, and even a sagging complexion (since water is what plumps up cells to make us look more radiant). So how do we avoid dehydration? There are countless ways for us to become dehydrated, and it's worth spelling these out so you can pay special attention by eating water-rich vegetables and fruits and drinking extra fluids whenever you're in any of these situations.

We all know that we lose water through sweat when we exercise, but did you know that you also lose additional water when you're at high altitude, when you're out in the sun and the wind, and even just through breathing? Another big culprit is consuming cooked foods. Heating food dehydrates it, which means that when you consume cooked foods, your stomach must draw water from other parts of your body to make up for the lack of it. This means that you're actually pulling water away from other organs that need it to function effectively.

This highlights yet another problem with the standard American diet: many of the foods that Americans eat on a regular basis are water deficient, such as potatoes, meat, and bread. The foods on that diet start out low in water content and then get cooked, which further dries them out. In addition, certain foods are diuretic, which means they cause even further dehydration. Coffee, alcohol, and salt are all common examples of diuretics. If you consume any of these low-water-content foods or diuretics, you need to drink more water and/or eat more water-rich foods to compensate for the toll of additional dehydration.

"Fruits and vegetables ... are filled with water. When food is cooked, especially at high temperature, it loses moisture and can even act as a sponge once consumed to pull water from the system, increasing your thirst."

— Brazier,
Thrive

HOW MUCH WATER DO YOU NEED?

I recommend that you consume between two-to-four quarts of water per day, depending on your activity level. Two-to-four quarts is a wide range, but you have to consider all of the hydration variables: exercise, sun, wind, higher altitude, diuretic foods, cooked foods, and non-plant-based foods.

Lower hydration status is related to slowed psychomotor processing speed and poorer attention and memory performance in healthy older adults, as demonstrated in a 2004 study conducted at Ohio University.

Another helpful formula is to take your weight in pounds, cut it in half, and use that number as the number of ounces of liquid you should drink. For example, if you weigh 150 pounds, you should drink approximately 75 ounces as a minimum baseline, without taking exercise into account. My own consumption depends not only on my exercise routine on any given day, but also on the types of foods I'm consuming. On a day when I eat seeds and nuts, I tend to need more water. If I'm eating only fruits and vegetables, I need less.

Keep in mind that you don't have to get all that water from drinking. If you are consuming a plant-based diet, you'll be getting plenty of water through your food (just think of all the water in a juicy orange). Some days I know that I'm getting so much water through my food that I hardly need to drink much extra water. When I make my vegetable juice in the morning, it is organic vegetable water. Blended salads are another fabulous and tasty way to hydrate. I regularly consume oranges and grapefruits, which are loaded with water. Grapes and melon are other super-hydrating fruits. So if you don't feel like drinking pints of straight water every day, there are lots of tasty alternatives that will do the trick. Another benefit of satisfying your water quota through organic fruits and vegetables is that you'll be getting water in its purest, cleanest form.

ESTABLISH A REGULAR WATER ROUTINE

It's important to establish a regular water routine to make sure your fluid intake is adequate. For instance, I drink about a quart of water or vegetable juice over the course of a half-hour when I wake up in the morning, then fruits and vegetables, and I drink water throughout the day. Others like to break up their water intake throughout the day. For example, they might consume eight ounces when they wake up, at midmorning, before lunch, in mid-afternoon, a double dose before dinner, then eight more ounces before bed. Spreading it out over the course of the day is a good idea, since gorging on water all at once will make you feel uncomfortable and bloated.

WHEN SHOULD YOU HYDRATE?

While staying hydrated is vital to your health, when you hydrate is also important. If you are planning to work out, hydrate before you exercise as well as after. And if you're exercising for more than an hour, take a few breaks and hydrate during your workout. Hydrating throughout your workout can help reduce fatigue, increase your athletic performance, help with muscle cramps and lightheadedness, improve your coordination, and help you avoid heat exhaustion. Keep in mind that staying hydrated during exercise doesn't limit you to just drinking water. Oranges, for example, are an especially revitalizing choice.

I generally avoid drinking with my meals. If you drink water while eating, you dilute important digestive enzymes and negatively affect the efficiency of your digestion. According to Dr. Mantena Satyanarayana Raju, a naturopath from India, drinking water while eating weakens the acids that are critical to digesting food, which triggers the creation of even more acid. Further, when water is mixed with food in your stomach, it is not absorbed as quickly as it should be. This leaves water and undigested food fermenting in the stomach, causing bloating, gas, and a sagging stomach.

Drinking a glass of vegetable juice or water a half-hour before my meal tends to work best. And since I'm always consuming raw high-water-

Thirst is not an accurate measure of hydration, because you're already dehydrated once thirst kicks in. Your goal is to stay ahead of your thirst at all times. A nutritionist once suggested to me that we drink four ounces of water every half hour. She believed that the body couldn't absorb more than that at one time.

content vegetables and fruits during my meals, I typically don't get thirsty when I'm eating. Here are some good general guidelines: wait at least a half an hour after drinking water/vegetable juice to have a meal and wait to drink one hour after a fruit meal, two hours after a vegetable meal, and four hours after a protein meal.

HOW DO YOU KNOW WHEN YOU'RE ADEQUATELY HYDRATED?

There are several ways to check your hydration level. First of all, your urine color should be clear to pale yellow, not dark. Second, count your pulse rate. If you're dehydrated, it's going to be elevated. It will go down when you've had enough, but not too much, to drink. You can also get a sense of how much water you've lost during a workout by weighing yourself before and after. Eventually as you tune into your body's messages, you'll be able to sense what your body needs and it will become intuitive.

Is it possible to drink too much water? Well, yes—if you are very extreme about it, you may be at risk of overconsumption. Forcing large amounts of water into your body at one time puts an unnecessary burden on your cardiovascular system and your kidneys. But barring extremes, it's better to drink a little too much than too little.

DRINK PURIFIED, FILTERED WATER

It's counterproductive to buy water in plastic containers since plastic leaches harmful toxins into the water that are bad for you and bad for the environment. These toxins, such as biphesmol A, have been linked with obesity and insulin resistance. I suggest that you drink filtered water that has been purified using a reverse-osmosis system, which effectively removes contaminants, parasites, sodium, and even lead. This makes water safe for Boomers facing high blood pressure, kidney or liver disease, or sodium restrictions.

Dr. Andrew Weil, in discussing the presence of antibiotics and other drugs in water systems around the nation, has another suggestion. He points out that reverse osmosis technology can be expensive, which is true. However, only reverse osmosis can remove antibiotics from water.

SHED POUNDS WITH PROPER HYDRATION

Staying hydrated can help shed pounds. Here's why: if you don't drink enough water, your body holds on to what it does have, which means that it isn't as effective at flushing out waste. If your body is not flushing out waste, the liver is called in to rid the body of extra toxins. The liver also metabolizes the fat in your body and turns it into energy, but it can't do that if it's busy cleansing toxins. If liver is not metabolizing fat, the fat builds up. So water can contribute to weight loss by making the body function more efficiently.

116

CHAPTER 8

SLEEP — THE GREAT BATTERY CHARGER

■ ■ ■

Sleep recharges the battery of the human machine, and
much like nutrition and exercise, it is vital to our well-
being. While important, good sleep can also be elusive
for two-thirds of Boomers. By developing good sleep
habits, you can improve the quantity and quality of
sleep you experience.

REALIZE THE VITAL TRUTH
ABOUT SLEEP

To become the Ageless Boomer version of yourself, it is vital that you adopt sleep habits now that will fill you with energy in body and mind. Most of us underestimate the importance of sleep. Thanks to the conveniences of the modern age, we live in a fast-paced world that provides a nonstop procession of activities at all hours of the day and night. Further, we have an array of stimulants at our fingertips from coffee to diet pills to keep us going at a breakneck speed. With the endless flood of stimulants and activities, we often disregard our natural fatigue and biological clocks so that we can keep up with our friends, our families, and the Joneses. To fully become Ageless Boomers, we must start listening to our bodies again and return to our natural circadian rhythms.

In our early years, our bodies functioned effectively, even after long, youthful nights of little-to-no sleep. In our middle years, we were still able to function on little sleep as career and family demands exacted their tolls. Now, as you get older, you may feel that all those late nights are finally catching up with you. And it is true. By trading sleep for work or play early on in life, we have risked the long-term consequences in the form of serious medical illnesses, such as high blood pressure, heart attack, heart failure, stroke, obesity, psychiatric problems, and the list goes on.

Let's face it. For many Boomers, a good night's sleep is only a daydream. In a 2002 survey by the National Sleep Foundation, two-thirds of Boomers reported that they have problems sleeping. Michael Vitiello, Ph.D., a professor of psychiatry and behavioral sciences at the University of Washington in Seattle reports that common sleep problems that plague older adults include lighter sleep, a decrease in the deep-sleep stage, and an increase in periods of wakefulness when compared to their younger counterparts. If you are in the 67 percent of Boomers who have a difficult time falling asleep and staying asleep, you have probably already seen a doctor and may have been prescribed medication. Vitiello states that not only are these medications unnecessary, but they also are habit-forming and can cause side effects and even worsen existing sleep disturbances.

But how do we obtain that restful sleep that we need? The good news is that by reading this book and actively applying the concepts within it, you are already on the road to better sleep, but there are also other things you can do. This chapter will explain why sleep is so vital to our well-being, what induces sleep, what we can do

"[Sleep is] one of the components of a three-legged stool of wellness: nutrition, exercise, and sleep. The three are synergistic. It's hard to lose weight if you are sleep deprived. It's hard to eat healthy if you are sleep deprived. It is hard to exercise if you're tired."

— Safwan Badr, a past president of the American Academy of Sleep Medicine and a sleep expert with Detroit Medical Center and Wayne State University

to improve our chances of getting a good night's rest, and how to determine if we are getting enough sleep.

Along with proper nutrition and exercise, sleep is the third essential component in the basic trifecta of achieving optimal health. The power of the whole (nutrition + exercise + sleep, along with proper breathing, detox, water, and sun) is much greater than the benefits of the individual parts. There is a complex but vital synergy between low-stress nutrition, exercise, and rest. If we only focus on one or two of these things but ignore the third, we lose many of the benefits. It is only by giving adequate attention to all three elements that we can achieve perfect harmony.

Much like nutrition and exercise, sleep is vital to our well-being. To give sleep the significance it deserves, first we must understand its importance. Let's start with the obvious: sleep is our chance to rejuvenate our minds and bodies. While your body recovers from the stresses of the day, repairing muscles and soft tissue, your mind uses this time to process memories and experiences from the day. It gives your brain a chance to recuperate so that it is more effective the next day. In addition to that, most muscle-tissue repair occurs at night.

Over the long term, sleep boosts your immune system, increases your prospects for good health, and reduces stress levels and symptoms such as high blood pressure and weight gain. According to the Centers for Disease Control and Prevention, sleep deprivation is associated with an increased risk of many serious health problems including obesity, high blood pressure, type 2 diabetes, depression, heart attacks, and strokes, as well as a reduced quality of life and productivity and even premature death. It is quite apparent that if you don't snooze, you certainly lose.

APPLY THE SCIENCE OF SLEEP TO GET A GOOD NIGHT'S REST

You've probably heard of the hormone melatonin. This hormone ebbs and flows over the course of 24 hours, and an increase in melatonin is what makes us groggy and ready for bed. Melatonin is triggered by darkness. It generally increases to its highest level at the end of the evening and decreases in the early morning when we wake up. The critical fact is that melatonin takes its cues from the light and dark. Interestingly, the hormone melatonin has very powerful antioxidant effects, which means it plays an essential role in our long-term health by repairing tissue and combating the effects of aging.

Before the invention of electricity, people rose at dawn and spent their days outside. The body received the signal from the sunlight that it was daytime, causing the melatonin levels to drop, and the body enjoyed a natural increase in energy. As darkness fell, the body reacted by triggering the release of melatonin. Without electric lights, TV, or computers to distract them, people went to bed earlier, following the rhythm prescribed by their natural surroundings.

A 2014 study from the University of Oregon published in the *Journal of Clinical Sleep Medicine* reveals that when middle-aged or older people receive six to nine hours of sleep, they think more effectively than those sleeping fewer or more hours.

Thanks to electricity, we have learned to circumvent the darkness and stay up all hours of the night. This means that our bodies' release of melatonin is thrown off course, and although our bodies may need to rest and recuperate, we push our bodies harder and harder instead. In the short term, people think that they can fight fatigue and get more done, but that's only an illusion. Fatigue interferes with our abilities to perform efficiently—as we progressively become more tired, we are in fact less productive, more forgetful, less lucid, and less clear-headed. As a result, it takes us more time to accomplish tasks.

Over the long term, it's a simple matter of diminishing returns. However, if we take the time to reconnect with our natural cycles and embrace the benefits of deep rest, we can recuperate energy, speed repair, and become more productive in less time.

Some nights it may seem like there are not enough sheep in the world to count. If you find yourself watching the clock and thinking to yourself, "If I just go to sleep now, I can get six hours of sleep"; and then after counting 6,709 more sheep, you check the clock again and think, "If I just go to sleep now I can get five hours of sleep," you probably have not taken the proper steps to set yourself up for sleep success. The key to improving your chances of getting a good night's sleep lies in the preparation. To ease your way to dreamland, you will need to first establish a regular sleep pattern and take specific, practical steps towards sleeping.

ESTABLISH A REGULAR SLEEP PATTERN

How do we establish a regular sleep pattern? Well, for starters, it's important to recognize that the body thrives on regularity. This means that you should try to go to bed and wake up at the same time every day. If you have to stay awake longer than usual, try to wake up at the same time—even if you're a little tired. The most important part of your routine is to wake up at the same time. That regularity will do amazing things for your body and tell it exactly what to do when. Tempting as it may be, sleeping in

throws your body into jetlag mode, and it will lose its place in the cycle of the day. Your body is a creature of habit, and it will benefit from a stable waking-sleeping pattern.

In a 2010 study published in the journal *Sleep*, researchers determined that the maintenance of daily routines is associated with a reduced rate of insomnia and an improvement in sleep quality for the elderly.

Help your body recognize day and night cues by exposing your body to daylight in the morning and dimming the lights in the evening. If you can, try to get outside during the morning hours. Go for a walk. Eat breakfast outside. Play tennis outdoors. Note that although you can achieve some of this effect with electrical lights, natural sunlight is always preferable. Then, when the sun sets, take it as a reminder that it's time to start dimming lights in your house. It's unlikely you'll go to bed at sunset, but do what you can to minimize exposure to bright lights. Invest in dimmer switches. Turn off lights you don't need. Minimize your screen time. Diminish stimulation. These steps will all trigger the release of melatonin.

You can also help your body prepare for sleep by developing certain pre-bedtime rituals. I like to read at night (generally light fiction at that hour to rest my mind). I also often take a hot shower followed by a bracing cold plunge. I do breathwork and meditate (both of which should be done on an empty stomach) in the morning and sometimes I also meditate in the evening, depending on the stress of the day. This might be a bit different for everyone, but remember that your body will take its cues from regular patterns. I also advise finishing your evening meal about three hours before bedtime so your body doesn't need to work at digesting as it tries to slip into a state of rest. You'll sleep more deeply if your body isn't toiling away on digestion.

Some people have trouble getting their brains to slow down when they turn out the light. A college professor of mine gave me sensible advice to address this problem: keep a pad of paper by the bed and write down anything and everything you are thinking about—whether it is something you are worried about or things you need to remember to do the next day. That way, you can let your brain relax. It's all there for you to look at the next day: it's on the pad and off your mind.

CREATE A GOOD SLEEP ENVIRONMENT

It also helps to make your surroundings conducive to rest. I keep my windows open because I sleep better in a slightly colder room. I advise keeping your room temperature in the low 60s. I like the fresh air no matter how cold it is. Some people, if they really can't take the cold, will air out their bedroom for 10 to 30 minutes before they go to bed so that at least they will go to sleep with some fresh air. I invested in an excellent mattress—neither too firm nor too soft. I wear an eye mask to eliminate visual stimulation. When we lived in New York City, we purchased a white noise machine to drown out the city noise. (Now I have the ocean, the real thing.) All of these things are signals to my body that I'm getting ready to go to sleep. As a result, once I turn out the lights, I tend to fall asleep very quickly.

Occasionally, I wake up in the night. But rather than get frustrated by it, I work on relaxing my body. I might do some breathing exercises. A favorite of mine is very simple: I inhale through my nose for a certain number of seconds, then exhale out through my nose for at least twice as long. It's remarkable how relaxing that can be. I might also employ progressive muscle relaxation (see chapter 16, "Meditation and Breathwork," for details), which shows the difference between tension and relaxation. And sometimes, I just get up and go work at my desk for an hour. The important thing is not to get stressed or anxious, which will make it harder to get back to sleep.

START POWER NAPPING

Napping is an excellent way to revitalize your body and sharpen your mental clarity. Even just a 10- to 20-minute catnap can increase your vitality. I often say it gives you two days in one. When I worked on Wall Street, I used to attach a "Do Not Disturb" sign to my office door, put on my eye mask, and rest for 10-20 minutes. I always woke up refreshed and ready to work. The important thing is not to nap for too long. According to James B. Maas, a professor of psychology at Cornell University and author of *Power Sleep: The Revolutionary Program That Prepares Your Mind for Peak Performance*, seniors shouldn't take naps of more than 15 to 20 minutes if they want to sleep well at night. But don't underestimate the power of a good nap if you want to increase your clarity of mind.

DETERMINE HOW MUCH SLEEP YOU NEED

As for how much sleep a person needs, that depends on the person. I recommend trying to get seven to eight full hours of sleep. A 2014 study from the University of Oregon published in *the Journal of Clinical Sleep Medicine* reveals that when middle-aged or older people receive six to nine hours of sleep, they think more effectively than those sleeping fewer or more hours. Experiment with varying amounts of sleep and track your energy levels to determine the best amount of sleep for you. To effectively accomplish this, you'll need to eliminate stimulants such as caffeine and nicotine and depressants such as alcohol and sleeping pills, all of which wreak havoc with natural sleep-wake patterns.

The point is to realign your body with nature's rhythm and not attempt to fight your body's desire for rest. Sleep is not optional. Every animal needs it. It's not in our best interests to set obstacles in the path to rest and rejuvenation.

In a 2002 survey conducted by the National Sleep Foundation, sleeping 7-9 hours is associated with more positive moods and outlooks, as well as more active and engaged lifestyles for older adults.

Think of this as an opportunity to reclaim some personal quiet time. Invest some time in coming up with pleasant pre-sleep rituals. Enjoy the process of slowing down as bedtime nears and succumbing to your body's natural rhythm. With better, deeper sleep, you'll enjoy renewed vitality and clarity of mind.

Remember that you should not eat or work out within three hours of going to sleep. Also note that the release of the stress hormone cortisol during the day could prevent your being able to get into the deeper stages of sleep at night. We'll talk more about methods for managing stress in Chapter 15.

Q: IS IT TRUE THAT YOU NEED LESS SLEEP WHEN YOU EXERCISE REGULARLY AND EAT WELL?

A: You're going to be more fit on this nutrition and exercise program. And if you're more fit, every aspect of your life is going to be more productive. Your movements will be more efficient because you will be stronger, so it will take less effort to do the same things you were doing before. Also, thanks to your diet, you are taking out most of the stress of digestion and will have less of cortisol to contend with. This means that when you sleep, you will sleep more deeply, and it will ultimately be more restful. As a result, you won't need as much sleep as before. So, yes, you will be able to get by with less sleep and get more done during the day. Note that I'm not advocating less sleep; I'm advocating more efficient sleep.

The model of diminishing returns also presents a vital lesson to exercisers. Overtraining and ignoring your body's demands for rest can tax your central nervous system and affect the quality of your sleep. If you're exercising too much, pushing too hard, and/or not giving yourself a chance to recover, you run the risk of injury or burnout. The fact is that you will achieve net gains in your physical well-being if you take care of your body and give it a chance to rest and rejuvenate.

CHAPTER 9

SUNSHINE — THE NUTRIENT WE DON'T EAT

■ ■ ■

Sunshine has gotten a bad rap in recent years. All we hear is that if we don't avoid it at all costs, we'll get skin cancer, age prematurely, and so on. However, there's more to this sunshine story than you've been told. And what you don't know has been hurting you.

The past few decades have seen the sun vilified and labeled a danger to be avoided at all costs. The result? We slather on sunscreen year round, cover up with hats and clothing, and avoid time outdoors. Now up to 85 percent of people are Vitamin D deficient, and the negative health effects are becoming known.

What you may not realize is that sunlight is a vital nutrient. Exposure to the sunlight is not only good for us—it's necessary for our general physical health as well as our mental well-being. Much of it has to do with Vitamin D, an essential nutrient that is produced in your skin in response to sun exposure. By avoiding the sun, we are also avoiding our daily dose of Vitamin D.

Older adults are particularly prone to low vitamin D levels, because they generally get less exposure to sunlight and because their skin is less efficient in producing vitamin D than the skin of younger adults. This puts them at an inherent risk for premature frailty and disability and for poorer physical performance, according to a study highlighted in the April 2007 issue of *Journal of Gerontology: Medical Science.*

So how do we avoid skin cancer and still get all the Vitamin D that we need? This chapter emphasizes the importance of and the body's myriad uses of Vitamin D and how to safely obtain it.

"The most natural way to get vitamin D is by exposing your bare skin to sunlight (ultraviolet B rays). This can happen very quickly, particularly in the summer. You don't need to tan or burn your skin to get vitamin D. You only need to expose your skin for around half the time it takes for your skin to turn pink and begin to burn. How much vitamin D is produced from sunlight depends on the time of day, where you live in the world and the color of your skin."

— *The Vitamin D Council*

SOAK IN THE IMPORTANCE OF VITAMIN D

So what's so important about Vitamin D? Isn't skin cancer a bigger risk? Well, it turns out that, no, skin cancer is a relatively small concern when you consider all the myriad benefits of adequate Vitamin D absorption.

Vitamin D reduces our chances of contracting a whole host of lethal diseases, ranging from heart disease, disorders of the musculoskeletal system, and various autoimmune diseases, to other more dangerous forms of cancer. Did you know that living at higher latitudes with less sun exposure increases the risk of dying from Hodgkin lymphoma, as well as breast, ovarian, colon, pancreatic, prostate, and other cancers, as compared with living at lower, sunnier latitudes? When you consider this multitude of cancers and diseases that Vitamin D can help prevent, melanoma contracted through sun exposure presents a relatively small threat in comparison.

In addition, malignant melanoma isn't associated with cumulative sun exposure, as Margaret B. Planta, M.D., explains in a 2011 article in the *Journal of the American Board of Family Medicine*. In the U.S., it's more common in northern states where people have less year-round sun exposure. And it's associated with sunburns, which occur when people suddenly get a lot more sunlight than they're used to getting. That's why I recommend that you increase your sun exposure slowly and methodically.

Aside from relatively rare malignant melanoma, most diseases linked to excessive sun exposure are fairly benign, according to Robyn Lucas, an epidemiologist at the National Centre for Epidemiology and Population Health in Canberra, Australia.

ABSORBING THE BENEFITS OF SUNLIGHT

Vitamin D has several crucial functions, but most importantly Vitamin D helps ensure that the body absorbs and retains calcium and phosphorus, both critical for building bone and for avoiding osteoporosis later in life. Recent Vitamin D research has also revealed correlations with lowering blood pressure, lowering cholesterol, controlling infections, reducing cancer cell growth, helping with a variety of skin conditions, and more.

Sun exposure also regulates your hormones, elevating key ones such as serotonin, your happy hormone. The sun also has proven warming effects on your mood, elevating your disposition, reducing depression, and generally helping you maintain your emotional equilibrium. According to research conducted in 2006 by Wilkins, Sheline, Roe, Birge, and Morris in a cross-section of older adults, vitamin D deficiency was associated with low mood and impaired cognitive performance.

That's not all. A 2008 article by M. Nathaniel Mead in *Environmental Health Perspectives* lists more potential benefits of sunlight: decreased auto-immune disease, increased endorphins, better melatonin and serotonin regulation, and more. Andrew Weil, M.D., has suggested that sunlight may benefit hundreds of our bodies' functions in ways that we don't yet know.

GETTING YOUR DAILY DOSE OF VITAMIN D

It is possible to get Vitamin D from three sources: sunlight, food, or supplements. So which is the best? To answer that question, you need to know that vitamin D is different from other vitamins because 1.) our bodies can produce it, and 2.) our bodies turn vitamin D into a hormone called calcitrol, which carries out a lot of different functions in the body, including binding calcium. But the only way our bodies can produce their own vitamin D supplies is through exposure to sunlight.

Our skin tissue contains Vitamin D receptors, a sign that our bodies evolved to get our Vitamin D directly from the sun. These receptors exist in other animals as well. What's more, the number of Vitamin D receptors we have increases when we expose our skin to the sun. The point is that our bodies are designed to be exposed to and make the most of the sun. This is especially important to Boomers, because as we age, we lose Vitamin D receptors. That sunlight is vital to replacing those lost receptors and ensuring that we continue to absorb adequate Vitamin D.

Some foods contain a small amount of vitamin D, but most of them are animal foods, so I don't recommend eating them. For those of you who live in a northern climate without access to daily sun exposure, you may need a high-quality Vitamin D supplement. Just be sure to take it with a meal that has a little fat in it so that your body can efficiently absorb the vitamin.

However, supplements should never be a first choice when there is a natural alternative. Supplements are never absorbed as well as whole foods or, in the case of Vitamin D, as sunlight. They do not increase the number of vitamin D receptors in your body. In addition, it's possible to overdose on supplements, which isn't likely to happen when you go with the natural sun source.

In the July 2000 issue of the *Journal of Human Evolution*, California Academy of Sciences anthropologists Nina Jablonski and George Chaplin wrote that dark skin requires about five to six times more sun exposure than pale skin for equivalent vitamin D photosynthesis.

AVOID SUNBURN

It's crucial to exercise moderation and caution when it comes to sun exposure. Too much exposure can cause sunburn and premature aging from free radicals, and sunburn has been linked to some forms of skin cancer. Being careful not to burn is critical. As with the rest of this lifestyle, you want to let your body adapt in stages. Be judicious and use caution. Begin by exposing your body to sunlight for five minutes at a time a few times a week (maybe less for very light-skinned people). Then build up from there once you've developed a good base. If you're dark skinned, you can spend a little more time in the

"The Skin Cancer Foundation [tells] consumers that 'sunscreen should continue to be an integral part of a comprehensive program' to prevent melanoma. That's what most people will likely hear from their dermatologists as well. What they won't learn is that dermatologists get much of their information from the SCF, and the SCF, in turn, is heavily supported by the sunscreen industry. (A sunscreen manufacturer even funded SCF's quarterly consumer publication, 'Sun and Skin News.')"

— Journalist Michael Castleman, Mother Jones

sun. If you're a fair-skinned redhead, increase your sun exposure at a slower pace. Eventually, your goal should be to expose as much of your skin as possible to the sunlight without getting burned.

Margaret Planta's article, "Sunscreen and Melanoma: Is Our Prevention Message Correct?" questioned the message that the health care community has been giving Americans about sunscreen. Planta explained that sunscreen, as used by most Americans, really only does one thing well—prevents (or delays) sunburn. (To achieve the results dermatologists recommend, you'd have to slather yourself in a thick layer of sunscreen every day. No wonder sunscreen companies recommend this approach too.)

Preventing sunburn is good, right? Well, as Planta explains, it's not: sunburn is one of the body's warning systems, telling you that you've been in the sun too long. Wearing sunscreen can give your skin enough protection to slow down the sunburn reaction, but you're still getting sun exposure. That's great for your Vitamin D levels, but it's not so good if your skin is trying to warn you that you're getting too much sun too fast.

Sunburns are associated with higher melanoma risk, but it's important to consider who gets sunburned. Planta points to numerous studies showing that people who have consistent, long-term exposure to the sun are less vulnerable than people with little regular sun exposure who get occasional sunburns. "When used improperly, sunscreen can potentially increase the risk for CMM [cutaneous malignant melanoma] by conferring a false sense of protection against sunburn. This false sense of protection can lead to more time spent in the sun, paradoxically causing a greater incidence of sunburns."

In other words, if you live in New York but you take a vacation to Florida in December, lying on the beach getting a tan puts you at high risk for dangerous sun exposure. Wearing sunscreen might prevent sunburn for a while, but sooner or later you'd likely burn.

So what do you need to know about using sunscreen? That using it once in a while doesn't prevent dangerous cancers. That putting on a thin layer doesn't do much of anything. And that you can't rely on sunscreen to keep you safe from the sun—you have to be smart about your sun exposure and consider your unique circumstances.

There's no single answer to how much time you should spend in the sun, as it depends on a variety of factors—your skin type, whether you already have a base tan, the time of day, having a history of sunburns, being in a high-altitude climate, and how much of your skin is exposed to sunlight when you go out.

One benefit of being on a raw plant-based diet is that it gives you a good amount of inner sunburn protection. Mead points out that antioxidants may be very protective against sun-related damage. It's certainly true for me: I absorb so many antioxidants and carotenes in my diet that they act like a natural sunblock. I spend approximately 30 minutes walking in the sun every day, usually before 10 a.m. and after 3 p.m., in only shorts or a bathing suit—and needless to say, I don't wear sunscreen—and never get a burn.

Recent research shows that it can be difficult to get sufficient UVB rays (the source of Vitamin D) if you aren't in the sun at midday, when the UVB rays are able to penetrate the atmosphere more effectively. So I currently try to spend a little time in the sun around noon, as well. If I am outside closer to noon, I spend less time in the sun.

"The relationship between sun exposure and bone health is so incontrovertible that even the antisun lobby increasingly hems and haws about this issue in the face of new findings. When its spokespeople are put on the spot, they usually mumble something along the lines of 'Kids gotta drink more milk.'"

—*Michael F. Holick, PhD, MD,*
The Vitamin D Solution

If you're not on a WFPB diet yet, you'll want to expose yourself to the sun in smaller doses. Also, note that alcohol speeds up the effects of sunshine on your skin. In any case, alcohol is best avoided—but especially so if you plan to spend more time in the sun. Before you start your new sun regimen, check with your health care provider to come up with a customized program tailored to your skin type. Read Holick's books to get a rounded perspective about the right approach for you.

CHAPTER 10

HOW TO EAT

■■■

I've told you all about what you should eat—does it really matter how you eat? Yes. While you'll get wonderful advantages just by consuming the right foods, you can increase and fine-tune those advantages by changing what you eat and when, and whether you eat the food whole, blended, or juiced. This chapter will give you several techniques for planning your food intake to maximize your energy and health.

GET YOUR FOOD FROM THE BEST SOURCE

Modern Americans are many degrees removed from the sources of their food. When you order a hamburger from a fast-food restaurant, you are consuming something that was assembled at that restaurant, but the parts were cooked or shaped at a factory before they arrived there. The ingredients used probably didn't come from a farmer—they likely came from another factory or slaughterhouse in some preserved form. How many more steps back to the food producer? You can't really say "farmer" because the products so often come from giant agribusinesses, and "farmer" implies an individual who cares about the quality of his or her crop.

We can't all be farmers, eating the fruits and vegetables of our own orchards and gardens. But we can get our food closer to the source instead of consuming the end result of a processed food assembly line.

Our food consumption hierarchy should follow this model:

> Home-grown
>
> Farmers' markets
>
> Health-food supermarkets
>
> Plant-based restaurants

Right now, we're often flipping this hierarchy, relying on restaurant-made food. When we do buy food to make ourselves, too often it's pre-processed, "heat-and-eat" convenience food. Fortunately, for most of us it's easy to access better alternatives. (The fact that millions of Americans are stranded in "food deserts," where even supermarkets are too far away, is a significant problem in this country.)

EAT SEASONALLY AND LOCALLY

One obvious way to introduce variety into your diet is to make sure you are eating according to the seasons. There are several good reasons to do this, but the first is that you'll naturally rotate through different types of fruits and vegetables throughout the year, ensuring that you don't tire of any one type and that you get adequate variety. As strawberry season wraps up, blackberries or a new variety of blueberry will be ripening. As peaches wind down, apple harvests begin, and so on. There's something satisfying about tying your eating rhythm to the seasons— you're in sync with Mother Nature in a way that you weren't before.

Q: HOW DO YOU STORE NUTS, VEGETABLES, AND SEEDS?

A: I just put vegetables in the crisper drawer of the refrigerator. I store seeds and nuts in mason jars in the refrigerator to keep the essential fatty acids from getting rancid.

Closely linked to eating seasonally is eating locally. There are lots of good reasons to do this, but an important one is that locally picked produce is almost always fresher, and fresher produce retains its nutrients better, which means you get more health benefits from cherries grown at a farm down the road than you do from cherries flown across thousands of miles from Chile. The produce is less stressed, the nutrients are more robust, and the planet benefits from the lack of shipping. Everyone wins.

I know it isn't always possible to eat this way, especially if you live in a cold-winter climate. Frozen, canned, and dried fruits and vegetables are not ideal—they don't have the intact enzymes and the wealth of micronutrients that fresh foods have—but if they are your only option, they are a far better choice than animal foods. In other cases, some foods like avocadoes just don't grow locally outside of California, Florida, and Hawaii, so if you want their benefits you have to buy food that has traveled across the country.

BUY ORGANIC AND BENEFIT FROM FARMERS' MARKETS

Another thing to look for when you shop for produce is whether it's organic. This word has come up a lot in recent years and with good reason. There is absolutely no good reason for us to be eating pesticide-infused foods. The only people who benefit are the commercial farmers, who manage to make sturdier, more bug-resistant products that stand up well to transport. But anyone consuming those pesticides pays a heavy price over the long term. Right now, organic foods are more expensive than "conventionally grown" foods. That's changing as more stores recognize the demand for organic produce and more farmers are seeing the financial benefit of going organic. While you may be reluctant to pay the higher price for organic, consider it a long-term investment in your health. You will almost certainly pay less in medical bills down the road if you've properly maintained your health along the way, and the best way to do that is to only put the most natural foods in your body.

Q. DO I HAVE TO INVEST IN ORGANIC FOOD, WHICH CAN GET PRICEY?

A. I firmly believe that you can't afford not to buy organic food. When you look at the long-term cost savings, you realize that it's not more expensive. Think of it this way: you'll get sick much less frequently, if at all, which will save on doctors, pharmaceuticals, stress, and time lost at work. If you eat an organic, high-raw, plant-based diet, you will be spending more initially, but over the long term, you'll save. You're investing in prevention rather than treatment.

This brings us to farmers' markets, which are popping up all over the place these days, and it's worth pointing out a few of the less scientific bonuses of buying direct from the farmers. First, farmers' markets build community. You're almost certain to run into neighbors and friends when you shop there. Second, it's always a good thing to know the people who grow your food. It will give you a newfound respect for farming. Third, you're almost sure to find new varieties of produce to experiment with—obscure heirloom varieties of apples or tomatoes, different kinds of blueberries, entirely new types of fruits and vegetables, such as persimmons or durian. Finally, you're eliminating the middleman, ensuring that the farmers in your community enjoy the maximum profit for their work. Farmers' markets are about as close as you can come to a celebration of all the plants in this diet.

When you can't get to a farmers' market, put the "super" in your supermarket shopping. Look for one of the many health food supermarkets that have opened in the past decades. These stores typically have a much better selection of organic produce and it's much better labeled. If you're in a conventional supermarket, stick to the produce section as much as possible, and look for organic foods. If your local market doesn't stock a lot of organic produce, ask the produce manager to start stocking more. You're probably not the only person who wants the organic option.

Remember that you will be eating a lot more fresh fruits and vegetables on this diet, so you will need to plan to buy more of them, store more of them, and shop for them more often. Buy lots of the foods you know you love to eat because you'll go through them quickly. When you buy a food you've never tried, don't buy more than you'll eat at one meal in case it doesn't appeal to you.

Q. WHAT IS A GMO?

A. GMO stands for Genetically Modified Organism, which describes any plant or animal that has had its genetic code changed in a laboratory by introducing genes from another organism. There is currently a huge movement against the corporations that make them. These unnatural foods are reputed to cause allergic reactions and affect you at the cellular level. When in doubt, choose nature over GMO foods.

The very best option of all is growing your own food. You'd be amazed at how satisfying it can be. You have a lot more control over how your food grows, the transit time and cost is eliminated, and the price beats anything out there. And nothing beats plucking your own apples off the tree and enjoying them on the spot.

You don't have a yard, you say? If you live in an apartment, try growing a pot of basil on your windowsill. If you have a sunny spot you can even nurture a small lemon or orange tree.

You don't have a green thumb, you say? The only way to become a better gardener is to practice. Many colleges and universities have extension campuses that teach gardening to members of the community—they can help you learn how to grow the right plants for your area. And nothing beats good know-how from a trustworthy local nursery.

Truly, growing your own food offers unique rewards, especially as you enter the extended third trimester of life. You get to provide for yourself and your family in a real way. You connect with the earth and the process of life and growth. You nurture other living things so that they may nourish you.

JUICING AND BLENDING

Juiced and blended foods are a staple of my diet. Many people want to know why I don't just eat whole foods all the time, but there are several good reasons for it. Although we all need fiber in our body (as I explained in chapter 6), I get an abundance of it from the many whole fruits, vegetables, nuts, seeds legumes and grain-like seeds I consume in addition to juice. I would never consume juices exclusively (except maybe on a short fast), but they are excellent when consumed as part of a whole foods diet.

Consider the example of Norman Walker, who discovered the benefits of juicing when he was ill and became an avid juicer, going on to write one of the first and still definitive books on the subject in the 1930s. Containing close to 100 recipes, it was initially called *Raw Vegetable Juices: What's Missing in Your Body?*, but later editions are called *Fresh Vegetable and Fruit Juices: What's Missing in Your Body?* Walker became so persuaded by the benefits of juicing that he included a section about the benefits in his book—going so far as to include juice formulas that he believed could prevent and reverse a specific disease more effectively than any medication. When Walker died of nothing at around 100 years of age; he did so during his daily nap after his usual walk! He was clearly on to something with his juicing regimen.

One important thing to understand about fiber is that it slows digestion. This is often a good thing. For instance, in the case of fruit, it helps slow the body's absorption of sugar, ensuring that you don't experience a sugar rush and a corresponding insulin spike (that's why you should **not** juice fruits). But it also slows down the absorption of nutrients and requires more energy to be digested. Juices allow for the fastest absorption of nutrients while diverting the least possible energy to digestion.

Q. WHAT ARE THE ADVANTAGES OF JUICING?

A. Vegetable juice is a simple way to get huge amounts of concentrated nutrition. You'll get an abundance of enzymes, vitamins, minerals, and phytonutrients, all of which help with athletic recovery and general well-being. I do not recommend juicing fruit because, without the fiber, you will get too much of a sugar rush.

THE VALUE OF VEGETABLE JUICE

I like to start out my day with vegetable juice so that I can get that infusion of energy. I do not recommend fruit juice—it creates too much of a sugar rush because there is no fiber to slow the absorption of the sugar. Although I usually drink straight green vegetable juice, when you're starting out you can make it a little sweeter by adding carrot and/or beet to it.

The other important benefit of juicing is that you can pack a lot of goodness into a very condensed form. My typical morning juice might include a bunch of kale, collard greens, bok choy, parsley, several stalks of celery, cucumber, spinach, and other leafy greens. I could never eat all of that without getting too full first (the fiber would make it too filling). This way, I get all of the nutrients from that big pile of vegetables but none of the drag of digesting them. I do get plenty of fiber from my whole-food, plant-strong diet. At times I'll work out first, then have a leafy-green vegetable juice immediately following.

Vegetables also contain an abundance of enzymes, which we discussed in detail in chapter 6. Green vegetables contain loads of

Green Morning Juice

Kale, collard greens, parsley, celery (several stalks), cucumber, bok choy, spinach, other leafy greens

Starter Juice

50% greens
50% carrots or beets

Vary your leafy green veggies based on what you have on hand, what's in season, and what you like.

chlorophyll—powerful antioxidants that banish free radicals, cleanse the system, improve oxygenation within the body, and help with muscle repair. I also get a good deal of protein from leafy greens, which my body can use to repair and rebuild my muscles after a workout.

My juice is the finest source of organic water available. That hydration is, of course, vital to the success of my workout and general equilibrium. You can put almost anything in your green juice—kale, collards, bok choy, parsley, chard, beet greens, even broccoli and sprouts. I vary mine depending on my mood, what fresh vegetables I have in the house, and what's in season. The combinations are endless.

Although I enjoy my straight green juice, those new to juicing might want to make theirs with up to 50 percent carrots or beets because they add sweetness and temper the intense flavor of the green vegetables. Beet juice is an especially good addition for athletes because it enhances oxygen intake. With the whole day ahead of me, including a workout and plenty of other tasks, I want to keep my energy available for those activities. Juice doesn't deplete me; in fact, because it is so densely packed with vital nutrients, it gives me a massive boost of energy and mental clarity.

BLENDED SALADS RETAIN THE VALUE OF THE FIBER

I am a fan of blended salads and throw almost any vegetable into them. What's a blended salad? Just what it sounds like: a combination of leafy greens and other raw veggies put into a blender and turned into a drinkable liquid. Although blended salads cannot be digested as quickly as juice (thanks to the fiber), they are still easier for the body to digest than whole foods since the plants' cell walls have been broken, ensuring easy bioavailability. Since the food has already been "chewed" into liquid form, your body doesn't have to do that work. So you're still experiencing a fairly significant energy gain when you consume blended salads.

The possibilities here are endless and endlessly satisfying. I am a big fan of medleys: celery, romaine leaves, spinach, lettuce, tomatoes, and avocado or ground flax seeds or hemp seeds. It's as delicious as anything you'll ever eat. Some people add a little water to their blended salads, but I prefer to add a tomato (or a bunch of little tomatoes) instead. Leafy greens and celery can be easily combined with other vegetables, so it's always okay to throw in a couple of neutral-tasting greens (romaine is a great choice) to get a little chlorophyll and protein boost from your blended salad.

Athletes especially should note the benefits of blended salads. Since blending breaks down the foods' cell walls, it's taking the first step toward digesting the food before you've consumed it. Since digesting blended salads requires much less energy, they are great post-workout drinks. Blend tomatoes with celery and lettuce for a great electrolyte-rich boost. It's far healthier than any sports drink you could find in a store that claims to be loaded with electrolytes (it may indeed have them, but it's also loaded with sugar). Sometimes I add ginger root and turmeric for its anti-inflammatory properties. You can make these blended salads as simple or as gourmet as you like, and there are unlimited tasty variations.

Blended Salad Medleys:

Celery, spinach, tomatoes, lettuce, ground flax seeds, hemp seeds, and nuts

Tomatoes, celery, romaine leaves, other leafy greens

Electrolyte Blended Salads:

Celery, lemon, water, ginger, and a handful of dulse

Celery and ginger

Celery, lettuce, water

Green leafy vegetables and celery

Avocado, tomato, celery, and spinach

GET THE RIGHT EQUIPMENT

Regarding equipment, you will want to have a good juicer and a good blender in your kitchen when you follow the Ageless Boomer diet. Along with your refrigerator and some good knives, they will be the most important food prep equipment you use. (Your stove will see a lot less use and your oven may turn into a storage area because you never use it.)

I use a Norwalk juicer. It's a stainless steel model that dates back to the 1930s, and I consider it to be the Rolls-Royce of juicers. Making the juice is a two-step process—first, you pulverize the vegetables, and then press them. But I highly recommend this investment. It's a much better option than the plastic juicers that employ centrifugal force to extract the juice. As the juice is whirled around at high speeds, it is exposed to the air and instantly begins to oxidize, which reduces the nutrients' value. By the time you drink it, the juice will have lost much of the vitality contained in the whole foods you started with. With the Norwalk, the juice is extracted by a pressing action, reducing oxidation tremendously.

When it comes to blenders, I use a Vitamix blender. I used to have the old glass model (which the company doesn't make at present—hopefully they'll bring it back), but I now use a plastic model that doesn't contain BPA.

There are many brands of juicers and blenders to choose from. I recommend purchasing the best possible model you can afford because juices and blended salads are a staple of this diet and you'll find yourself using them on a daily basis. Consider their value as you would for any major appliance.

You can make an infinite variety of blended salads, from simple, nourishing, two-ingredient concoctions to elaborate nutritional powerhouses, depending on what you're in the mood to consume. It all comes down to personal taste. Here are a few tips and suggestions to help you get started:

- Leafy green blended salads are an excellent way to get your fiber and minerals. Adding avocado or seeds/nuts to your green blended salads will make them not only more palatable, but will also increase the bioavailability of all the nutrients, including essential fatty acids and protein. I always grind flax seed down in a nut grinder before adding it to the blender.
- Use your blender to make some of the best salad dressings ever (for your non-blended salads); see recipes below.

Rod's favorite salad dressing:
Tomatoes, celery, cucumber, avocado, garlic and/or onion, and superfoods (hemp seeds and flax seeds). Sometimes I add soaked almonds.

OMG Walnut Sauce
(adapted from My Beef with Meat):
Walnuts (1 cup), garlic (2-4 cloves), water for consistency

Delicious Dip:
Avocado, lemon, and cilantro

- Add any of the superfoods to your blended salad (see Appendix A for a list of superfoods). I sometimes mix Pure Synergy with water and add that in. I also like to add maca, goji berries, bee pollen, and so on.
- Use tomatoes (either organic cherry tomatoes or heirloom varieties) as a base. These have a high water content, and you may find you don't need to add any water at all if you use tomatoes. Then add leafy greens, cucumbers, bell peppers, celery, and/or garlic and onion. Finish by blending in an avocado, which will give your blended salad a rich, creamy texture.
- Try to use a variety of greens. Different leafy greens have different amino acids. Here are my favorites, in alphabetical order: arugula, beet greens, bok choy, broccoli, carrot tops, celery, chard, cilantro, collard greens, dandelion greens, frisee, kale, mustard greens, parsley, radicchio, radish tops, romaine (and all green and red leaf lettuces), spinach. Do not use iceberg lettuce. Note that I include the tops of root vegetables on this list, e.g. beet greens. These are packed with nutrients. They can be bitter but are a great choice if you work up to them gradually.

EXERCISE AND
WORKOUT NUTRITION

You may not think of yourself as an athlete, but you are—you use your body every day in many diverse ways that you don't even consider. Standing, sitting, and walking all place different types of stress on your body. More importantly, if you're going to become an Ageless Boomer, exercise is going to become part of your daily life. As a result, you need to think about how to eat to best fuel your pre- and post-exercise nutrition. If you pay close attention to your post-workout meal, you will speed your recovery.

Getting the right nutrients is absolutely essential to athletic recovery—it can make all the difference in an athlete's ability to reach peak performance—and yet very few athletes give adequate thought to what kind of fuel will really enhance their performance. They know about carbo-loading. They know about protein powders. They know to drink water. But post workout nutrition, the single most important meal for an athlete in training, has gotten precious little attention. After a workout, many athletes feel tired and simply fill up on whatever they want. But this "whatever" they're consuming can impede recovery by forcing the body to divert energy from muscle repair to digestion.

Brendan Brazier's *Thrive* approach was the result of his desire to maximize the value of the rest and recovery phase of his workouts. He found that eating plant-based foods made a huge difference in the speed and effectiveness of his recovery time. In this section, I'm going to give you details about *which* plant-based foods can give you the most effective recovery.

If you pay special attention to that post-workout meal and all other meals, you will be able to get in more workouts because you'll recover more quickly, and therefore you will be able to exercise more, should you want to. This chapter will explain why this first post-workout meal is so important and give you some examples of optimal meals.

WHAT YOUR BODY NEEDS

So let's begin with an explanation of what is happening inside our bodies when we exercise. Muscles store glycogen, which is basically the way the body stores glucose. Our muscles burn that glycogen as fuel during a workout. After a workout, the body is depleted of glycogen and needs to restore its supply as quickly as possible, in order to be ready for the next burst of exercise. Glycogen comes directly from glucose. So, the very best thing you can do for your body is to give it a shot of glucose within 30 to 45 minutes of your workout.

Interestingly, your body's ability to convert that glucose into glycogen increases dramatically right after a workout (it can convert up to 50 percent more). So the sooner you get that into your body, the more efficient it will be at replenishing its diminished reserves. Your muscles are similar to a vacuum at that point, singularly focused on restoring the proper balance. This means that your body will be ready to work out again sooner. If you wait too long (more than 45 minutes), your body won't convert that glucose as efficiently. As a result, your recovery will take longer. So the very simplest, best thing you can do to ramp up your training is to take advantage of that window with proper, easy-to-digest foods and make the most of that first meal after a workout.

THE OPTIMAL POST-WORKOUT MEAL

I highly recommend making a vegetable juice with leafy greens or a blended salad with some celery and leafy greens in it. It takes just a few minutes, contains all the nutrients I need, and tastes absolutely delicious. For instance, I'll throw in whatever vegetable is in season, some lettuce leaves, a stalk or two of celery, and sea vegetables and blend them all together. The leafy greens add minerals, and the celery and sea vegetables add sodium, which is another key nutrient after a workout (when we've lost sodium through our sweat).

Sometimes I crave a monomeal, which means that I eat only one kind of food for the entire meal. After an especially intense workout, I've been known to eat several bananas or oranges. Consuming a single food is much easier on the body and doesn't tax your digestion. So it's much like eating a blended salad. Listen to your body and don't hesitate to give it what it craves. It's working hard to restore itself as quickly as possible. The main point with all of these options is that you want to get these essential nutrients into your body quickly, and you don't want to stress your body and digestive process with a lot of other kinds of food.

The last thing you should do after a big workout is sit down and indulge in a high fat, high complex-carb meal. That just means you're taxing your body doubly: it is trying to recover from your workout and diverting energy to digestion at the same time. In addition to that, high fat foods slow down the rate of absorption of glucose into the bloodstream. So your muscles aren't getting those much-needed replenishments when they need them most. You also don't need a lot of protein right after working out. Protein is not a fuel and takes more work to be digested and assimilated. While your muscles do need protein for muscle repair, high quantities of protein are not the ideal food right after a workout. Some nuts or seeds two hours after a fruit meal and one hour after green vegetable juice are great. I've heard it said that digestion of a heavy meal takes more energy than running a marathon. So if you want to recover quickly, stay away from foods that take a lot of time, effort, and stress to digest.

A: No. You'll find that your energy level goes up considerably. Importantly, your recovery time will decrease significantly, and your strength-to-body weight ratio will be much more favorable. You'll be stronger for your body weight.

If you plan to be working out for a long time (over an hour), it's a good idea to replenish those glycogen reserves sometime during your workout. I often consume an orange or two during my longer workouts (over an hour) just to keep my energy up. Fruit is ideal because it contains both glucose and fructose. The fructose gives me an immediate kick start and the glucose supplies my body with a slower, more sustained energy boost. That means I can work out harder and longer than if I waited until the end of my long routine.

You also want to get hydrated quickly after a workout. The good news is that if you eat whole fruit, you'll be getting plenty of water through that—it's killing two birds with one stone. So stay away from dehydrating foods.

If you follow this regimen, you'll enjoy another benefit that is especially important for people over 40—fewer if any injuries. Your body will be better able to repair muscle tissue and therefore be better up to the task of performing as your training sessions become more rigorous. Even if you don't follow this approach in order to exercise sooner, recovering faster will give you more energy to play with your kids and/or grandchildren.

DETOXIFY YOUR BODY WITH THE PROPER APPROACH

"Detoxification" is a general term to describe the process of cleansing or ridding your body of chemicals, organisms, or substances that interfere with optimal physical function. You can detoxify at any time, but this process is especially important when you're starting the Ageless Boomer lifestyle.

There are important steps you can take to make detoxification progress more smoothly. If you're in relatively good health, this renewal may take only a couple of weeks. For people who have eaten a lot of processed foods over the years, or those who are ill, it could take somewhat longer. Everyone's experience will be different, since each person is bringing his or her own personal nutritional history to the equation, and every body responds differently to change. That's why I'm offering several suggestions for how to go about this transition.

As your body gets lighter as you detox, pay attention to how you feel after your meals and feel free to modify your routine accordingly. You can then learn to listen to the signals your body is giving you and gradually introduce more flexibility into your dietary plan as time passes. The other good news is that your body basically wants to heal itself. It's programmed to do the work of cleansing and restoring balance if you give it the proper tools. The better the tools you give it, the better the results.

Start by introducing more raw enzyme-rich fruits and vegetables into your diet. Do this in the form of whole foods and also in the form of vegetable juices and blended salads. These are rapid-transit foods, which have several benefits. First of all, the body digests them quickly (particularly vegetables and their juices) and eliminates them rapidly. This means that the body is not diverting a lot of extra energy to digestion and can instead channel that energy toward detoxification. Second, these foods do not create more toxic buildup. The body recognizes them, absorbs their nutrients, breaks them down with the help of their own enzymes, and eliminates any waste from them quickly. Finally, they are nutrient-dense, which means that the body has the building blocks for repair and healing. As you remove toxicity from your body, your body will start absorbing those nutrients more effectively, so you won't feel as hungry as before. For those consuming cooked foods, note that lentils, beans, quinoa, buckwheat, and whole grains don't add toxicity, but they are slow to digest.

Another important step is to eliminate caffeine from your diet. It's a stimulant, but a phony one. It takes more energy than it gives, resulting in a net energy loss. It doesn't really restore your natural energy, but just creates a temporary illusion of increased energy. It's a mask: you haven't really addressed the real reason for your lack of energy in the first place. You may experience fatigue at first, but persevere, and you will be free of your coffee addiction forever. Once you've kicked the habit, you'll look back and realize what a drain it was on your natural energy. You'll have no regrets once you realize that you can just bounce out of bed in the morning without any help.

"Common detoxification symptoms include headache, bloating, diarrhea, nausea, fatigue, and sleep disturbances. It's important to remember that detoxification involves cleansing symptoms. Severe symptoms, however, are an indication that you should reduce the rate at which you are implementing the change. Keep in mind, though, that the worse you feel initially, the more there is to be gained."

— Brazier,
Thrive

Fasting, colon hydrotherapy, and rebounding are three ways to speed up the detoxification process. They are not for everyone, but, if they are done properly, they can be good solutions for those who want to jumpstart and speed up detoxification.

Consult with a health care professional before going on a fast. Don't try to do it on your own.

FASTING

One way to detoxify more quickly is to go on a fast. Note that you should only do this under the supervision of an experienced person. Don't try to undertake this on your own. Go to a health practitioner and explain you want to do a fast for detoxification. They may suggest several short fasts or one longer fast, depending on your condition. If you decide to go ahead with this, be sure to do it when you've got the time to do it right. You need to stay in bed as much as possible and be exposed to very little outside stimulation in order to maximize the amount of energy going toward your cleansing. Note that you will lose weight during your fast, but you will gain a good portion of it back afterward. You may do light workouts in order to not lose muscle mass (see the SMRs in the workout section of this book). I explain fasting in more detail later in this chapter.

COLON HYDROTHERAPY

Another option is colon hydrotherapy. This procedure is performed by a specialist who helps you to flush out your colon rectally. It is different from an enema in that the water goes much farther up the colon, so it is much more effective. (I've heard that one colonic is the equivalent of 15 enemas.) The procedure generally lasts about one hour, and it is recommended that you schedule two sessions the first week. I recommend the gravity method of colon irrigation, which is the safest method. Should you decide to give it a try, be sure to find a reputable specialist, ask plenty of questions, and get a list of referrals before you commit.

Colon hydrotherapy is somewhat controversial. Some say that it might adversely affect the electrolyte balance of the body. Others worry that it gives people an excuse to eat whatever they want, since they figure that all of the bad stuff will be cleaned out anyway. Another small group believes that the body will forget how to do the work of cleansing on its own. On the other hand, people have been having enemas for thousands of years, and believers are very enthusiastic about the results. It is true that it will ease the detoxification symptoms because it will flush the toxins out of your system quickly. I have tried it and have mixed feelings about it. Ultimately, it is a highly personal decision, and you are the only one who can judge whether it is the right way to go. I think if you're doing everything else right, it's probably not necessary, but you should definitely know it's an option.

REBOUNDING

Another way to speed up detoxification is through rebounding, one of my favorite exercises, which involves bouncing on a mini-trampoline. This simple bouncing motion does the body a world of good and aids in the detoxification process by helping to strengthen cells. The process of acceleration, deceleration, and gravity also helps flush out the lymphatic system, aids with digestion and elimination, improves balance and coordination, circulates more oxygen to your tissues, and keeps bones strong. It's also a wonderful form of relaxation. In fact, it's so meditative that I often incorporate gentle rebounding (meaning feet don't leave the mat) into my pre-sleep ritual. Last but not least, it's FUN! Read more about rebounding in chapter 15.

Rebounding is a great exercise because it stimulates the whole body. A 1980 study published in the Journal of Applied Physiology concluded that for comparable levels of heart rate and oxygen use, "the magnitude of the biomechanical stimuli is greater with jumping on a trampoline than with running." In other words, as your body accelerates and decelerates in response to gravity, you engage every cell in your body.

| FOOD COMBINING

Eating the right foods is a good start, but if you want to reach optimal Ageless Boomer results, you need to learn about proper food combining. To experience the greatest energy gain and maximize the benefit to your body, you need to learn how to properly combine the food in this diet. Not all nutrition experts agree with food combining, but based on my experience, it's a worthwhile practice. I want you to know how it works so that you can decide for yourself whether to practice food combining.

The good news is that once you understand a few basic principles of how our body digests food, the whole business of when to eat what will become quite intuitive. And the even better news is that you'll feel an astonishing lift in energy right away. Proper food combining also helps with detoxification when you're in transition (see the "Food Combining in Transition" section later in this chapter for more details). If you combine properly, you don't end up with a digestive backlog, which means that food moves through your system quicker without buildup. Once your transition period is over, you can start combining foods in any way that does not cause digestive stress.

For a detailed list of food families and rules for food combining, see Appendix A.

So what is food combining all about? It is, very simply, about helping your body digest food as efficiently and quickly as possible. If your body is not taxed with the hard work of digesting food, that extra energy means more energy for you. You'll enjoy greater clarity of mind, increased vigor, and fewer dips in energy.

Let's revisit what happens when you eat something. When food enters your stomach, digestive enzymes get to work breaking it down into smaller bits. The nutrients then get extracted and sent off into the bloodstream, which carries those nutrients to various organs and muscles that need them. The most important thing to understand is that the digestive process works most efficiently when it is not overly taxed. We can avoid overtaxing it by eating foods that don't force us to withdraw more enzymes or divert blood from other parts of the body for long periods of time. Digestion requires energy, and blood flow in the digestive system reduces the amount of oxygen our muscles get, which drains our energy and slows the pace of recovery. The best approach is to eat until you're about 80 percent full.

GUIDELINES TO EFFICIENT DIGESTION

In this section, we'll look at the various ways you can avoid taxing your digestive process. There are a few general guidelines here. First, eat smaller, more frequent meals than on the standard American diet. Plan to eat every three or so hours (or more if you're truly hungry). Just be sure those meals are small and nutrient-packed. Don't add lots of empty calories. By eating smaller quantities at any given time, your body won't get as worn out trying to process them. If you don't want to eat a lot of small meals, you can do what I do: have vegetable juice in the morning or after your morning exercise, and then eat until you're 80 percent full for your next two meals. You won't experience the wild dips and peaks in energy that result from eating three big, complex meals a day.

Second, eat mostly foods that are easy for the body to digest—fruits and vegetables. Fruits are practically predigested and enter and exit the digestive system in a very short time, requiring that very little energy be diverted in order to break them down. All kinds of melon, including honeydew, watermelon, and cantaloupe, are the fastest-digesting fruit.

Third, consider eating only one type of food, such as only oranges or bananas, at a time. Monomeals, or single-food meals, are much easier for the body to digest. If you like variety, consider consuming different fruits about 20 to 30 minutes apart. Start with a few kiwi, then wait, enjoy some grapes, wait some more, and have an apple. Sometimes I'll combine two foods (bananas and grapes or apples and fresh dates), but I try to have at least half of my daily meals in the form of rapidly digested monomeals. My post workout meal almost always consists of a monomeal (unless I'm drinking a blended salad or juice, which is easy to digest for other reasons). After my workout, I generally consume a monomeal of oranges or combine only two fruits within 30-45 minutes of working out. If I didn't have my vegetable juice beforehand, I have it as my first meal after my workout. This gets the nutrients I need into my bloodstream right away and doesn't detract from my recovery by forcing my body to spend a lot of energy on digestion.

If you do want to combine foods, limit the combinations to a few foods and make sure they are foods that are similar in terms of acidity. For instance, you can combine acid (as in acidic-tasting, not acid versus alkaline) fruits (oranges, pineapples, and grapefruit) or sub-acid fruits (apples, pears, cherries, peaches, and plums) or sweet fruit (fresh dates and bananas), but use care in combining fruits from different groups if you want to maximize the efficiency of your digestion. Sub-acid fruits can combine with acid fruits or sweet fruits, but acid fruits and sweet fruits should not be combined. Melons you should always eat alone because they digest almost immediately. I'll give more examples of what combines well later in the chapter.

If you're interested, you can test the transit time of your food. Just eat a few kiwi, which have easily identifiable black seeds, and see how long it takes for you to eliminate the seeds. If it takes less than 24 hours, the transit time is good. If it takes longer than that, you should take a close look at your diet and consider making some changes.

Fourth, embrace juicing and blending vegetables to eliminate a lot of work for your digestive system. In the case of juicing, you've already extracted all the nutrients and are sending them into your system in a form that is very easy for the body to assimilate. In the case of blended

salads, the blending breaks down the foods before you even consume them. As I explained earlier in this chapter, you're still getting the fiber, but much of the work is done.

Finally, progress from the least-dense foods (vegetable juices and whole fruits) to the most-dense foods (avocadoes, seeds, nuts, and beans) over the course of the day. I remember hearing that you should eat breakfast like a king, lunch like a queen, and dinner like a pauper. I couldn't disagree more. If you eat dense food early in the day, you'll start the day with an energy drain. Eat the fastest digesting foods during the day when you need access to all your energy reserves. Then consume slower-digesting foods at your evening meal when you need less energy, and have your final meal of the day at least three hours before bedtime.

Earlier in this chapter I mentioned that I eat a big green salad in the evening. When I want to combine a lot of different whole, unblended foods in one meal, or consume a lot of legumes, I

Eating Principles

Eat smaller, more frequent meals

Eat plant-based foods, mostly fruits and vegetables

Eat monomeals (one type of food at a time)

Juice and blend veggies

Progress from the least-dense foods in the morning to most-dense foods in the evening

eat that meal late in the day so that I'm not splitting my energy between digestion and high-energy activities.

To give you a sense of how all this works, here's a typical day for me.

I always start by drinking some water (about a quart over a 30- to 60-minute period) when I wake up. (See chapter 7 for more details on why this is a good idea.) I do some light warm-up exercise—range of motion dynamic stretches, health bounce on my rebounder, slow-motion resistance, and so on. After that I make my vegetable juice.

As far as I'm concerned, there's no better way to start the day than with vegetable juice. You get the benefit of a massive enzyme boost, the digestive system isn't overworked, and you've got a powerhouse of nutrients coursing through your bloodstream. I often juice a mix of different leafy greens (a combination of kale, collard greens, spinach, beet greens, bok choy, and parsley) and throw in some celery (for a little natural sodium). I consume my juice slowly, about an average of an ounce a minute, and swirl each sip in my mouth before swallowing (blending the juice with my saliva further speeds up the digestive process). All of these steps mean that I have the maximum possible reserve of energy to devote to my morning workout and activities. If I'd eaten a typical American breakfast, all that energy would have gone toward digesting it, and I would have felt depleted. This way, I'm rearing to go. If making fresh vegetable juice is too time consuming, I recommend eating a monomeal of fruit—nothing else.

After my workout (which you'll learn all about in the next few chapters), I generally consume a monomeal (or combine only two fruits) within 30 to 45 minutes of finishing. This is the most important meal for anyone in training. The point is to avoid derailing my recovery, so I keep this meal very simple. Oranges are a personal favorite with some leafy greens and celery. Occasionally I'll make a banana blended salad (just bananas, spinach, celery, and some water in the blender). A heavy meal right after a workout is the absolute worst thing you can do to your body. It'll be working double-time to recover and digest, and you'll feel sluggish instead of invigorated by your workout.

I have a couple more easy-to-digest snacks over the course of the afternoon. As a rule, I avoid mixing fresh and dried fruits because they digest at different rates (the dried fruit takes longer). Combining seeds and nuts with leafy greens, celery, or tomato is effective and helps with the acid/alkaline balance. I also continue to work from least dense food to most dense.

> "The body's biochemistry works in the most efficient manner when the proper food combinations are applied, and this is the main reason I advocate this approach—I want your body to be working in the healthiest way, which will give the most beneficial lifestyle change."
>
> — Fred Bisci, PhD, nutritionist and endurance athlete,
> Your Healthy Journey

Later on, for my evening meal, I might have a blended green salad. I'll often throw leafy greens and celery into the blender with avocado, cucumber, peppers, tomato, and sometimes a little spirulina, chlorella, and sea vegetables. This is easy to digest because the blending has already pulverized the vegetables and broken their cell walls. Other times, I'll make a blended vegetable mix with tomatoes as a base, flax seeds, hemp seeds, pistachios, Brazil nuts, lettuce, celery, bell pepper, and cucumber. It's delicious. Sometimes, I'll make a big salad with a mix of leafy greens, peppers, tomatoes, and cucumbers, with an avocado or blended seed/nut dressing. If I eat avocado, which is a denser food, I may not eat nuts that day. I save the avocado or seeds and nuts for my evening meal, when I'm less concerned about extremely rapid digestion.

> "If you fail to follow the principles of food combining and sequencing, and if you overeat, you may not immediately notice the negative consequences on the body, but they will be occurring nevertheless."
>
> — Bisci,
>   Your Healthy Journey

SET THE RIGHT MOOD FOR EATING

No matter what I'm eating, or when, I strive to create a relaxed ambience so that my body can unwind and focus on doing its job. I take my time eating. I may set some time aside for meditation or light rebounding (gently bouncing on a mini-trampoline) before my meal. The point is to make sure you're not bringing any outside tension or stress to the table with you. It will inhibit proper digestion and reduce the optimal uptake of nutrients into your system.

COMBINE FOOD EFFECTIVELY DURING TRANSITION

Following some strict rules on food combining during your transition from your current diet to an Ageless Boomer diet will help your detoxification process immeasurably. The more strictly you combine at first, the more energy you'll have and the less digestive stress you will experience.

Remember that the idea is to avoid backing up your system. You want to consume foods in such a way that they can be digested and make their exit as quickly as possible. Your goal should be to consume the fastest-digesting foods first, then leave time for your body to break them down and eliminate them before moving on to denser foods. For instance, if you eat a quick digesting fruit after consuming legumes, the fruit has to sit in your system and wait for the slow-digesting beans to be digested. In the process of waiting, it begins to ferment, irritates your system, slows the digestion of not only the fruits but also the beans, and backs up your system, resulting in slower elimination and wasted energy. Ideally, eat the fruit first, wait at least a half hour (two to three hours is optimal) to let it pass through your system, then eat something else.

As your body adjusts to eating more raw foods, you can start to let yourself be more flexible with your food combinations. For instance, many people don't think that dried fruits and nuts combine well, but I have no problem with them. Others think that you shouldn't combine seeds and nuts with other fats, but I have no trouble digesting flax and hemp seeds that are occasionally sprinkled on my avocado-dressed salad. This is different for each person, and you'll learn to listen to your body and know whether different combinations work for you.

As a general guideline, you want to eat the foods that are easiest to digest earlier in the day, since they will give you a positive energy gain. Save the slower digesting foods for evening when you are less likely to need extra energy and your body can devote more energy to digesting them.

People respond differently to different combinations. Many nutritionists consider trail mix (a mix of dried fruit and nuts) to be one of the worst food combinations, but I like it and my system handles it well. The high fat, high protein seeds and nuts slow down the release of the sugar in the fruit so that you don't experience as much of a spike and enjoy more prolonged energy. I also like combining seeds and nuts in my blended salads (tomatoes, celery, and lettuce with ground flax seeds and/or nuts). The point is that you should experiment with your own combinations, listen to your body, assess the results, and adjust your quantities and combinations accordingly.

BOOST YOUR ENERGY LEVELS

If you give food combining a try, it won't take long for you to experience a quantum leap forward in your energy levels. The standard American diet incorporates the most slow-digesting, energy-draining, processed food in the world—protein with starch—and meat has no fiber, so it takes lots of work for your body to eliminate it. I promise you that if you can break free of this pattern, you'll tap into whole new reserves of vitality.

A person who has good digestive strength can relax these rules and eat outside of general food combining principles. However, if you are exercising a lot or under other stresses, stay closer to the strict food combining rules in order to have as little stress as possible in your digestive process.

Fasting has a long history in many cultures across the world, for good reason. Fasting is not only good for detoxifying and flushing out your system, but it also can help heal all manner of diseases. This makes sense when you consider what fasting means for your body. By giving your digestive system a rest, your body can divert that extra energy to wherever it is needed most. If your body is trying to overcome some type of illness, that extra energy boost can make all the difference. Before modern medicine, this was a very common healing technique. Today, even with so many medicines on the market, I recommend fasting because it allows your body to heal itself, which, to me, is always a better option than whatever the pharmaceuticals and their side effects can do.

When you're making changes to your diet, fasting may seem like the last thing you want to do. I don't want you to feel hungry when you switch to WFPB eating. However, if you make sure to eat small, frequent meals that include fiber, you won't feel hungry. You may have sugar or caffeine cravings for a few days as you eliminate them, but you won't feel hungry if you're eating properly. Once you have established your nutritional rhythm and you're not feeling hungry, you can try fasting for the many benefits it provides.

"Promising and exciting research suggests that occasional fasting could have profound immune-boosting benefits for healthy individuals and those undergoing chemotherapy. By simulating an energy shortage with a few days of fasting, we can jumpstart the immune system's natural self-renewing capacity, exchanging old immune cells for new ones."

—Fuhrman,
"Taking the 'Fast' Track to Improved Immunity"

Even when you're not sick, a fast is a good way to reset your system. A fast recalibrates your body, restores balance, detoxifies, and restores clarity of mind. It gives your body a much-needed chance to recuperate, heal, and recover from daily stresses. It enhances all of your senses. Food tastes better afterward. The sunshine on your skin feels wonderful. Your outlook becomes more positive, and you'll likely enjoy a renewed sense of lightness and optimism.

TYPES OF FASTING

Juice and water fasting both have proponents: I've done both and think there are benefits to each kind. Ultimately, the choice is up to you, but here are some of the variables to consider as you figure out which is right for you. The biggest difference is one of intensity. A juice fast doesn't slow down your metabolism in the same way a water fast does. This means that you can still function somewhat normally: you can go to work, exercise moderately, and so on.

With a water fast, you really should rest. You need to plan to spend as much time as possible relaxing, including meditation and breath work. Because it is more intense and more mentally and physically challenging, it can be harder to maintain. That said, the benefits of a water fast can also be greater. It accomplishes its goals quicker, so you'll detoxify more rapidly and heal more deeply. You also lose more weight on a water fast, though I don't think that fasting is a great method for weight reduction, since much of it comes back when you start eating again; less

weight comes back if you're eating a WFPB diet. If you decide to go on a water fast for any length

"Fasting promotes accelerated healing and is a valuable treatment for a variety of medical conditions. In fact, my colleagues and I have published a series of case reports that showed remission of autoimmune diseases following fasting."

—Fuhrman,
"Taking the 'Fast' Track to Improved Immunity"

of time, be sure to consult your health care professional and undergo the fast under experienced professional supervision. If I'm doing a water fast I try to spend as much time relaxing as I can.

PLAN A FAST CAREFULLY

It's important to plan a fast carefully. What you consume pre- and post-fast are as important as the fast itself. Starting one to two days before, you should plan to eat only raw fruits and vegetables. Skip the seeds, nuts, and beans. This allows your body to begin to transition and starts giving it the rest it needs. Alternatively, consider consuming monomeals as a pre-fast diet—only oranges, for instance.

Then it's time to start the fast. I often have my last meal (a simple salad with no fat-rich foods—no avocadoes, no nuts, no seeds) at dinnertime. Then I fast for 36 hours, consuming only vegetable juice and/or water during that time. During the fast, I tend to drink exclusively

green juices. If I'm doing a water fast, I try to spend most of that time lying down, napping, and resting as many senses as possible. I read, but I don't watch television or use the computer. I basically try to eliminate as many forms of stimulation as possible.

Some people say you shouldn't exercise during a fast. When I go on a vegetable juice fast, I do only a light amount of exercise. If you're sick and want to focus on letting your body repair itself, skip the exercise. Get plenty of rest and let your body do its job. Some people may feel a little hungry, but generally, people have a sense of overwhelming well-being. They feel revitalized, balanced, and calm. They enjoy increased mental focus and clarity. Their pulse rate goes down, and they sleep better.

I break my fast slowly with my first meal two mornings later. As with your pre-fast, consume only fruits and vegetables for a day or two. It's very easy to sabotage all the benefits of your fast if you don't break your fast carefully. In fact, how your fast is broken will determine its success or failure. Some people consider the breaking of the fast to be the most important part of fasting. You can undo all the good you've done very quickly if you reach for a cheeseburger as your first meal—but then again, you should never reach for a cheeseburger. So begin by consuming small amounts. Be a little bit hungry when you stop eating. Don't overwhelm your system. Do your digestive system a favor and chew slowly and thoroughly. The slower the transition, the better. If you fasted for one day, break it over the course of a day; if you fasted for two days, break it over the course of two days.

I believe that a one- to three-day fast is ideal and that you should try to fast at least once every three months. I wouldn't recommend anything more than a week. No matter what you do, you should double-check with your health care provider if you plan to fast for any longer than a day and come up with a program tailored to your specific goals and health condition.

PART 3

CHAPTER 11

EXERCISE WILL POWER YOU FOR THE REST OF YOUR LIFE

■■■

To get your body to an Ageless state, you have to tune it
and move it daily. It's not complicated and it's not
strenuous. That doesn't mean it won't be hard—
changing ingrained habits is always a challenge. But
the rewards—strength, flexibility, energy, and a fit
physique—will amaze you.

EXERCISE AND NUTRITION
COMBINE TO MAXIMIZE HEALTH

In his excellent book *The Exercise Cure*, Dr. Jordan Metzl writes that the one thing you can do today to live longer is to exercise. A little exercise (such as brisk walking plus strength training), he explains, can add years to your life.

Of course, we want those years to increase in quality as well as quantity. But the beauty of exercise is that it increases our life quality by almost every measure. Metzl writes, "It makes bones stronger and muscles less likely to be injured. In older people, [exercise] aids in mobility and prevents falls." As I mentioned in part one of this book, it also decreases your risk of dementia, cancer, heart disease, diabetes, strokes, and more.

Metzl spends the first half of his book addressing the ways exercise cures a host of problems: cardiopulmonary problems, psychological problems, musculoskeletal problems, and many others. (He also describes the warning signs that a problem is serious enough to require a doctor's care.) In almost all these cases, a preventive dose of regular exercise will prevent them from ever arising.

As life-changing as exercise can be, exercise alone can't create a healthy body—healthy nutrition is critical. That's why I spent the largest part of this book describing the foods you need and how to eat them. By the same token, good nutrition alone can't create a healthy body—a healthy human body needs to move frequently in order to stay strong, vital, and flexible.

And together? In combination they have the power to be truly transformative. I wish I could point you to all the studies demonstrating the power of this combination, but truthfully, modern science has only scratched the surface. Studies show that diet plus exercise can lead to faster, more effective weight loss. Dieters who also exercise keep more muscle mass, so they have a higher metabolic rate and burn more calories even when they're not exercising. But researchers are still investigating the benefits of these powerful preventative tools.

I can point you to my own experience and my own good health. By combining a whole-foods, plant-based diet with consistent, comprehensive exercise, I have maintained peak health and fitness well into my seventh decade of life. You can do the same.

"As time goes on priorities change. Your physical fitness goals change. You fight the battle of staying physically fit, but you are also fighting the battle of getting older and the effects that gravity and wear and tear have on our bodies...The main thing is, you stay positive. You do what you can do for that day and what makes you feel good, and what gives you energy to carry your tasks out for that day. You don't waste yourself or drive yourself. It is the journey, not the destination that is important."

— Greg Newton,
John Peterson's Transformetrics Forum

SITTING IS THE NEW SMOKING, SO GET OUT OF YOUR CHAIR

Here's a simple test of your physical fitness: choose your favorite sedentary activity (watching TV, reading the newspaper, browsing the Internet) and try doing it standing up. How long does it take before you feel like you need to sit down? A minute? Five minutes? If it's a good half-hour before you notice anything, congratulations, you're already on the right track. If it's less, then your body is telling you that you're too used to sitting.

Sitting is like junk food—when we get used to it, we start to crave it all the time. And like junk food, it's a pleasure trap. The feel-good feeling we get from taking a load off isn't actually good for us.

A sedentary lifestyle ages us and puts us at greater risk of premature death. A study from Sweden's Karolinska University Hospital showed that older adults (in their late sixties) who spent most of their time sitting had shorter telomeres than active individuals of the same age. What are telomeres? They're the caps at the ends of your DNA, and other studies have established a connection between short, frayed telomeres and disease, premature aging, and early death. Yes—too much sitting will kill you, and it shows in your DNA.

"Taking regular exercise is the most effective single lifestyle choice people can make to reduce their risk of dementia, according to one of the most extensive studies yet into people's long-term health outcomes.

"The 35-year investigation, carried out by researchers at Cardiff University, found that consistently following just four out of five key behaviours could reduce dementia risk by 60 per cent, while also cutting the chance of heart disease and stroke by 70 per cent."

— The Independent, December 9, 2013

Dr. James Levine, director of the Mayo Clinic/Arizona State University Solutions Initiative, calls sitting "the new smoking," and based on his research, that comparison is no exaggeration. In his book *Get Up! Why Your Chair is Killing You and What You Can Do about It*, he explains that for every hour of sitting, you could be taking two hours off your life span. He quotes Martha Grogan, a Mayo Clinic cardiologist, "For people who sit most of the day, their risk of heart attack is about the same as smoking." If you're not sure how much time you spend sitting, Levine has a handy "chair test" on his site, juststand.org.

As an alternative, Metzl recommends practicing NEAT—non-exercise activity thermogenisis—which is a fancy way of saying movement that isn't exercise. Stand up at meetings, talk on the phone while walking or standing, park farther from your destination, walk more on your errands, and so on. Find any reason to move around instead of sitting. And as *The Week* reported in June 2015, "Researcher Gavin Bradley tells the Washington Post that the key is to avoid sitting for more than 30 minutes at a time. He advises 'taking your calls standing; walking around; pacing; holding standing meetings; walking over to a colleague's desk instead of sending an email; using the stairs instead of the elevator. Eventually, Bradley says, people should aim to increase their standing time from two to four hours. 'However you do it, the point is to just get off your rear end.'"

Q: WHAT'S THE BEST TIME TO EXERCISE?

A: Basically, whatever time works best for you, as long as you work out. Dr. Andrew Weil's site drweil.com cites a National Sleep Foundation poll that shows people who work out get better sleep. The poll showed no difference in the sleep quality of late-day exercisers vs. early morning exercisers.

Many of you will remember Dr. Laurence Morehouse's bestseller *Total Fitness in 30 Minutes a Week*, first published in 1975. Morehouse was well ahead of his time with this book, which explained a simple, accessible plan for fitness for any person. (Just so you know, his program takes more than 30 minutes a week—that claim got people to buy the book, but in reality it takes several hours spread throughout the week.) He laid out five very simple requirements for minimum physical maintenance:

- Limber up by reaching arms, twisting trunk, bending waist, and turning trunk.
- Stand for a total of two hours during the day.
- Lift something unusually heavy for five seconds.
- Walk briskly for at least three minutes to stimulate your cardiovascular system.
- Burn up 300 calories a day in physical activity.

Morehouse made this suggestion for increasing total daily movement: "Don't lie down when you can sit. Don't sit when you can stand. Don't stand when you can move." And researchers today are telling us exactly the same thing.

Levine suggests, among other things, that we simply spend more time standing. Like Morehouse, he says don't sit when you can stand. Look for a standing desk so that you can use your computer while on your feet.

Movement *plus* exercise is critical. Metzl also cautions against too much sitting: "Recent

"One of the reasons it's so tough to maintain good posture at a desk is that your ligaments and other soft tissues start to deform after about 20 minutes in the same position, gradually giving your body a permanently chair-shaped appearance. Fight this tendency with 1- to 5-minutes breaks for every 20 minutes you're at work: stretch, breathe, focus your eyes on a distant object. You'll come back to work refreshed and recommitted."

—Metzl,
    The Exercise Cure

research suggests that sitting for 11 hours a day or more increases your chances of dying from any cause by a stunning 40 percent—and that's independent of all other factors, including age, education, and physical activity." Note that last item—even if you exercise often, you can undo the benefits of exercise by spending the rest of your time sitting.

Sitting versus standing is almost always a matter of habit. Remember that little test I just suggested? When you felt like sitting down, was it because you were in pain? Out of breath? Exhausted? If you're an able-bodied adult, probably not. You probably just got a hint of muscle fatigue in your thighs or your back, and your habit—which you don't even think about—is to sit down when you feel that hint of fatigue. You can retrain your brain so that instead of sitting down, you can tighten your abdominal muscles, tuck in your tailbone, and continue standing comfortably.

While standing may be our most basic weight-bearing exercise, just standing more won't get you to the Ageless Boomer fitness state we're after. You'll need aerobic exercise and, above all, strength-training exercise. But it's important to remember that if you want to retain the benefits of your exercise, you have to stay off the couch and, as much as possible, off the office chair. After I've been sitting for a while, I'll go over to the rebounder and do several minutes of health bouncing.

POSTURE PROVIDES THE FOUNDATION OF HEALTHY MOVEMENT

Another victim of our sedentary lifestyles is posture. As Phil and Jim Wharton explain in *The Whartons' Back Book*, "When most of us sit, we tend to sort of settle into a puddle … We roll our shoulders forward, stressing the upper back and caving in our chest muscles. This posture might feel fine for a little while, but if you're in for the long haul, you're in trouble."

As the Whartons point out, the back is a flexible and fluid system, designed to give us a wide range of motion and to balance out our forward-focused, upright stance. Sitting too long, even in a back-friendly position, is bad for our posture, and sitting the way many people do, curled up in a slouch, is terrible.

Good posture isn't just for girls at finishing school balancing books on their heads—it's for everyone. It reduces back and neck pain, helps you breathe better, and helps digestion. Bad posture brings many problems, as explained in an October 2012 *Prevention* article: worsened depression, constipation, and higher stress levels. Good posture makes you look taller, thinner, younger, and more confident, too—the finishing school girls knew that decades ago.

"Taking short work breaks every 20 to 25 minutes, changing your sitting position often, and staying physically active throughout your day—and not just during your workout—will … go a long way toward improving posture."

—Metzl,
  The Exercise Cure

What does good posture look like? As the Whartons explain, "When you stand in perfect alignment with perfect posture, your earlobes line up directly over your shoulders. Your shoulders line up directly over the points where your femurs (thighbones) connect to your pelvis. Those points on your pelvis line up directly over the midpoints between the fronts and backs of your knees. And your knees line up directly over your anklebones."

As you start exercising more, you need to be very aware of your posture. Bad posture can increase your risk of injury, even during low-risk exercise like walking or body-weight strength training.

Posture is another reason why strength training using the SMR exercises I explain in this book is important. These twelve exercises not only increase your strength, they also increase your flexibility and improve your overall posture and alignment. They'll help you develop good, healthy posture—but make sure you don't sabotage it by spending too much time sitting!

PRACTICE AGELESS BOOMER EXERCISE

Life offers us a variety of terrific exercise opportunities: biking, swimming, dancing, skiing, snowshoeing, playing ball, running, rowing; you name it, we do it. If you have a favorite exercise, by all means keep doing it. *Exercise should be fun.* And we've lost sight of that truth because too often we think of movement as work, or worse, as punishment.

When I talk about nutrition, I admit that I have some pretty strict rules. (I won't say it's a strict diet because I truly believe it's brimming with delicious options.) When I talk about exercise, though, my rules are really flexible. The most important rule is that you should listen to your body—your body will tell you what you can do.

These days, a lot of popular exercise programs want you to push you body to its limit and beyond. Boot-camp gyms, mixed-martial arts trainers, and other hard-core fitness programs encourage people to "push past the pain," "take it up a notch," and "give it everything you've got." Orthopedic surgeons I know tell me they love these kinds of programs because the injuries they cause pay for the surgeons' lifestyle. Don't get me wrong: I like to push myself and test my limits. But pushing your body without paying attention to its limits is a one-way ticket to injury.

> "Unless you work at it for a long time, the visible changes you get from aerobic training are fairly subtle: You're a little leaner, a little more toned. But most people who begin regular strength training—and work hard at it—see some pretty substantial improvements in how they look after just a few weeks."
>
> —Metzl,
> The Exercise Cure

Morehouse recommends using your pulse as a barometer. Check your pulse at a baseline before you start exercising, and then check it during exercise. See how long it takes for your pulse to go back to pre-workout level. If it takes more than a minute or so of rest for your pulse to slow back down to baseline, slow down and don't push yourself as hard.

This part of Ageless Boomers will introduce you to simple, effective exercises that will sharpen and strengthen your body and mind. They aren't strenuous and they won't increase your risk of injury. Like the nutrition approach I recommend, you just need to do them for a few weeks and you will see the dramatic results. And you'll want to keep doing them for the rest of your much longer life.

SMR STRENGTH TRAINING — YOUR STRENGTH BUILDS YOUR STRENGTH

SMR stands for "slow-motion resistance." In SMR exercises, your muscles are the agonists and antagonists, two muscle groups working at the same time to provide resistance to one another.

The beauty of slow-motion resistance exercises (SMRs) is that they are perfectly tailored to your body and your fitness level. You don't pick up weights that are too heavy when you're doing SMRs because you're pushing against your own muscles. An increase in difficulty is built in—as you get stronger in one muscle group, the opposing group gets stronger as well, increasing the challenge at a pace that's perfectly suited to you.

The twelve SMRs in this book, designed by my friend John Peterson, engage your "kinetic chain," the musculoskeletal connections stretching from your head to your feet. You'll work each major muscle group, moving each one in a full range of motion, thereby increasing your flexibility. By working through your kinetic chain, you improve alignment and posture, and you decrease the chance of injury that can occur when we exercise muscle groups in isolation.

Just so you know, almost any movement can be an SMR. These twelve are foundational exercises, but any multi-joint functional exercises can be turned into an SMR. You can even do SMRs while walking and kill two birds with one stone.

"Dr. Kenneth Cooper, the doctor that coined the term 'Aerobics' in 1968, has changed his viewpoint considerably as relates to strength training … I have a hard cover copy of his original book and back in 1968 the good doctor all but criticized strength training as though it prevented people from becoming healthy. Dr. Cooper changed his beliefs considerably and recognized the importance of strength training during the 1990s when he saw some of his early patients become too weak to continue aerobics due to skeletal injuries."

—John Peterson
in his Transformetrics Forums

Certain exercises—push-ups, pull-ups, squats, lunges—have remained popular for decades. Trends come and go, but these remain because they are simple, effective, and have low risk of injury. *Men's Journal's* list of "The Only Eight Moves You Need to be Fit" includes lunges, push-ups, pull-ups, chin-ups, squats, and rows because they're terrific, simple body-weight exercises that you can do anywhere with little to no equipment.

More importantly, these are all functional, multi-joint exercises that mimic the kind of movements we perform in real life. And functional fitness is our ultimate goal.

John Peterson and I wrote a book together called *Ultimate Push-ups for the Awesome*

Physique. As you can guess from the title, it celebrates the amazing results you can achieve from one simple exercise: the push-up.

Now, I know push-ups seem scary to a lot of you. Maybe they remind you of gym class and the physical education teacher you hated. But they don't need to be. If you can't do a push-up from the floor, don't worry: you can do it leaning against your wall. I'll take you through the steps so that you can progress from standing push-ups to counter push-ups to full push-ups. If you never get to a full push-up, that's OK—but if you keep at it, I bet you will.

"Push-ups activate a chain of muscles — particularly in your arms, shoulders, chest, and back — that are key for everything from getting up off the ground to shoving something heavy into the back of an SUV. The humble push-up beats the bench press for developing this functional push strength because the push-up doesn't take your back and legs out of the movement."

—Men's Journal, "The Only Eight Moves You Need to be Fit"

REBOUNDING—LOW IMPACT ON YOUR JOINTS, HIGH IMPACT ON YOUR HEALTH

Go bounce on a trampoline. How's that for fun fitness advice?

Seriously, though, rebounding—working out on a mini-trampoline—is one of the most effective exercises you can do for your whole body. Gravity is the reason: as you bounce up and down on a trampoline, you're changing the g-forces affecting your body. Those changing g-

forces cause more oxygen to flow through your cells (NASA researched it for astronauts). Acceleration, deceleration, and gravity work together to give you the most complete exercise around.

Rebounding also works your core because you're maintaining balance while moving in an irregular way. It works your legs as you bounce.

It's good aerobic exercise with minimal joint stress and thus reduced risk of injury.

And best of all, it makes you feel like a kid again.

WALKING — THE WORLD'S EASIEST, MOST ACCESSIBLE EXERCISE

Walking is your key to great fitness. Start walking every day, even for just half an hour every day, and you will unlock the door to Ageless living.

Mark Fenton, author of *The Complete Guide to Walking*, cites studies that show a small amount of walking improve cardiovascular health, increase bone density, and reduce cancer risk. People at risk for developing diabetes could slash their risk by 58 percent by walking at least 30 minutes a day, five days (or more) a week. That's a pretty big benefit from a small change in lifestyle.

All of the changes I've mentioned in this book are important: eating right, getting good sleep, strength-building exercise, meditation, and more. All of them build your Ageless picture of health. *But walking is the key.* When you start

walking regularly, you're going to want healthier food that gives you consistent energy rather than blood-sugar spikes. You're going to start sleeping better. You're going to have less stress. You're going to notice your need to hydrate. You're going to be out in the sun, getting vitamin D and all the other benefits of being in the sun.

You can change your life today, and you can do it by putting on some comfortable shoes, stepping out your front door, and taking a walk.

"Vigorous walking can give you the same total energetic high and cardiovascular fitness as any other single activity, with far less damage to your body."

— Mark Fenton,
The Complete Guide to Walking

MEDITATION — EXERCISE AND STRESS MANAGEMENT FOR YOUR MIND

Stress is a killer. Our bodies produce cortisol in response to stress, giving us the fight or flight kick we need to combat danger. But we live in a world where we're bombarded by stressors that don't need a fight or flight response, and that leads to chronic stress and long-term damage on all our systems.

One of the best practices for combating stress is meditation, which I use in combination with breathwork (see below). A huge body of research has shown the benefits of meditation, including reduced risk of dementia, delayed progress of dementia, reduced anxiety, better cardiovascular health, and so on.

Some people in our generation still raise their eyebrows at the idea of meditating because they associate it with New Age philosophy or Buddhist monks. It's time to let those prejudices go. Meditation is part of Western and Eastern traditions, and it has stayed around for millennia for a reason.

I've said it before, I'll say it again: meditation=push-ups for your brain. Try it daily for several weeks and you'll never doubt again.

"Until recently, I thought of meditation as the exclusive province of bearded swamis, unwashed hippies, and fans of John Tesh music ... But then came a strange and unplanned series of events, involving war zones, megachurches, self-help gurus, Paris Hilton, the Dalai Lama, and ten days of silence that, in a flash, went from the most annoying to the most profound experience of my life. As a result of all this, I came to realize that my preconceptions about meditation were, in fact, misconceptions."

— Dan Harris, journalist,
10% Happier

BREATHWORK — STRENGTHEN YOUR BRAIN AND CALM YOUR BODY BY CONTROLLING YOUR BREATH

Breathwork and meditation work hand-in-hand—or should I say, breath-to-breath? In Kundalini yoga, breathwork is a form of meditation. Learning to control your breathing gives you a powerful tool in combating stress. You can't control your heart rate when your heart starts to race, but you can control your breath, and slowing your breath can help bring the rest of your body back to a state of calm. If you want a long, vital life, you have to take charge of your stress levels, and learning new ways to breathe will help.

READINESS: MAKE SURE IT'S SAFE FOR YOU TO BEGIN

While I adamantly believe that not exercising is far more dangerous than exercising, I don't want to recommend that you try anything that will endanger your health. The exercises I recommend in this book are designed to let you progress at the pace that best suits your body—no lifting 100-pound barbells or going for ten-mile runs in the heat.

Before you start a new exercise routine, you should talk to your health care professional. At the very least you can get some benchmark measurements like blood pressure and cholesterol levels that will show you where you began. If you stick with the exercise plan I recommend, you are going to see those numbers get healthier with every visit.

WARM UP
THE RIGHT WAY

On one hand, you already know you should warm up before you exercise. On the other hand, you may not know how to warm up the right way. As Metzl explains, "If you're a dedicated stretcher, you may be surprised to learn that standard, reach-and-hold flexibility exercises before a workout aren't necessarily a great idea. Numerous studies have shown that those types of moves actually reduce your strength and power temporarily. More effective in prepping you for a … workout is dynamic stretching, moves that look very similar to old-school calisthenics." When I refer to stretching, I mean range of motion dynamic stretching, not static stretching where you stretch and hold a particular position. A good warm-up will get your body moving and will improve your range of motion.

In addition, you need to think about general warm-up exercise and specific warm-up exercise. General warm-ups include everything in this section, as well as jumping jacks, lunges, and other calisthenics—they get your entire body warm and limber. Specific warm-ups depend on the exercise, but in general you do a modified version of the actual exercise. For example, if I'm getting ready to do push-ups, I might do wall push-ups to warm up.

The following general warm-up exercises come from several sources, including John Peterson's book *Pushing Yourself to Power*. They're easy, comfortable dynamic stretches that warm up your whole body, getting you ready to exercise. I do dynamic stretches like this every morning as soon as I get out of bed, and I do more of them as I'm getting ready to work out. I'll also do them throughout the day to stay flexible and comfortable. You can do some of these while you walk, while you rebound, or during breaks from your daily activities.

- Six-way Neck Movement
- Neck Circle
- Shoulder Roll
- Arm Circle
- Maximum Amplitude Arm Circle
- Y Arm Movement
- T Arm Movement
- W Arm Movement
- L Arm Movement
- I Arm Movement
- Wrist Rotation
- Torso Twist
- Torso Rotation
- Forward Bend
- Hip Rotation
- Knee Bend
- Knee Rotation
- Ankle Rotation
- Heel Raise

You don't need to limit yourself to these dynamic stretches, of course. Your amazing body is built to move in hundreds of ways, and you can stretch in all of them. Just make sure to take it slow—don't pull long and hard in any one direction. Don't "bounce" or "pulse" during your dynamic stretches—those short, jerky movements are very bad for your muscles. Instead, focus on slow, consistent movements that expand your range of motion, breathing smoothly and deeply throughout the movement. Each dynamic stretch recommends that you do it ten times, but if they feel good, you can do more.

As you'll see in chapter 13, SMR exercises are wonderful for stretching your body and expanding your range of motion. You can incorporate low-tension SMRs into your dynamic stretches at any time.

SIX-WAY NECK MOVEMENT

Range of motion in the neck is one of the biggest problems among people over 50, and this neck warm-up as well as the Neck Circle can really help improve your range of motion.

1. Stand with your shoulders relaxed. Turn your head as far as comfortable to the right, then turn it as far as comfortable to the left. Repeat ten times.
2. Tilt your head down (chin toward your chest) as far as you comfortably can, then tilt it back (chin toward the ceiling) as far as you comfortably can. Repeat ten times.
3. Tilt your head to the right as far as comfortable, bringing your right ear toward your right shoulder, then tilt it to the left as far as comfortable, bringing your left ear toward your left shoulder.
4. Repeat ten times.

SHOULDER ROLL

1. Stand with your shoulders relaxed. Raise your shoulders up (toward ears), back, and around, for ten slow reps.
2. Reverse and raise shoulders up, forward, and around, for ten slow reps.

ARM CIRCLE

1. Put your arms out to form a T with your body.
2. With your arms straight, move your hands forward in a circle, making the circles progressively larger, until you have done ten.
3. Move your hands back in a circle, making the circles progressively larger, until you have done ten.

MAXIMUM AMPLITUDE ARM CIRCLE

1. Stand with your feet shoulder-width apart and your hands at your sides.
2. Slowly raise your arms outward and upward, inhaling deeply, stretching as much as possible while rising up on your toes.
3. Continue moving your hands upward in an arc until they cross at the top.
4. Continue moving your hands inward until they cross at the elbows while simultaneously exhaling forcefully. (If you can't cross your arms at the elbows yet, start by crossing your forearms.)
5. Repeat ten times, then reverse direction and repeat ten times.

"Muscle mass is the engine of youth: Sedentary adults typically lose it at a rate of about 1 percent per year after the age of 40."

—*Metzl,*

The Exercise Cure

The Y, T, W, L, and I arm movements help warm up your arms, shoulders, chest, back, and hands. Each movement works the muscles in a slightly different way, so doing all five gives you a well-rounded warm-up.

Y ARM MOVEMENT

1. Stand with your feet hip-width apart.
2. With your arms straight and your shoulders down (squeeze your shoulder blades down and back), raise your arms overhead, palms facing one another, until your body forms a "Y" shape. Let your arms go backward as far as you comfortably can.
3. Pause in the top position, then lower your arms.
4. Repeat ten times.

T ARM MOVEMENT

1. Stand with your feet hip-width apart. Extend your arms directly out to your sides, parallel to the floor, palms down. Don't shrug your shoulders.

2. Squeeze your shoulder blades down and back, then bring your palms together in front of you. Return to the starting position.
3. Repeat ten times.

W ARM MOVEMENT

1. Stand with your feet hip-width apart. Keep your arms straight, parallel to the floor, with palms facing the floor.
2. Rotate your arms so that your thumbs point up. Bend your arms so that they create a W with your head as the center point. Your thumbs will now be pointing back.

3. Squeeze your shoulder blades down and together. Pause and then return to the starting position.
4. Repeat ten times.

L ARM MOVEMENT

1. Stand with your feet hip-width apart.
2. Bend your elbows 90 degrees, palms facing upward.
3. Keeping your elbows close to your sides, rotate your upper arms outward so your palms travel backward slightly, as shown in the photo.
4. Squeeze your shoulder blades down and together, pause, and return to the starting position.
5. Repeat ten times.

"In addition to offering immediate feedback, well-lubricated pain-free joints allow you to enjoy life to the fullest and dramatically lessen your susceptibility to injury if you have to move suddenly or if you participate in an activity that is not part of your daily routine."

—John Peterson,
  Pushing Yourself to Power

I ARM MOVEMENT

1. Stand with your feet hip-width apart.
2. With your arms straight and your shoulders down (keep your neck long), raise your arms as high as possible overhead, palms facing one another, until your body forms an "I" shape.

3. Pause in the top position, squeeze your shoulder blades down and together, then lower your arms.
4. Repeat ten times.

1. Stand with your feet hip-width apart and your hands in front of you, elbows bent.
2. Rotate your wrists toward each other (right wrist moving counterclockwise, left wrist moving clockwise) ten times.

3. Reverse the movement and repeat ten times.

These two torso dynamic stretches are terrific if you have back pain. Just be careful, move slowly, and pay attention to how your back responds as you stretch.

TORSO TWIST

1. Stand with your feet shoulder-width apart or slightly wider. Extend your arms out from your sides, forming a straight line across your shoulders.
2. Keep your arms and shoulders in one solid line, as if you had a straight pole attached to them, and twist your upper body to the right as far as you comfortably can (see photo). Keep your hips facing forward as you twist your upper body.

3. Slowly reverse the movement, twisting your upper body as far to the left as you comfortably can. Don't let your hips swing as you twist—keep them facing forward.
4. Repeat this twist to both sides ten times.

TORSO ROTATION

1. Stand with your feet slightly apart and your hands on your hips.
2. Bend forward until your torso is at a 45-degree angle to your legs.

3. Start moving your torso to the left, around back, then right, and back to the starting position. Keep your lower body stationary from the waist down and only move your upper body in a circle.
4. Repeat the rotation ten times going to the left, then reverse direction and rotate ten times to the right.

FORWARD BEND

1. Stand with your feet about hip-width apart. Raise your arms straight over your head.
2. Gently bend back from the small of your back. Bend forward, trying to touch the floor between your feet while keeping your legs straight as you can without locking your knees.
3. Stand up, raising your arms over your head. Repeat ten times.

UP, OVER, AND DOWN

This exercise should be one smooth, continuous movement. You should exhale each time you bend down and inhale as you stand up and change sides. Don't worry if you can't touch your toes right away—as you practice you will gain the flexibility.

1. Stand with your feet shoulder-width apart or slightly wider. Extend your arms out from your sides, forming a straight line across your shoulders.
2. Swing your right arm up and over your head. Continue moving your arm down across the body while bending from the waist with your legs straight. Try to touch your left big toe.
3. Reverse the movement, swinging your arm back up, past the starting position, over your head. As you bring your arm overhead, gently bend back from the waist.
4. Repeat with your left arm, moving across your body to the right, and trying to touch the right big toe with your left fingers.
5. Repeat ten times on each side.

The hip rotation can be a little tricky when you start out. Remember to keep your knees bent and your lower back relaxed so that your hips can move freely.

HIP ROTATION

1. Stand with your feet shoulder-width apart and your hands on your hips. Bend your knees slightly.
2. Circle your hips ten times clockwise.
3. Reverse the direction and circle your hips ten times counterclockwise.

This exercise is a great warm up and cool down for walking, rebounding, strength training, and more.

KNEE BEND

1. Stand with your feet shoulder-width apart in front of a chair.
2. Squat down until your butt touches the chair lightly, then stand up.

Eventually you won't need the chair!

KNEE ROTATION

1. Stand with your feet close together and bend over slightly to place your hands on your knees. Bend your knees slightly.

2. Slowly rotate your knees in a circular movement clockwise ten times and then counterclockwise ten times. Range of motion is limited, so don't push it too far.

ANKLE ROTATION

1. Sit on the floor with your legs straight out in front of you.
2. Rotate your ankles, moving your feet toward each other (right ankle moving counterclockwise, left ankle moving clockwise) ten times.

3. Reverse the movement and repeat ten times.

HEEL RAISE

1. Stand with your feet hip-width apart.
2. Push yourself up until you are standing on the balls of your feet, then lower yourself down. Repeat ten times.

Standing on a book or stair will increase your range of motion. Be careful, though—if you're on a stair don't go to the point of pain.

SOOTHE YOUR MUSCLES WITH FOAM ROLLER EXERCISES

One of my favorite ways to stretch and massage my muscles is to use a foam roller. Foam rollers are available at almost any store that has a sporting goods department, and they're very affordable. Metzl writes, "If you only buy one piece of exercise equipment for the rest of your life, make it a foam roller … The foam roller is a piece of dense, industrial grade Styrofoam. It's also the most convenient, reliable, and inexpensive massage therapist money can buy."

173

Using a foam roller is really easy and simple. You just position the roller under part of your body and roll your body back and forth over it for at least 30 seconds. It may not sound impressive, but you'll find that the results are incredible. "Once you learn how to do it," Metzl writes, "a full foam-rolling routine lasts only a few minutes, and you'll notice immediate changes in your ease of movement, posture, and mobility. Without stretching at all, you'll feel looser and more flexible—as if you've developed a healthier body almost instantaneously." He goes on to explain that foam rolling massages the fascia, a web of tissue that surrounds and penetrates the muscles. Fascia is very adaptable and changes to reflect the kind of physical activity we do— which, for many people, is sitting in a chair. Foam rolling loosens and moves the fascia so that it can realign itself around your muscles.

Whatever the specific mechanism may be, you'll find that foam rolling makes you feel great.

"A little proactive self-care goes a long way toward keeping you pain-free and active for a lifetime."

— Sue Hitzmann,
manual therapist and creator of the MELT foam roller method.

"The best time to roll is before activity as this helps to unlock stuck tissues that aren't gliding properly."

— Dean Somerset,
a University of Alberta—trained physiologist and exercise expert, as quoted in Men's Journal

I would add that you can do foam rolling at any time, as often as you like. It's also good after a workout, and you can do it anytime you have a kink in your body you want to work out.

This section includes the following foam roller exercises:

- Shoulder-Blade Roll
- Upper Back Roll
- Lower-Back Roll
- Iliotibial-Band Roll
- Groin Roll
- Glute Roll
- Hamstring Roll
- Quadriceps and Hip-Flexor Roll
- Calf Roll

I learned these exercises from Jordan Metzl's books, *The Exercise Cure* and *The Athlete's Book of Home Remedies*, as well as from Sue Hitzmann's MELT method book. I prefer Hitzmann's MELT roller to other foam rollers I have tried because the foam is softer.

SHOULDER-BLADE ROLL

1. Lie on your back with a foam roller positioned under your shoulders (at the tops of your shoulder blades). Bend your knees and keep your feet flat on the floor. Cross your arms over your chest.
2. Tighten your glutes and lift your bottom off the floor. Using your legs to push, roll your torso back and forth over the roller, letting it massage your shoulder blades, upper back, and mid-back. Do this for about 30 seconds.

"'Your body's going to tell you where you need it,' says Karl Knopf, author of the Foam Roller Workbook. *Meaning, when you find a knot, you want to pause, relax the muscle, roll through it, and apply pressure.*

— Matt Fitzgerald,

writer, athlete, and trainer, Men's Journal"

UPPER BACK ROLL

1. Lie on your back with a foam roller positioned under the middle of your back, near the bottom of your shoulder blades. Bend your knees and keep your feet flat on the floor. Put your hands behind your head and pull the elbows toward each other.
2. Lift your bottom off the floor slightly. Relax your back muscles and let your back bend over the foam roller. This should feel fantastic—if it doesn't, only bend as far as you comfortably can.
3. Tighten your abdominal muscles and straighten your back out. Use your legs to roll your torso down few inches so that the roller is high up on the back.

4. Repeat step 2, relaxing your back over the roller. Again, only bend as far as comfortable. Repeat steps 2 and 3 for at least 30 seconds.

"[A foam roller] can be used as a strength-training tool, helping to engage key muscles you want to tone, like your arms, abs, thighs, and butt. Because the foam roller is a curved, unstable surface, it can . . . improve your balance and fire up your core muscles."

— Jen Ator,

fitness director of Women's Health magazine

LOWER BACK ROLL

1. Lie on your back with a foam roller positioned under the middle of your back. Bend your knees and keep your feet flat on the floor.

2. Tighten your glutes and lift your butt off the floor. Using your legs to push, roll your torso back and forth over the roller, letting it massage your lower back, for at least 30 seconds.

ILIOTIBIAL BAND ROLL

1. Lie on your right side with a foam roller positioned under your right hip and your right forearm on the floor for support. Place your left foot on the floor in front of your right knee (as shown above).
2. Using your left foot to push, roll the side of your thigh back and forth over the roller from your knee to your hip, letting it massage your iliotibial band. Do this for at least 30 seconds.
3. Repeat on the left side.

"When you start foam rolling, you'll probably find that [the iliotibial (IT) band] tissue is one of the most sensitive areas that you can roll over … Remember, pain means you need to roll it. Make this a priority because over time, if your IT band is too tight, it could cause knee pain."

—Metzl,

The Exercise Cure

GROIN ROLL

1. Lie on your stomach with a foam roller positioned parallel to your body on your right side. Use your forearms, forming a triangle with your forearms and hands, for support. Bend your right leg and bring your thigh up toward your torso, then place your thigh on the roller (as shown in the photo).
2. Using your left leg and arms to push, roll your thigh back and forth over the roller from your knee to your pelvis, letting it massage your inner thigh muscle. Do this for at least 30 seconds.
3. Repeat on the left side.

"While you will benefit from a general, full-body foam-roller program once a day (before and/or after workouts), it is best to target trouble spots, rolling the offending area for about 20 seconds at a time, and repeating until you lose the tightness."

— Fitzgerald,

Men's Journal

GLUTE ROLL

1. Sit on the floor with a foam roller positioned under your hips where your leg meets your buttock. Put your hands on the floor for support. Cross your right leg over your left thigh, resting your ankle on the thigh (as shown above). You'll tilt to the right a little, which is good.

"Adhesions in the fascial web [around your muscles] resemble knots in a bungee cord, inhibiting its ability to extend fully. A knotted cord still stretches, of course—it just stretches a whole lot better if you get the knots out first. Over time, foam rolling will do that for you."

—Metzl,

The Exercise Cure

2. Using your left foot and arms to push, roll your buttock over the roller from the starting point to your lower back. Roll back and forth for at least 30 seconds to massage the muscle.

3. Repeat on the other side by crossing your left leg over your right thigh.

HAMSTRING ROLL

1. Sit on the floor with a foam roller positioned under your knees and your legs straight, with your hands on the floor for support. Keep your abs contracted and your back stable.

2. Using your hands to push, roll your thigh back and forth over the roller from the bottom of your glutes to your knee, letting it massage your hamstrings. Do this for at least 30 seconds.

Variation: You can do one leg at a time if you want a more intensive massage. Just cross the inactive leg over the active leg as you did in the Glute Roll.

QUADRICEPS AND HIP FLEXOR ROLL

1. Lie on your stomach with a foam roller positioned just above your knees. Use your forearms for support; keep your abs contracted and your back stable.

2. Using your arms to push, roll your thighs back and forth over the roller from your knees to the tops of your thighs, letting it massage the quadriceps and hip flexors. Do this for at least 30 seconds.

Variation: To massage one leg at a time, cross the inactive ankle over the active ankle, placing all the weight on the active thigh.

"Hit a tight spot? Roll directly onto it and hold for 30 to 60 seconds. This activates your muscle's proprioceptors (which monitor upticks in muscle tension) and prompts the muscle to reflexively relax, easing the pressure."

—Ator,

Women's Health

ROLL OUT CELLULITE

According to Sue Hitzmann, author of The MELT Method, you can do a move similar to this one on the backs of your thighs to reduce the appearance of cellulite. On her blog, she explained, "Fat loves to live in the tiny compartments called microvacuoles (bubbles) of our connective tissue. Once they are there, it damages the collagen as water should be in those spaces. If fat lives there, collagen collapses and intertwines the fibers with the fat—and fat cells can not only get bigger, they can multiply. This is the onset of cellulite." But using a foam roller helps those bubbles expand and take in water, smoothing

177

out the "lumps and bumps" in the skin. It takes time and daily practice, but foam rolling can help smooth out stubborn cellulite.

---

1. Sit on the floor with your legs straight and a foam roller positioned under your ankles. Keep your hands on the floor for support. Keep your abs contracted and your back stable.
2. Lift your hips off the floor and, using your hands to push, roll your calves back and forth over the roller from your ankles to the backs of your knees, letting it massage the calf muscles. Do this for at least 30 seconds.

Variation: To massage one leg at a time, cross the inactive ankle over the active ankle, placing all the weight on the active leg.

"After you get the hang of this routine, it will take you less than 10 minutes and leave you feeling fantastic."

— Metzl,
The Exercise Cure

FUNCTIONAL FITNESS: YOUR FOUNTAIN OF YOUTH

The exercises in this book engage all 620 muscles of your body in a functional way (mimicking your daily life). If you use all your muscles you are telling your body that you still need each and every muscle. Using your body prevents muscle cell death. If you don't use it, yup—you lose it.

To prevent atrophy, send a message to your cells: I still need these muscles because I'm using them every day. By engaging your muscles, you will tell your DNA, "Hey, keep this muscle alive because I still need it." Fire up your body and tell your mitochondria (the

"All parts of the body which have a function, if used in moderation and exercised in labors in which each is accustomed, become thereby healthy, well developed and age more slowly, but if unused they become liable to disease, defective in growth and age quickly."

— Hippocrates

powerhouses of your cells) "I'm using you, not losing you."

You can prevent cell death, atrophy, and lousy posture. Don't let your body decay through inactivity. Without daily exercise atrophy and inflexibility set in. With atrophy our bodies bend over and we have poor posture. By exercising, you are choosing to stay youthful with an abundance of health, energy, and vitality.

Yes, we have control over how fast we age. Regular exercise means an energetic life full of strength and mobility. A life free from fatigue, pain, and dependence. Should you choose not to exercise every day, you will probably age with speed and painful injuries. If you're weak, you'll always be tired and full of pain due to muscle atrophy. Keep Father Time at bay. Relish your independence.

You have a choice to allow the aging process to take over or defy the "normal" aging process. Me, I'm gonna stay forever young. Vegetables, fruits, nuts/seeds, clean water, deep restful sleep, and exercise. The way of youth.

Your daily exercise will keep your muscles strong and pain-free. Feel young, not old. Be healthy, not sick. Choose vitality and health.

By being active you are choosing to enjoy life and all its wondrous adventures. Have fun 'til the day you check out. Fire up your life force (chi) and your body will respond by growing younger. This is the fountain of youth.

Get stronger, muscular, full of energy, with flexibility, balance, and great circulation. Decrease or eliminate the need for prescription drugs. Decrease back, knee, shoulder, hip, and foot pain. Alleviate or reverse arthritis and osteoporosis. Decrease falls that can lead to inactivity, lack of mobility, and a life dependent on others.

Experience the joyful pleasures of movement in your life. Bring back that light in your eyes and that youthful spring in your step. The time you spend exercising will give you an exponential return in your quality of life.

The exercises in this book will enable you to experience the vitality of youth at any age. Use your body as the vehicle to live longer, better, healthier, and happier. Keep these mantras in mind:

- Slow aging with strength training
- Challenge your muscles every day with exercise
- Do functional exercises
- Sitting means rusting
- It's never too late to get back to moving like a youngster
- Keep (or regain) your independence for life
- Muscle cell loss is the consequence of inactivity and not age
- Move like a kid by revitalizing your life with these exercises

CHAPTER 12

WALKING — CHANGE STARTS IN THE SOLES OF YOUR FEET

■ ■ ■

Humans were born to walk. It's the world's most basic,
most natural, and most accessible exercise.
Unfortunately, people don't believe walking alone can
make them healthy and strong. They couldn't be more
wrong.

YOU WERE
BORN TO WALK

One of the unfortunate legacies of the fitness boom is the idea that exercise isn't exercise if it isn't "work." Too many people believe that being fit means huffing and puffing, getting red in the face, dripping with sweat, and worst of all, "feeling the pain." In fact, these conditions may mean you're working too hard and putting yourself at risk.

We need to start thinking of exercise the way we thought of it when we were kids: play. Joy. Fun. Done right, exercise should *feel good*. When exercise feels good and joyful, you won't think of it as work or punishment, and you'll want to do it every day.

That's why I strongly recommend walking. Physically, your body needs more than just aerobic exercise like walking—strength training is essential, and I'm going to give you lots of ideas about how to build strength. Psychologically, however, walking may be the most beneficial form of exercise because it will help you start to be active and stay active.

Numerous studies confirm walking is the best exercise to help you "form a habit of daily activity," as Mark Fenton explains in *The Complete Guide to Walking*. (Fenton's book is a terrific resource and I highly recommend it.) He points out that yes, you already know how to walk—the goal of his book is to help readers incorporate walking into their daily lives. Many health care professionals say, "Find a form of exercise you enjoy" because you're more likely to keep doing it if you enjoy it. If you're very sedentary, though, you may not **have** a form of exercise you enjoy, so you give up before you begin. You can walk, though, and if you start slowly and build your stamina, you will discover that you enjoy it. Really!

Walking is the key to becoming an Ageless Boomer because you're not likely to quit, get bored, or get hurt, and as you start taking a daily walk, you'll start noticing benefits—more energy, better sleep, better mood, and better muscle tone. Your body will experience loads of benefits you won't notice but your doctor will: lower cholesterol, lower heart rate, healthier blood pressure, and stronger bones.

One of the biggest knocks against walking is that it isn't really effective because it isn't hard. That's nonsense, and it's another result of the "no pain, no gain" myth. People who have exercised all their lives may dismiss walking because they don't think it will do anything for them, and people who are sedentary may dismiss it because they don't think it will make a difference. They're all wrong. Walking can be great no matter your current fitness level. All of us were born to walk.

You—the bank branch manager who spends all day on her feet but can't chase her grandchild for more than a few minutes. You were born to walk.

You—the researcher whose back aches every night from hunching over equipment and computers. You were born to walk.

You—the high school gym teacher who's in pretty good shape but feels like he's losing a step. You were born to walk.

You—the former marathon runner who wants to stay fit without aggravating her injured ankle. You were born to walk.

If you're sedentary, walking is the best thing you can do to improve your health (after changing your diet, but by now you know that!). If you're already active, walking will be terrific for you, too. This chapter has loads of suggestions for increasing the challenge level of your walking exercise, so you will be able to maintain and increase your fitness level.

I encourage you to walk more every day in two different ways: one, walk so that you spend less time in your chair; two, walk to get your blood pumping. Both types of walking are important, so I'll explain each one separately.

WALKING PART 1: GET MOVING

As I explained in Chapter 11, each of us needs to get up and moving more often during the day. Too much sitting can negate the value of any exercise regimen. The "10,000 steps a day" goal comes up frequently when people talk about walking more, but when it comes to your activity level throughout the day, the frequency of your movement may be more important than the specific number of steps you take. You don't want to spend long stretches of time in a chair—

take a few minutes at least once an hour to move around.

Look for opportunities to stand instead of sit. If you're working in an office, walk to a water cooler or bathroom that's farther from your desk. Follow Laurence Morehouse's suggestion from *Total Fitness in 30 Minutes a Week* and make sure you're on your feet at least three hours out of every day.

WALKING PART 2:
TAKE A DAILY WALK

Walking to get your blood pumping is a little different but just as important. First, you should take a walk every day for at least 30 minutes. Why 30 minutes? Because it's a short enough time that you'll find a way to fit it into your day, but it's a long enough time that you'll get the benefits. (If you are very sedentary, you can start with shorter walks and work up to 30 minutes of walking.) Keep in mind that this is a starting point—as you gain stamina, you'll need to walk longer or faster to raise your heart rate, as I'll explain in this chapter. More importantly, you can't neglect strength training because it makes such a huge difference for your whole-body health.

"A number of recent articles on pedometers confirm the idea that activity spread throughout the day offers health benefits. For example, women in a six-month study, who increased their daily steps from 5,400 to 9,700, averaged an 11-point drop in blood pressure and lost three pounds."

— Fenton,

The Complete Guide to Walking

Second, your goal with this kind of walking is to increase your heart rate. Morehouse called it "pulse-rated exercise," by which he meant exercise that raises your pulse rate by a small increment over your normal rate (when you're standing and relaxed, for example).

Fenton uses the phrase "walking purposefully": "…walking as if you're trying to get somewhere, not just sauntering along smelling the flowers or window-shopping." When you're starting out, this simple idea is perfectly adequate; when you walk, do it briskly to get your blood pumping. He suggests an easy, "slow-fast-slow" approach to your beginning walks:

1. For 3-5 minutes, walk at a comfortable pace.
2. Walk briskly and purposefully for most of your walk—if you're doing a 20-minute walk, walk briskly for 10 to 15 minutes of it.
3. Return to your comfortable pace for 3-5 minutes to cool down.

This program is a super-easy starting point. If this is a little too easy, try a 10-minute warm-up, a 30-minute walk, and a 5-minute cool down. And if that's not enough, don't worry. I'll give you lots of suggestions to increase the challenge level of your walks later in this chapter.

It's that simple, and if you do nothing but maintain that walking habit for the rest of your life, you're going to give yourself enormous health benefits. As Jordan Metzl wrote in *The Exercise Cure*, "More walking is almost always a good idea, and if you like, it can become your primary mode of aerobic exercise, now and forever. I can't recommend it enough—or enough of it."

A: Yes. As Fenton explains, people often quit exercise because of discomfort, and walking in the wrong shoes can be uncomfortable. Fenton points out that even good athletic shoes lose their cushioning after about six months of regular wear. If you'll be walking mostly on roads and sidewalks, he recommends a lightweight walking shoe with a lot of flexibility in the ball of the foot, a low heel, and a top that stops below your ankle. If you're going to be walking on uneven trails or ground, consider a light hiking boot instead.

WALK OUTSIDE WHENEVER POSSIBLE

An average American suburb is filled with small sensory wonders: the smell of a juniper bush as your knee brushes its branches, the brightness of light shining off a puddle of water, the sound of rain or of snow melting, or the feel of the wind on your face. These wonders are accompanied by the rhythmic slap of your feet on the concrete or asphalt, or the rustle of your shoes moving through the grass. Sure beats the grinding sound of the treadmill motor and the sight of a TV across the gym, right?

We spend so much of our lives inside, and in the process we rob ourselves of the huge benefits we get from being outdoors. As you take up the habit of daily walking, take your walk outside so that you can multiply the benefits of this simple practice.

SOAK UP THE SUN

After reading Chapter 9, you know how I feel about sunlight: it's an essential source of nourishment because it's the absolute best source of Vitamin D. Vitamin D helps regulate your body's use of calcium and phosphate, giving you strong, healthy bones. It keeps your blood pressure down in the safe, healthy range. Vitamin D levels (particularly low levels) have been shown to play a role in the development of autoimmune diseases such as multiple sclerosis, asthma, and rheumatoid arthritis. Getting enough sun may help you stave off such diseases.

"But what about skin cancer?" you ask. It's less of a bogeyman than it has been portrayed to be. Professor Martin Feelisch, a professor of clinical and experimental sciences at the University of Southampton, stated in November 2014, "We have to balance the benefits (of Vitamin D) with the detrimental effects for the greater good of the entire population. The current public health advice is dominated by concerns about cancer...That may be very important for a high-risk group, but that high-risk group comprises the minority of the population."

The bottom line? Yes, you need to exercise caution so that you don't burn, but you need adequate sun exposure to get plenty of vitamin D in your body. (See "Chapter 9: Sunlight" for more suggestions.)

"We have to balance the benefits (of vitamin D) with the detrimental effects for the greater good of the entire population. The current public health advice is dominated by concerns about cancer...That may be very important for a high risk group, but that high risk group comprises the minority of the population."

—Martin Feelisch, PhD,
    University of Southampton

BOOST YOUR MOOD, CLEAR YOUR HEAD

Exercise is one of nature's greatest mood boosters, and you can increase that boost by exercising outside. Over the decades many studies have confirmed that "green exercise"—doing some physical activity in a natural setting—has positive mental health effects. However, in 2010 a study published in the journal *Environmental Science & Technology* demonstrated that even a little green exercise can do a lot for you. The authors found that as little as five minutes of exercise, from walking to gardening to cycling, in a green space (including a city park) can boost mood and self-esteem.

Green exercise is also great for your mental sharpness: just the presence of plants helps office workers and college students perform better on mental tasks. Taking a break from your work to get out and walk in a green space can help you focus and reduce your mental fatigue. Individuals with dementia and Alzheimer's disease showed better mental faculties after time spent gardening.

We know that exercise helps to stave off dementia; I suspect that green exercise is even better.

The authors of the *Environmental Science & Technology* article also found that "green and blue spaces"—natural spaces with water present—gave an increased boost to mood. That's probably no surprise to you: almost everyone enjoys spending time around oceans, waterfalls, lakes, brooks, and rivers. And there's a reason: moving water increases the amount of negative ions in the air.

Negative ions are actually a positive thing for people. They're negatively charged molecules

"Negative air ion treatment for mood disorders is in general effective ... Roughly one-third of the population seems to be particularly sensitive to negative-ion depletion."

—Olimpia Pino, PhD,
    "There's Something in the Air," Research in
    Psychology and Behavioral Sciences

(i.e., they have more electrons than protons) that exist for a few minutes at a time. Research has demonstrated that large concentrations of negative ions make people feel happier and calmer and may even boost immune response. Spaces near waterfalls, rivers, and especially oceans have very high concentrations because moving water creates the negative ions. Our urban environments often lack these sources of negative ions, and what's more, they contain many devices that produce positive ions (air conditioners are a particularly big source). As a result, urban environments are frequently depleted of negative ions. You can buy negative ion "generators," but even if they work, they can't produce the volume of ions you'll find near an ocean or a waterfall. However, even getting away from the city to the country will get you closer to those negative ions—rural spaces usually have many times more negative ions than urban spaces.

So step outside for a breath of fresh air as often as you can. And try to make your way to an open, water-rich environment whenever you can so that you can breathe in negative ions.

INCREASE THE CHALLENGE LEVEL OF YOUR WALKS

When you've been walking daily for a while your body will get used to it. For many people, that's just fine—they just want to maintain a basic level of fitness and get the many benefits of walking. Other people may get a little frustrated, particularly if they're trying to lose a significant amount of weight or get ready for a physically taxing event like a day-long hike.

Once your body has gotten used to your walking pace, you have to change things up a little to increase your heart rate. Increasing your heart rate is the key, as Morehouse explains: "The heart [like any other muscle] needs [an increased workload] if it is to be conditioned. To achieve this 'overload,' you must pursue an activity that pushes your heart rate to a level a little higher than you get in everyday routine activities."

"It's not the physical performance that matters, it's the exertion it takes to perform. [Your purpose] is not to beat some person, or lift some heavier weight, or run faster than [you] ever have. It's to get [your body] fit."

— Laurence Morehouse,
   Total Fitness in 30 Minutes a Week

After a few months (or even weeks) of regular walking, your baseline pulse rate will drop—that's a sign of a strong, healthy heart. As a result, you have to gently increase the challenge level to hit that "overload" zone during your walk. In Start Strong Finish Strong, Drs. Ken and Tyler Cooper suggest the following target ranges for your heart rate depending on your age and the amount of time you exercise (on the following page):

Exercise time	Age				% Max Heart Rate
	40 years	50 years	60 years	70 years	
20 min	145 bpm	135 bpm	130 bpm	120 bpm	80%
30 min	135 bpm	125 bpm	120 bpm	115 bpm	70%
40 min	115 bpm	110 bpm	105 bpm	100 bpm	65%

bpm=heart beats per minute

You can see that they recommend a higher heart rate if you're exercising for a shorter period of time and a lower heart rate if you're exercising for a longer period. (If you're doing intervals, which we'll discuss shortly, your heart rate will go between those ranges.)

Fenton recommends three basic changes: "longer," "faster," and "stronger." Take longer walks which will burn more calories; walk faster, at "a challenging but still comfortable pace," which will make your body work harder in the same time or distance; and do strength training to build your overall muscle mass. Like Fenton, I recommend strength training for everyone, and I believe you should do strength training at least three times a week (a full body workout every other day). Not only does strength training give you stronger bones, better metabolism, and healthy muscle mass, but it also increases the effectiveness of your aerobic exercise.

I'll discuss strength training in depth in the next few chapters; in the meantime, let's look at some other ways to increase the physical challenge of your walks. And remember, as you start increasing the physical difficulty of your exercise regimen, talk to your doctor to make sure it's safe for you.

But before we get into the specifics of how to increase the intensity of your effort, we need to talk about how you gauge the intensity of your effort. After all, how do you know if you're making a difference?

Like Morehouse, Fenton explains that the best indicator of intensity is heart rate. You can use a heart-rate monitor (see sidebar) or you can take your pulse periodically during your workout. Depending on your fitness level, your target pulse rate may vary, but in general 120 beats per minute is good during your moderate-intensity walking: "Your goal is to get your pulse up to 120 and hold it there for a few minutes—every day, if possible," according to Morehouse.

Q. DO I NEED A HEART-RATE MONITOR?

A. No, but it can be a useful tool. Fenton points out that in the beginning, a heart-rate monitor can tell you if you're increasing your intensity enough to give yourself a workout. However, many people find that once they've been walking for a while, they can tell when they're working hard just by feeling the degree of exertion. If you like fitness gadgets and you can afford one (some are available for under $100), then you might consider investing in a heart-rate monitor.

Another useful measure is the Rate of Perceived Exertion (RPE). You may have encountered the recommendation that when you're exercising with moderate intensity, you should be able to talk but not to sing. Fenton describes the "talk test" a little differently, "If you can talk when necessary but you'd find it hard to maintain a non-stop conversation, then you're walking at a challenging but safe speed." The talk test is a way to measure how hard you're working as you walk based on your own perceptions of your effort. Physiologists have developed a detailed tool to measure RPE at all different levels, but for most of us, if we pass the talk test then we know we're exercising in a productive, challenging zone. And it's perfectly tailored to you—two different people might

"If you've been diagnosed with cardiovascular disease, work with your doctor to set up a smart and, most importantly, safe exercise plan."

— Metzl,
The Exercise Cure

experience the same degree of exertion with one walking at 3 miles per hour and the other at 4.5 miles per hour. The talk test helps you gauge your intensity based on where you are now, and it still works as you get stronger.

CHALLENGE ONE: GO LONGER

The easiest and most obvious method to increase the workload of a walk is to walk for a longer time and a longer distance. See if you can make it over the next hill, around the next block, or past the next bend in the road. Try to maintain a consistent pace, and check your pulse to make sure that you push yourself enough to raise your heart rate.

As you begin walking longer distances, you may find it helpful to wear a pedometer or use a smart phone app to keep track of your distance and pace. You can find very simple, inexpensive options or very elaborate and expensive ones. If you have a smart phone with GPS, you can use a free application such as RunKeeper to track your route, distance, and speed. Or do as I do—walk your distance one day and try to exceed that distance the next day in the same amount of time using a stopwatch to gauge the time.

189

The biggest downside of taking longer walks is the time commitment: you have to spend more time walking to get the same degree of physical conditioning. If you have lots of leisure time, that may be no problem at all, but if you need to increase your challenge without doubling or tripling your daily walking time, you'll want to add another type of challenge to your walks.

CHALLENGE TWO: CLIMB HILLS

My favorite way to increase my challenge level is by tackling hills. My neighborhood is built on a hill, and so it's filled with steep little side streets. When I go out for a walk, I use the main street as my basic route, but then I turn on every side street because there's a hill on every side street. When I'm walking down the hill, I'm getting active rest—it's not vigorous work, but I'm still moving. When I'm walking up the hill, I'm getting a vigorous, pulse-boosting workout.

If you can't go walking in an area with a lot of hills, look for steps: even the flattest cities have outdoor steps if you look for them. Morehouse wrote that climbing stairs may be the best all-around exercise in existence. You may end up walking up a fire escape on a nearby building or half a flight of concrete steps in a city park or beach. That's fine, although you may need to go up and down that flight of stairs a few times to get your heart going. If you have pain or injury in your knees, be careful with stairs and talk to your doctor before using them for exercise.

CHALLENGE THREE: QUICKEN YOUR STEPS

"There are plenty of ways to boost your heart rate and burn more calories during a walk," Fenton writes, "but speeding up is the most straightforward and natural." The idea is to increase your step rate, the number of steps you take in a minute.

Just like measuring your pulse rate, you measure your step rate by counting the number of steps you take in one minute. Fenton has a chart that helps you calculate your miles per hour based on your step rate, but you don't really need that—measure your step rate when you're walking slowly, moderately fast, and really fast, and you'll get a good idea of your personal range.

"Faster walks are a great way to get more out of the time you invest in exercise: more bang for your buck. You burn a lot more calories as you increase your walking speed — especially as you approach 4.5 miles per hour and beyond."

— Fenton,
   The Complete Guide to Walking

190

But how do you know if you're walking fast enough? Remember the RPE, Rate of Perceived Exertion? Fenton recommends that you walk fast enough to get to a 7 on a scale of 1 to 10, where 1 equals doing nothing and 10 equals your all-out exertion. A 7 is moderately hard work that you would be hard-pressed to maintain for more than 40 minutes.

Fenton emphasizes that you should not try to increase the length of your stride: "Focus on taking faster steps, not longer steps. As you speed up, your stride will naturally get longer." In addition, he reminds us to keep our heads up, backs straight, and shoulders relaxed but not slouched. He recommends keeping the abdominal muscles "gently contracted" so that you don't get "shelf butt"—where your behind is sticking out and putting stress on your lower back.

CHALLENGE FOUR: TACKLE THE TERRAIN

As I explained earlier, walking outside gives you loads of mental and physical benefits, and you can increase both if you step off the sidewalk and onto the earth itself. The uneven ground of a mountain, beach, or even an open field gives your body extra physical work and gives your mind the joy of exploration. Remember that the extra work and pleasure comes with a degree of risk— you must watch your footing to avoid holes, slippery surfaces, and other unexpected terrain features.

If you live close to a beach, try walking in the sand. The uneven terrain of sand requires more than twice as much effort as walking on an even surface, according to a 1998 study. If you go barefoot, it also gives your feet a terrific therapeutic massage, but check the sand about 20 feet ahead to make sure you don't step on anything sharp (remember, you need to keep your head straight). Keep in mind that your legs are doing a lot of work with this kind of exercise, so listen to your body and find a comfortable pace so that you don't injure yourself. Some arthritis experts discourage walking in sand because of the challenge, and diabetes experts discourage all barefoot outdoor walking because of the risks of foot injury. Talk to your health care professional to make sure beach walking is safe for you.

GET YOUR ARMS INVOLVED: NORDIC WALKING

Nordic sticks—basically ski poles designed for use while walking instead of skiing—are a great tool for intensifying your workout. (You don't want to use actual ski poles, mind you, since those are designed for snow and Nordic sticks are designed for dirt.)

Nordic walking can use about 20 percent more calories, according to Fenton, because your upper body is moving the poles with each step. I think they can also be a lot of fun, and they're great for use on trails or uneven terrain. You get a little aid to your balance as you're negotiating rocky paths. Fenton even notes that they can be helpful for people recovering from stroke or injury (in such cases, you must talk to your doctor before trying them out).

Fenton suggests easing into Nordic walking with a few steps:

1. Carry the poles in your hands by the middle of the shaft to get used to the weight.

2. Let the poles drag along with you by putting your hands through the wrist straps.

3. Hold the poles as you would a ski pole. Let the tips of the holes poke into the earth with each step, and "gently push backward on the ground as you step forward with the opposite foot."

4. As you get more comfortable with the motion, you can increase the force of your push, which will engage your arms, back, and shoulders.

Nordic sticks are available online and at many sporting goods stores.

CHALLENGE 5: INTERVALS

Interval training is a simple idea—you take a baseline, low- to moderate-intensity pace and insert small bursts of high-intensity work. Your baseline pace is your "active rest," which means that you're still working but at a pace that will let your heart rate come down from the high-intensity speed.

It's also extremely effective: research indicates that interval training may burn fat more efficiently than a single steady pace, may increase your endurance, and may improve your cardiovascular fitness. It's a great way to break out of a rut if you feel like your routine is getting stale.

As I explained earlier, I use hilly terrain as interval training, with the uphill portions being

"People who find long, slow cardio dull may get a surprising kick out of interval training. Children rarely jog for long periods, but they sprint all the time — because it's fun. You'll probably agree."

—Metzl,
   The Exercise Cure

my high-intensity intervals and the downhill segments being my active rest. You can also vary your speed—when you go this route, it's helpful to have a good idea of your step rate at different paces so that you can set a good target for your intervals.

You can develop an interval workout just about any way you want. Fenton outlines several in his book. You can find lots of interval training plans online as well. Or you can make up your own based on what feels right for your body right now. In every case, let your heart rate be your guide—when you're raising your pulse to 120-140 beats per minute, you're doing a strong, fat-burning interval.

SOME CHALLENGES AREN'T WORTH THE RISK

Some people, including Metzl, suggest adding weight, but I don't recommend it. You're artificially boosting your body weight and putting additional stress on your joints. In some situations, extra weight makes sense: if you go for a hike you're probably going to carry a loaded backpack, and if you walk to the store and back you may be carrying groceries for your return trip. Even in these situations, though, ease into it—don't carry 40 pounds of gear or groceries if you aren't used to it. Start with 5 pounds and work up to more, and be careful about how you carry the weight so that you don't injure yourself.

You should absolutely not use ankle weights—as Fenton explains, they can throw off the way you walk and put your knees at risk for injury. Even hand weights carry some risk: you could injure your shoulder or elbow joints and even cause a spike in blood pressure from the action of gripping the weight.

MORE EFFORT
ISN'T ALWAYS BETTER

"If walking is good, isn't running better?" you may ask. In a word, no. Fenton describes a study he helped with that took two groups through a 28-week training regimen. One group walked, the other ran, each for 40 minutes a day, four days a week. In the end, their aerobic fitness was essentially equal, but the runners had missed on average 11 days due to injury, where the walkers missed a day and a half, on average.

More is not necessarily better. Exercise is essential and overwhelmingly beneficial to our bodies—up to a point. Once we start working ourselves too hard, we may actually harm ourselves.

Most people remember that the word "marathon" comes from the historical run of a Greek messenger from the battle of Marathon to

"Anyone who is physically capable of activity should try to 'reach at least 150 minutes of physical activity per week and have around 20 to 30 minutes of that be vigorous activity,' says Klaus Gebel, a senior research fellow at James Cook University in Cairns, Australia."

— "The Right Dose of Exercise for a Longer Life," Gretchen Reynolds, The New York Times

Athens. They may even remember his name: Phidippides. They may not remember what happened to Phidippedes after he delivered the message—he dropped dead on the spot.

Tragically, some modern runners are experiencing the same fate. Micah True, a 58-year-old endurance runner who became famous through Chris McDougall's book *Born to Run*, was an experienced endurance athlete who completed 50-mile runs on a regular basis. One day he went out for a 12-mile run and died while running. The cause, according to his autopsy, was heart disease.

How is that possible? True was an incredibly fit man whose biggest indulgence was a rare scoop of vanilla ice cream. How could he die during an easy run? Unfortunately, endurance exercise has problematic long-term effects.

Q. BUT WHAT IF I LIKE RUNNING?

A. Even if you run, you may benefit from slowing down. Matt Fitzgerald, author of *80/20 Running*, has developed a training plan that helps runners improve race speed by having them run at a slow, easy pace 80 percent of the time but then run fast intervals 20 percent of the time.

Cardiologist James O'Keefe led a study that examined the long-term effects of endurance exercise on the heart. He found that marathon runners and other endurance athletes had significant damage to the heart muscle that put them at risk for heart attacks.

"As great as exercise is, it's like a powerful drug," O'Keefe told *Time* magazine. "More is better up to a certain dose, but after that there is a point of diminishing returns, and it may actually detract from [heart] health and even your longevity."

In a 2012 TED talk, O'Keefe reminded the audience that Phidippedes was an experienced runner who had been a messenger his whole life. "I'll bet he was the fittest guy in Athens the day he died," he said. Today his name has been given to a cardiac condition observed among endurance sport athletes: Phidippedes cardiomyopathy. (Note: Micah True's autopsy did not give this form of cardiomyopathy as an official cause of death, but several cardiologists have pointed out the similarities between the state of his heart post-mortem and the symptoms of this disease.)

What does O'Keefe suggest instead? Walking. Or, for those who want to run, run slowly for a moderate amount of time. As he told *Time*, when his patients want to run a marathon, he doesn't tell them not to, but he tells them to make it a one-time event, something they can cross off their bucket lists. Don't make endurance running an exercise habit.

"We're not born to run ... we're born to walk," O'Keefe said in his TED talk. "We need to be walking more today. We need to be strolling. You need to be moving your body instead of sitting. Every chance you get, move." He recommends vigorous activity too, but in small doses: intervals of high intensity broken up by stretches of low- to moderate-intensity exercise.

WALKING IS CONNECTION

The greatest thing about walking may be its ability to connect us to the world around us. With each step, we're touching the planet we live on, even if it's through layers of concrete or asphalt. We're moving through the neighborhoods that surround our homes, engaging with our neighbors, even if it's just a wave or a smile. We're connecting with our environment, whether that environment is urban, rural, or something in between.

Finally, walking, like any exercise, helps you connect your mind to your body. It forces you to take notice of the skin you live in, the strength of your legs, the swing of your arms, the pound of your heart. It helps you balance mind and body, making both stronger in the process.

"More walking helps reconnect the fabric of our communities. Those too old and too young to drive can still walk. Neighbors greet neighbors, streets feel safer, and local businesses thrive."

— Fenton,
   The Complete Guide to Walking

CHAPTER 13

STRENGTH THROUGH SLOW-MOTION RESISTANCE

■ ■ ■

Strength training is essential! (Ladies, strength training is especially important for you. I'll explain why in this chapter.) Slow-motion resistance (SMR) is an elegant, ancient exercise method that has gained new popularity. It can give you lean, strong muscle without pain and injury.

YOU MUST
STRENGTH-TRAIN

If you want to be an Ageless Boomer, living through all your years with vibrant good health, you must practice strength training as part of your exercise routine. But if you're cringing at the thought of pumping iron, stop right now: I'm going to teach you how to strength-train in a natural, simple, comfortable way that scales up or down based on your body's needs and abilities.

Benefits of strength training:

Arthritis relief

Better balance

Fewer falls

Stronger bones

Weight maintenance

Better glucose control

Better mental state

Better sleep

Healthier heart tissue

— Centers for Disease Control

As I told you in the last chapter, walking is vitally important to your health, but the biggest value of walking comes from its impact on your psyche, your heart, and your lungs. It's not going to be your primary muscle builder—it's not even going to be your primary calorie burner. Muscle is your miracle calorie-burning machine, and strength training is the way to build it.

If you want to maintain your physical ability to function in daily life as you age, strength training is the way to go, according to Mark Peterson, Ph.D., a research fellow in the University of Michigan Physical Activity and Exercise Intervention Research Laboratory. "The most important factor in somebody's function is their **strength capacity**. No matter what age an individual is, they can experience significant strength improvement with **progressive resistance exercise** even into the eighth and ninth decades of life," he says (emphasis mine).

Peterson and his colleagues published an article in *The American Journal of Medicine* showing that after an average of 18-20 weeks of progressive resistance training, an adult can add 2.42 pounds of lean muscle to their body mass and increase their overall strength by 25-30 percent. I want to note a couple of things in that statement: first, in four to five months you can increase your overall strength by 25 percent or more. You can do one-quarter *more* with your body—like lifting a 50-pound child instead of a 40-pound child—in just a few months through strength training. Second, the term "progressive resistance training" is very important. You have to slowly and incrementally increase the amount of effort your muscles put forth in order to see gains.

"But Rod," you might ask, "doesn't that mean lifting weights?" Nope. In fact, I never want you to lift weights or use a weight machine. The strength training I recommend is SMRs as well as body-weight exercises such as push-ups (don't worry—I have pushup variations that will take you from easy to challenging). I'll show you how to use your own body as your gym.

DITCH THE DUMBELLS, IGNORE THE NAUTILUS

"The concept of fitness is implicit in the word: fit for what?"

—Laurence Morehouse, M.D.,
 Total Fitness in 30 Minutes a Week

It seems like every commercial for a wacky fitness device tells you that it's great because it "isolates" some particular muscle group—the abs, the thighs, the biceps, whatever. Gym machines operate on the same principle: they keep your torso and limbs locked into a particular position so that you're moving a limited set of muscles as you perform the exercise.

And they act like this is a good thing! It's not. When you train your muscles in this rigid, unnatural way, you may be making them bigger and stronger, but you're not making them better. You're not making them *fit*. As Laurence Morehouse asked in *Total Fitness in 30 Minutes a Week*, "The concept of fitness is implicit in the word: fit for what?"

WOMEN NEED STRENGTH TRAINING TOO!

To my female readers, if you think that strength training is just for men, you need to change your thinking right now. In fact, it may be more important for you to strength-train. All adults lose muscle mass as they age (unless they strength-train), but women can lose it faster than men. That means you're losing all the benefits of muscle mass faster than a man of your same age and state of health.

To make matters worse, women are naturally at a greater risk of osteoporosis than men. Strength training will help you keep your muscle mass so that you have balance, strength, and control, and body-weight exercise will help to build your bone density and strength. And don't forget that the number one killer of American women is heart disease. By maintaining a healthy ratio of muscle to fat, you'll see your heart disease risk plummet.

Not convinced yet? Are you concerned about "bulking up" or looking "muscle-bound"? Well stop worrying about that right now.

As former Navy Seal Mark Lauren explains in *Body by You*, testosterone is what builds big, visible muscles. Women don't naturally produce enough testosterone to build huge muscles, so unless you take a testosterone injection, you're not going to get big. Instead, you'll build lean, evenly distributed muscle mass that will give you a healthy, athletic body.

John Peterson, author of *Pushing Yourself to Power*, *The Miracle Seven*, and co-author of *The Ultimate Push Up for the Awesome Physique*, is my friend and my mentor, and I learned the SMR exercises in this chapter from him. John is always scrupulous about giving credit to the people who taught and inspired him, and I'm happy to do the same for him.

Functional fitness is critically important. By functional fitness, I mean movement that mimics the way you move in everyday life and everyday tasks. It trains you for everything you need to go through life injury-free. And to get functional fitness, you can do the simple exercises I'm laying out in the book. You have to strengthen your body in such a way that when you need it to lift a child, carry a box, or catch yourself when you trip, it will perform for you.

Be conscious and mindful of what you do throughout the day so that you'll see the kind of movements you need in exercise. If you're teaching a child to ride a bicycle, you have to run behind that bicycle. Are you squatting down to pick things up? Are you pushing boxes onto a shelf or pulling them down? These movements form the foundation of good functional fitness training.

Muscles don't operate in isolation. Many muscles are involved in every motion or every task you do. Tell me one movement in life that would require a leg extension or a bicep curl. The kind of exercises that I've outlined will give you the fitness and strength you need for everyday life—when you're running late for a meeting,

when you're lifting something heavy, or when you're reaching for something high on a shelf.

Exercises that increase functional fitness engage multiple muscle groups. If you're standing as you exercise, you're engaging your core for balance while you're strengthening your arms. If you're working on a shoulder exercise, you're also engaging your chest, back, and arms. You're training your body to move in a coordinated, cohesive way so that when you need to apply your strength in daily life, your body will respond.

"But Rod," you may ask, "if I'm not using weights or machines, how will I get stronger?" The answer is already in you—your own muscles and your own body weight. In this chapter I'll be taking you through a revolutionary yet ancient system of exercise that will build your strength through slow-motion resistance (SMR) of your muscles against each other. In the next chapter I'll give you a system of body-weight exercise to augment and complement SMRs. They also provide great benchmarks for your SMR training, e.g., you may be able to do one pushup when you start doing SMRs, but after a few weeks or sooner, you can do more. You'll have a good measure of your progress.

My friend John Peterson, the modern master of SMR exercise, says, "Protective exercise [like SMRs] will build your muscular strength while sculpting a lithe, lean, athletic body that is perfectly matched to your own bone structure. Protective strength is developed in direct relationship to your own body, and each workout will end well within your training capacity."

A functional fitness program like this one is protective. Programs based on machines or

weights are too often destructive. As John explains, "Destructive exercise … always pushes one to the edge of his capacity and oftentimes beyond, and that is when injuries happen. Destructive exercise will ultimately be the source of all pain and no gain as injured joints, ligaments, and tendons make productive exercise a virtual impossibility. At that point everything that was gained will be lost with the exception of pain, which you will always have."

SMRs are all gain, no pain. You control the movement and the tension, so you can't hurt yourself by pushing your limits. You're doing multi-joint, multi-muscle exercises that prepare you for the real-world tasks you face daily.

What we're doing is training your entire body for real life.

WHAT IS SLOW-MOTION RESISTANCE?

As John explains, SMRs are "nothing more than stretching (extending and contracting) with great tension." The diagrams on the following pages will show you the correct motion; you will tense (contract) your muscles as you perform those motions.

SMRs are not isometric exercises—an isometric exercise does require you to tense your muscle, but it also requires that you keep the muscle still. SMRs are a type of isotonic exercise, where you contract your muscles while moving. A push up is also an isotonic exercise, but with a push up your body weight provides the resistance. In an SMR, you're giving internal resistance. In John's system, Transformetrics, they're called dynamic visualized resistance (DVR) or focused muscular tension (FMT) exercises.

Simple, right? You tense your muscles and move your body, and you're exercising. At this point you might be wondering whether reaching up to get a can off the top shelf is an SMR. In a way, yes—*any* movement can be an SMR. That's the whole point. These exercises should be natural and functional and familiar. For example, if archery is your sport, mimic pulling a bow. If you're a golfer, you can mimic your golf swing in slow motion without the club. It will help your flexibility and power.

Even though you can do SMRs anytime, anywhere, and with any motion, I have given you a system to follow. This system will help you make sure that you're working all your major muscle groups, that you're giving yourself enough challenge to get stronger, and that you're using the right techniques to make these exercises as effective as possible.

Before we get into the exercises, though, I'd like to give you a little background on SMRs.

A BRIEF HISTORY OF SELF-RESISTANCE AND BODYWEIGHT STRENGTH TRAINING

You may already be familiar with practices like chi kung and yoga that strengthen your mind and body through slow movements. SMRs, like those

Even though you may never have heard of this type of exercise, it has a long and storied history, and you'll probably recognize some of the characters.

practices, draw from movements that have been part of our lives since prehistory.

EARLY MAN AND ANCIENT PRACTICE

In 1953, Selvarajan Yesudian and Elisabeth Haich brought their book *Yoga and Health* to the United States. This book was the first introduction many Americans received to the practice of yoga. In their chapter "The Miracle of Slow Motion Exercise," they explain:

> Early man did not need to be taught any physical exercises. His simple way of living and his out-door activities: hunting, fishing, climbing trees, throwing stones, swimming, fighting off wild animals, throwing spears, etc.—were far better than our modern sports and gave him the most perfect exercise with the maximum concentration of his attention… From dawn until late at night his day consisted of constant exercise.

This description of early man isn't perfect—for example, as was common in the fifties, early

"The daily routine of the occidental office worker is a crying sin against health."

— Selvarajan Yesudian and Elisabeth Haich,
Yoga and Health

woman is absent from the picture. The important idea is that our bodies evolved to be in motion for most of our waking hours, performing a wide range of physical tasks.

Yesudian and Haich then explain that the problem of civilized life for our bodies is that we specialize our movements—we no longer move our whole bodies daily. What's worse, in this day and age we spend way too much time not moving at all. As Yesudian and Haich say, "The daily routine of the occidental office worker is a crying sin against health."

As a simple alternative, they offer slow-motion exercise. "All we need is a mirror and 15 minutes a day. With this system of slow motion exercises … combined with strong mental concentration, powerful muscles are developed in a very short time."

After describing a simple arm SMR, they explain, "After a few weeks of diligent practice of this simple physical exercise, combined with mental concentration, we suddenly realize that our arm muscle has grown as if we had been doing hard work for several months."

Slow-motion strength building is nothing new; in fact, its longevity is a testament to its effectiveness. It just works. If you don't believe me yet, consider the stories of some of America's most famous strongmen.

In the late 1800s and early 1900s, Americans began to take an interest in physical development and "physical culture," which is similar to our interest in physical fitness today. In the days before television and radio, the ideas of physical culture spread through traveling shows and mail-order bodybuilding courses. The pinnacle of that interest came in the form of ads featuring a skinny little guy at the beach who turned himself into an intimidating physical specimen. It began many decades earlier with the rise of a farmer turned wrestler.

FARMER BURNS

Martin "Farmer" Burns was born in 1861 in Iowa, and rose to fame as a "catch as catch can" wrestler. ("Catch" wrestling is a hybrid style; several modern wrestling and fighting styles have roots in catch wrestling.) He was also known for his feats of strength, including being dropped by a hangman's noose and living through it without injury. Burns became even more famous, however, as a trainer, developing an exercise style that he and his students used to build tremendous strength and agility.

Burns opened a gymnasium in 1893 and spent decades training hundreds of wrestlers. He trained even more starting in 1914, when he first published a mail-order course called *Lessons in Wrestling and Physical Culture*. Burns was not a weight lifter: his lessons include a heavy emphasis

"[Burns] was teaching in the late 1800s and early 1900s what most people today would consider 'Eastern' martial arts principles."

—Matt Furey,
    author and martial artist

on deep breathing, body-weight exercise, and full-body training. One of the SMRs in this book is a variation of a Burns breathing technique—he calls it a breathing technique, but as you'll see, it's an amazing core strengthener.

One of Burns' modern disciples, Matt Furey, points out that Burns' lessons display his knowledge of several martial arts styles. "He was teaching in the late 1800s and early 1900s what most people today would consider 'Eastern' martial arts principles."

203

EARLE E. LIEDERMAN

As John Peterson writes in *Pushing Yourself to Power*, "After conducting a thorough and intensive research into the foundations of modern bodybuilding, I'm convinced that the man who was most instrumental in creating and elevating the American public's awareness of strength and physical conditioning was Earle E. Liederman."

Liederman was a famous strongman who toured the country as part of the vaudeville circuit from 1910 to 1919. During this period he met Angelo Siciliano, also known as Charles Atlas. Liederman didn't train with weights—almost all his exercises were free hand, using either his own resistance or his own body weight.

By 1919, as the age of vaudeville was ending, Liederman started selling a 12-week bodybuilding course by mail. He listed Atlas as his student (although Atlas was already a bodybuilding star when they met). The course was hugely successful and made Liederman a millionaire.

"I'm convinced that the man who was most instrumental in creating and elevating the American public's awareness of strength and physical conditioning was Earle E. Liederman."

—John Peterson

One of the attractions of Liederman's course was the fact that it didn't require weights or exotic equipment. He had a few exercises that used a chest expander, but otherwise, all his exercises used body weight and self-resistance to build considerable strength.

Unfortunately, Liederman lost his fortune during the Great Depression when the bottom fell out of the mail-order market. He went on to have a successful career in radio and writing, however, always keeping physical fitness close to the heart of his work.

CHARLES ATLAS

Charles Atlas, born Angelo Siciliano, is not just a giant among bodybuilders, he's a giant in American culture. Even if you aren't old enough to remember seeing the advertisements for his course in comic books and boys' magazines, you've seen them or heard of them in the years since. The skinny teenage boy at the beach with a pretty girl gets sand kicked in his face by a bully. Humiliated, he goes home and orders the Charles Atlas Dynamic Muscular Tension course. Six weeks later he goes back to the beach with a new muscled physique and shows up the bully who embarrassed him, impressing the girl in the process. The ad and the story have become a permanent fixture in American popular culture.

You might not know that Charles Atlas *was* that teenager. He was a "97-pound weakling," he often explained. That advertisement was drawn from one of his own life experiences, one of the incidents that pushed him to try to build up his body. He tried weight lifting but to his dismay it had no effect.

Here's where dynamic muscular tension, the phrase Charles Roman developed to describe Atlas's system, enters the story. The teenage Atlas was at the Brooklyn Zoo watching big cats stretch and flex their muscles when he discovered something amazing. "Does this old gentleman have any barbells, any exercisers?" he explained to his biographer, "And it came over me....He's been pitting one muscle against another!"

As Jonathan Black explained in *Smithsonian* magazine, "Atlas threw out his equipment. He began flexing his muscles, using isometric opposition and adding range of motion to stress them further. He tensed his hands behind his back. He laced his fingers under his thighs and pushed his hands against his legs. He did biceps curls with one arm and squeezed his fist down with the other." This is what John Peterson describes as dynamic self-resistance.

As Atlas built his strength with these slow-motion self-resistance exercises, he added classic calesthenics like push-ups, sit ups, and knee bends to his regimen. Within a few months, he had built an impressive physique, and one of his friends compared him to the statue of Atlas on top of the Atlas Hotel in New York. He later combined Atlas with his nickname "Charlie" to coin his famous name.

The rest is history—Atlas worked as a vaudeville strongman alongside Earle E. Liederman for years. He was discovered as an artists' model in 1916, modeling for dozens of sculptors and artists. He won a "World's Most Beautiful Man" contest in 1921 and "World's Most Perfectly Developed Man" contest in 1922. By 1928, he had a mail-order bodybuilding course for sale, and when he partnered with advertising executive Charles Roman, it exploded into the biggest mail-order fitness course of all time. (Roman came up with those unforgettable comic book advertisements.)

One more note about Charles Atlas—he was a great example of an Ageless Boomer. After his beloved wife died in 1965, Black explains, Atlas retired to Florida, where he "kept up a morning

> "Does this [lion] have any barbells, any exercisers? And it came over me....He's been pitting one muscle against another!"
>
> — *Charles Atlas*

routine of 50 knee bends, 100 sit-ups and 300 push-ups. Occasionally a photo of him appeared, bronzed and flaunting his godlike chest, his measurements almost exactly the same as [they were in 1940]."

The Charles Atlas Dynamic Muscular Tension course is still around—you can order it online for $49.95, not much more than it cost back in 1930. The principles behind Atlas's approach are as sound as they have ever been, and you'll put them to use as you practice SMRs.

TODAY'S SMR MASTERS: JOHN MCSWEENEY AND JOHN PETERSON

Despite the boom in gym memberships, fitness machines, treadmills, weight rooms, and every other fitness trend around, slow-motion resistance and body-weight exercises have continued to draw followers. It's hard to argue with the results, and the sheer convenience of weight training without a gym or a set of dumbbells will keep this method alive forever.

More importantly, though, today's modern Atlases know that using slow-motion resistance and body-weight exercise won't leave you "busted up," a term bodybuilders use to describe each other when they've lifted too much and injured themselves. In fact, as many former weight lifters have discovered, slow-motion resistance can help you restore function in joints and muscles that you could once barely move.

JOHN MCSWEENEY

John McSweeney was a martial arts grand master and one of John Peterson's teachers who practiced until his death in 2002 at age 74. McSweeney taught John Peterson the seven "Tiger Moves" that form *The Miracle Seven* as well as six of the SMR exercises in this book.

As Peterson explains, during his long career McSweeney tried just about every kind of exercise on the planet. He felt that the seven tiger moves were the very best. He explained to Peterson the one thing he felt Earle Liederman and Charles Atlas could have done better with their exercise systems:

> It doesn't matter whether you're talking about Charles Atlas, Earle Liederman, or any of the great mail-order instructors of the past. They all had good information, but they never taught anyone the essential key of how to gain the most from their respective systems of exercise. That key was how to think into and powerfully contract every muscle group at will. Without this specific understanding, you're missing the greatest benefit completely.

This understanding is part of John Peterson's system as well as this one. I've explained the

techniques you need to begin "thinking into" your muscles later in this chapter.

JOHN PETERSON

In many ways, John's story resembles Charles Atlas's story—he was an underweight kid who used dynamic tension and body-weight exercises to develop into a powerfully built young man. In one way his journey was easier: he had Atlas's techniques as well as two mentors in his grandfather and his Uncle Wally to guide him. In another way, however, his journey was much harder: John's body had been damaged by polio when he was four years old, and he had a long way to go to build the body he has today.

"I took to the Atlas exercises with a vengeance. I didn't have any muscles, so I just practiced smiling like Atlas did in those famous ads … But what I lacked in muscle I made up for in determination, and it wasn't long before I was packing on some serious muscle."

— John Peterson

John began his fitness journey with the Atlas system, but of course he didn't end it there. In addition to being a martial artist and teacher, he is also a writer, and his inquisitive mind and outgoing attitude has led him into friendships with Laurence Morehouse, John McSweeney, Matt Furey, and many other modern legends of physical fitness. He is always researching and testing the methods available, looking for ways to improve his own methods.

As a teacher and writer, he took his experience and shared it with others through his Transformetrics system. Transformetrics combines elements of the Atlas Dynamic Tension system, the McSweeney Tiger Moves, Furey's

Combat Conditioning (which builds on Farmer Burns's techniques), and more to create a system that allows anyone to build great strength and flexibility without injury or pain. Throughout it all, John's enthusiasm for self-development and self-improvement provides motivation. After all, when you consider that this man overcame his struggle against polio and its aftereffects, you have to believe that you can overcome your struggles too.

I had the good fortune to co-author with John the book *The Ultimate Push-Up for the Awesome Physique*. I have experienced the transformative power of Transformetrics myself—in particular, the Tiger Moves. I had a nagging shoulder injury for years and I was in constant pain. The doctor I saw about it told me that my only option was surgery, but I wasn't ready to go that route.

About that time I ordered *Pushing Yourself to Power*, and when I read it I thought, "This is what my father taught me," because he was a Charles Atlas student. I got *The Miracle Seven* right after I read John's first book, and I started practicing the Tiger Moves every day.

After two weeks of doing the Miracle Seven, my wife asked me, "How's your shoulder?"

I thought about the constant pain, and said, "It's gone." The pain was gone.

My experience is not unusual. Many, many people have told John how the Tiger Moves, especially the High Reach, have helped them heal injuries that nothing else seemed to help.

In this chapter you'll see a number of quotes from John's Transformetrics Forums, an internet community of people who use Transformetrics and want to discuss it. I've included these quotes because these people are Boomers—some in their fifties, some in their seventies. But they're great examples of Ageless Boomers who use SMRs to maintain great physical fitness.

FUNDAMENTALS OF SMR

As I told you earlier, SMRs are very simple exercises. You might be wondering why I am now giving you several pages of directions on how to perform them. It's because if you do them with the right techniques, they are tremendously effective at building strength. If you don't do them with the right techniques, you'll just be moving your body around like you do in your day to day life. That's not a bad thing— movement is good for you, as I said in chapter 11—but it's not strength training. It's not overloading your muscles so that you build strength.

You need to apply the following fundamentals when you perform SMRs:

- Breathing
- Posture/Form
- Tension
- Visualization
- Frequency of practice
- Range of motion

Don't be intimidated by this list. It may take you a few tries to apply them all, but once you get the hang of doing SMRs, all of these techniques will become second nature.

BREATHING

Healthy, deep breathing is essential during SMR exercise. As John once told me, "Deep breathing is an excellent exercise in and of itself … it speeds recovery by itself." You must keep your blood oxygenated through these long muscle contractions by supplying your lungs with deep breaths of air. Breathe in through your nose and out through your mouth. Exhale in a forceful way on the hardest part of the exercise with your lips slightly parted so that it makes an "ssss" sound as the breath comes through your teeth.

When you do SMRs, your breathing should follow the rhythm of the exercise—exhale as you perform the most strenuous part of the exercise, inhale as you perform the easier part. For example, you should inhale as you go down in a knee bend and exhale as you come up. You should exhale as you press up through a calf raise and inhale as you come down. With some exercises, for example the high reach, your level of exertion is fairly even. In those cases, you can decide when the inhalation and exhalation feel right to you, as long as you follow the rhythm of the exercise, changing from one to the other as you change the direction of the movement.

When you get to the point of performing SMRs with very heavy tension, you will be performing them very slowly. As a result, you may need to inhale and exhale more than once during a single repetition. If you do, make sure that your breaths are long and deep, not short and shallow.

POSTURE/FORM

Yesudian and Haich recommend performing slow-motion exercise in front of a full-length mirror. Charles Atlas recommended the same

"Deep breathing alone has made many a sick man well, and many a weak man strong."

— Farmer Burns

thing to his students. You need to be able to see your body to make sure your form is correct. It helps you "think into" the muscle. I do recommend that you wear snug-fitting clothing or as little clothing as possible when you do SMRs, at least as you get started. And I strongly recommend that you exercise in front of a full-length mirror. Once you've learned the exercises well enough that you can do them perfectly without a mirror, you can do them anywhere, anytime.

Watching yourself as you exercise will really help your posture, form, and amount of tension. Even though you're not lifting weights as you do

SMRs, you need to develop good form and posture. If you train your body to have good form/posture, then when you lift something heavy in a real-life situation, your body will protect your joints.

Good posture means that your spine is elongated so that you're not swaybacked. If your belly is sticking way out, you need to tuck in your bottom and tighten your abdomen so that you're lengthening your spine rather than compressing it. You should keep your head lifted and your shoulders back; you don't have to be military-style rigid, but you don't want your shoulders and neck to slump. Use this posture when you exercise and correct yourself any time you find yourself slouching.

Most of the SMR exercises will have you stand with your feet shoulder-width apart. A few of them will have you stand with one foot "about one step" in front of the other foot, which means about 12 to 18 inches for most people. This stance will help you really feel the movement through your core. In either case, your stance should feel very solid and balanced.

"At age 76 I do 3 sets of 10 Tiger Moves 5 or 6 days a week at 80 to 90 percent tension and I feel great both physically and psychologically."

— Andy,
Transformetrics Forum Senior Member

Tension is the key to success in SMRs. You use tension instead of weights; more accurately, you replicate the tension of lifting, pulling, and pushing heavy weights without actually lifting, pulling, or pushing them. You can visualize those weights and move your muscles accordingly.

Replicating that labor is a big mental challenge for many people. Some people just can't believe that it's possible to build muscle this way. As John would say, "Bull roar!" Remember, you're doing the same work with your muscles. You control them the same way. The only difference is that you're not straining your joints with the force of the weight.

"I get it a lot. People don't believe I am 54. Part of it is genetics. Part of it is being health conscious. But, McSweeney's Tiger Moves also play a part.

"I got my EMT student ID yesterday. I pulled out my driver's license picture from 2008. I actually looked younger. The unsung hero here is McSweeney's Tiger Moves and other tension type exercises."

— Greg Newton,
Transformetrics Forum Legacy Member

You will need to learn how to apply different amounts of tension as you perform SMRs. These exercises are designed to build your strength, so you will need to learn to increase the tension to make your body work harder.

Self-created tension is a fluid spectrum, and it's very difficult to put a specific measure on the amount of force you use. The good news is that you don't have to—your "light tension" will be different from my "light tension," and that's OK. The system is designed to work with your body where it is today and where it will be in the future.

RANGE OF TENSION

I'll be talking about four levels of tension: light, moderate, heavy, and extremely heavy. These levels will vary depending on your body and your current level of fitness, so you will need to figure out your own benchmark for each level of tension. (The following technique is borrowed from John Peterson's training approach.)

Let's start by figuring out your range. Wherever you are right now, extend your left arm straight out to the side with the palm facing up. Without doing any special flexing, bend your elbow and bring your hand to your shoulder in a basic bicep curl.

How did that feel? Try it again just to get familiar with the sensation. Got it? Good. That is your baseline, zero tension benchmark.

The next step is to define your upper limit benchmark. You may want to put down your book, roll your shoulder a little, and shake out your arm before you start.

When you're ready, extend your arm out in front of you again. Flex your muscles—hand, arm, shoulder, and back—as hard as you possibly can. Very slowly bend your elbow and bring your hand to your shoulder. It should take you much longer because you're flexing very hard. It should take you at least six seconds to perform the motion. If it takes less, try again with more tension.

OK, you're done. Shake out your arm. You've established your "extreme tension" level—the level at which you can only do one repetition of any given exercise. You should feel like you're "moving with the brakes on," as John puts it.

Will your extreme level be different for different exercises and different parts of your body? It's certainly possible. Many people will be much stronger in one range of motion than another. You will have to experiment to find your upper limit for each exercise.

LEVELS OF TENSION

Now you need to break down different levels of tension within your range. As I mentioned before, this isn't an exact science; you're going to break down the levels that feel right to you. The important thing to remember is that each level should increase the amount of the challenge.

Put your left arm out to the side again. This time, place your right hand on top of your left bicep. Tense your muscles just a little bit, just enough that you can feel them contracting. One of the things that is key in an SMR is to contract your muscles before you begin the movement. Contract them strongly and then ease up to the degree of tension you want to use for that set. Maintain that tension as you bend your elbow and bring your hand up to your shoulder and then back down.

Repeat this action a few times. You should feel like you could do it a dozen times without fatigue. (Go ahead and do a dozen if you want—your muscles should feel warm but not tired by the time you're done.)

If you can do this action with this level of tension 10-12 times, then you are using *light tension*. You should not feel tired after one set at light tension. If you do, then you need to use less tension—start from your zero baseline and see how many you can do. (If you can only do 10-12 at your zero baseline, you should start there, but you should not try to go beyond light tension until you have built up a little more strength.)

If you've been very sedentary or have never done any strength training, you may not go beyond light tension for a while. That's fine—the goal of this program is to build strength, not cause harm. When you can do the whole program at light tension and not feel fatigued, then you'll know you need to start using more tension.

As you get stronger in each exercise, you'll find that you want to use more tension so that you can continue to build your strength.

Let's try *moderate tension*. Flex your left arm again with your right hand on your bicep. You should feel like your muscle is working but not straining. It should feel very warm. You should be able to do 8-10 repetitions at moderate intensity.

Finally, try *heavy tension*. Flex your left arm (with your right hand on your bicep again). Go slowly, as if you were lifting a very heavy weight in your hand. Don't flex so hard that you can only do one—you want heavy tension but not extreme tension. You should be able to do 6-8 repetitions at this level.

The feeling of your muscle under your hand can also help you determine your level of tension.

With light tension, the muscle should feel firm. With moderate tension, it should feel hard. With heavy tension, it should feel very hard. With extreme tension, it should be very hard and will probably shake or quiver a little.

You'll need to experiment a little to find the right levels for you for each of the exercises. And as you get stronger in each exercise, you'll find that you want to use more tension so that you can continue to build your strength. Don't worry about trying to be perfect—just try to find levels that feel right to you and that you can apply consistently.

TENSION, REPS, AND SETS: AS YOU RAISE THE TENSION, REDUCE THE REPS AND SETS

For the first three months or so of your strength training, just use light to moderate levels of tension. As you build your strength you can start increasing the intensity of your effort.

As you increase tension, you decrease *speed* and *number*. As you tense harder, you naturally move through the exercise slower. You also reduce the total number of repetitions (reps) and sets of each exercise. The following table gives

you a good set of guidelines for reps and sets at different levels of tension.

When you do the SMRs, aim to complete at least three sets as long as you're not doing heavy tension sets. If you're just starting out, keep it at

General Guidelines

Repetitions (reps)= Number of times you perform an exercise without rest

Sets= A group of repetitions; you usually perform multiple sets

Reps+rest=1 set

Intensity	Reps	Sets
Low	10-12	3-4
Moderate	8-10	3 max
Heavy	6-8	2-3
Very heavy	3-5	2 max

light tension for two sets and then increase to moderate for the last set. When that feels really easy and comfortable, do one light, one moderate, and one heavy.

Basic 3-Set SMR Workout

Do 1 set each of all 12 exercises, then move up to the next level

	Intensity	Reps
Set 1	Low to moderate	8-12
Set 2	Moderate to heavy	6-10
Set 3	Heavy to very heavy	3-5

Accelerated Tension SMR Workout

1 Set=3-12 Total Reps

Intensity	Reps
Low	3
Moderate	3
Heavy	3
Very heavy	3

John recommends doing one set each of all 12 exercises at one level of tension, then doing another set at a higher tension, and so on. The following table shows you a basic 3-set workout that will help you bump up your intensity. You will perform one set each of all 12 exercises at low to moderate tension, then one set each of all 12 at moderate to heavy tension, and then one final set of all 12 at heavy to very heavy tension.

When you get to the point that you want to increase the challenge level of your SMR workout, you can try one of my favorite techniques, the accelerated tension technique. In this technique you're only doing one set of each exercise, but in each set you're ramping up the tension several times during the set. It's great because it has a built-in warm-up, but it also gives you a tremendous workout (it will leave your muscles shaking). The following table explains what to do.

When you do the accelerated tension workout, your last rep should take as long as the other 11 put together. You should move so

"[The Accelerated Tension Technique] works better than any single technique that I have worked with so far. And I use it daily as my morning wake up series. It literally 'resets' the muscles for the entire day and delivers a very pleasant muscular pump that borders on euphoric."

— John Peterson,
Transformetrics Forums

slowly that it's almost isometric. It's like moving with the brakes on.

You can also choose to do multiple sets at a single intensity. Later in this chapter I've created a daily schedule that uses this approach. It will give you another option for changing up and experimenting with your routine.

SMRS AND STRESS RELIEF

Another great benefit of SMRs is stress relief. It may seem strange that tensing or contracting your muscles would lead to relaxation, but that's exactly the basis of a stress management technique I discuss in Chapter 16 called "progressive muscle relaxation."

Dr. Edmund Jacobson developed this technique in the 1920s; it requires you to tense one group of muscles and then relax them, letting all the tension melt away. It's amazingly relaxing. SMRs follow the same basic formula—you contract your muscles one group at a time and then relax them. The primary difference is that you'll spend more time contracting when you're doing an SMR. The relaxing result is exactly the same.

VISUALIZATION

For many people, visualization is the hardest part of SMRs, but it's critically important to make the exercise as effective as possible. You must "think into" the muscle as you are exercising it with tension.

"Clench your fist as tight as possible. Pretend you are gripping a 100-pound dumbbell so hard your knuckles are turning white. Then slowly … curl your fist to your shoulder, feeling the muscles of your forearm and upper arm contracting with maximal force… This is what is meant by *Dynamic Visualized Resistance.* You literally visualize you are working against an imaginary heavy resistance."

— John Peterson,
   Pushing Yourself to Power

"Rod," you say, "that sounds crazy. What does 'think into' the muscle even mean?"

It means you use your mind while you use your body. As crazy as it sounds, research confirms that concentrating on your movement while you exercise can make a big difference in your results. As early as 1972, researcher R.N. Singer said, "There is growing evidence that the learning and performance of motor skills can be greatly enhanced through the use of mental practice, particularly when such practice is used in conjunction with [physical] practice."

This finding would have been no surprise to Martin Burns or Charles Atlas. Nor would it surprise great athletes like Jack Nicklaus who use visualization in their sports. Nicklaus wrote:

I never hit a shot even in practice without having a sharp in-focus picture of it in my head. It's like a color movie. First, I "see" the ball where I want it to finish, nice and white and sitting up high on the bright green grass. Then the scene quickly changes, and I "see" the ball going there: its path, trajectory, and shape, even its behavior on landing. Then there's a sort of fade-out, and the next scene shows me making the kind of swing that will turn the previous images into reality and only at the end of this short private Hollywood spectacular do I select a club and step up to the ball. (1974)

In an SMR, you're not swinging a golf club, you're moving your body. But as you move your body, whether it's your arm or your head or your foot, you're going to concentrate on that

214

movement as much as you can. It's very similar to meditation in this respect.

The easiest way to visualize in SMR exercise is to imagine that you are lifting or pulling a heavy weight during each exercise. For example, if you're doing the High Reach, you can imagine lifting a heavy object on the way up and lowering it—slowly!—on the way back down. If you're doing light tension, you can imagine lifting something that weighs a few pounds, like a brick. If you're doing moderate tension, you can imagine lifting a gallon of milk, And if you're doing really heavy tension, you can imagine lifting a 40-pound bag. Like everything else in SMRs, you can modify it to fit your needs—if you want to imagine that you're Superman lifting cars, go for it. Just imagine different sizes for your different levels of tension.

VISUALIZATION EXERCISE

Try this exercise to practice visualization techniques:

1. Find a firm, small object around your home—a ball, a stone, a can—that is small enough to fit in your hand but large enough that you can't close your fingers around it.
2. Close your eyes and squeeze the object with your hand for a few seconds. Concentrate on the sensation of pressure in your hand; don't concentrate on the object itself. Notice the amount of tension in your muscles. Stop and set the object down.
3. With your eyes closed, repeat the squeezing motion as if you still held the object in your hand. Concentrate on the muscles in your hand. Try to recreate the pressure and tension you used when you were holding the object.

This exercise will be difficult at first, so repeat it a few times with the same object. Try different objects as well.

Recreating the tension of an imagined object is "thinking into" the muscle. It's not the only way to do it, but it's the easiest place to begin. As you gain more experience and comfort with visualization, you'll be able to concentrate on your SMR muscle contractions without imagining an object.

Many people like to imagine something flowing into their muscles as they work—some people like to imagine concrete things like blood or oxygen while others like to imagine ideas like energy or strength. Yoga practitioners like Yesudian and Haich use the word *prana*; many martial arts practitioners use the word *chi*. Some of you will find this form of visualization very energizing; others will find it very difficult. If it helps you, use it; if not, just concentrate on your muscles contracting and relaxing.

You should do some form of strength training three to four times per week. If you want to, you can do SMRs every day, but you don't have to. If you're just starting out with strength training, stick to the SMRs. They're perfect for building up your strength. In fact, I recommend you do SMRs only for the first three months of strength training (as does John Peterson) before you start introducing body-weight exercise and circuit

Change up your routine periodically so that you don't get bored. SMRs are flexible — you can try different routines and play with levels of tension. And you can do them anywhere. Do them outside. Do them during your walks. Do them on the rebounder. Have fun!

training. And if you want to do only SMRs for the rest of your life, that's fine. They will keep you strong all by themselves.

When you begin strength-training with SMRs, start with light tension, and do them with light tension seven days a week. Once you've learned the exercises well and you've begun to increase your strength, you can increase the level of tension and decrease the number of reps per set (see the "Tension" section).

If you decide to start mixing circuit training in with your SMRs, that's great. The two types of strength training complement each other very well. For example, you can do light-tension SMRs as a warm up for body weight exercise. When I'm doing calisthenics, in between every set

I do a set of one of the tiger moves at light to medium intensity with deep breathing.

Whatever approach you choose, make sure that you're doing some strength training three to four days a week and vary the tension day to day.

GREASE THE GROOVE: WORK OUT THROUGHOUT THE DAY

One of the great things about SMRs is that you can do them any time, any place, so you don't have to do all your sets at one point during the day. You can do a set in the morning, a set before lunch, and a set before dinner, as long as it feels good to you. You do need to warm up before you start, but the warm-up dynamic stretches take only minutes. And if you've been doing something else active—say, rebounding or taking your daily walk—you can start your SMRs because you're already warmed up.

The goal with "Greasing the Groove" is to infuse the body with highly oxygenated, nutrient-rich blood and deliver it to the muscles throughout the day. This method works perfectly with moderate tension SMRs and deep breathing. You may decide to use light to moderate intensity for 12 reps, and then increase it incrementally on

Looking for a great combination workout? Do SMRs while rebounding! You can do all of the upper-body SMRs while you're bouncing.

Use your rebounder for active rest between sets of SMRs — do the health bounce to keep your blood flowing and your lungs working.

the last half dozen until you get to 18 so that your muscles feel reasonably taxed. For example, if you performed 12 to 18 reps several times throughout the day of the tiger moves, it would enhance the blood flow and healing process.

John starts his day with SMRs, doing them as soon as he gets out of bed. He says it gets him energized for the rest of the day. I will often do the Farmer Burns Stomach Flattener before I even get out of bed.

This approach is great for your mood and your mind. It gets your blood pumping and your juices flowing, leaving you relaxed and ready to take on your daily challenges. If you're injured, greasing the groove can really enhance the healing process by giving you long periods of rest in between your exercise sets.

"To improve is to change. To be perfect is to change often."

— Winston Churchill

A WEEK OF SMRS

You can modify your SMR workout to fit your lifestyle and your level of fitness; as long as you're doing it every day, that's great. The following table offers you a possible schedule. Since it includes very heavy tension sets, the beginner will want to reduce the intensity of this schedule. Don't do two days of heavy tension in a row. Vary the stress—don't overdo.

	Tension	Reps	Sets
Monday	Light	8-12 reps	3 sets
Tuesday	Heavy	8-12 reps	3 sets
Wednesday	Medium	8-12 reps	3 sets
Thursday	Very heavy	8-12 reps	3 sets
Friday	Light	8-12 reps	3 sets
Saturday	Heavy	8-12 reps	3 sets

RANGE OF MOTION DYNAMIC STRETCHES

Always warm up your muscles before you start your strength-training workout. The range of motion (ROM) dynamic stretches in Chapter 11 will warm up your muscles completely, getting you ready to start the SMRs. They take only a few minutes, and they feel great.

THE AMAZING VALUE OF THE TIGER MOVES

"[Tiger Moves] are the perfect exercise system for men and women of all ages. Repetition for repetition, they deliver more benefits than virtually any other form of exercise. And while they can certainly build a powerful and beautifully developed physique or figure, they do so without any of the usual joint and tendon injuries associated with heavy weightlifting. But even more importantly, they accelerate healing while dramatically slowing the aging process. This is due mainly to the fact that Tiger Moves teach you how to conserve and powerfully use nerve force to your best advantage. …Weightlifting causes severe compression of the lower spine; this in turn inhibits the flow of nerve force not only to the muscles but also to all of the vital organs of the body. As a result, premature aging is accelerated through the use of excessively heavy weights."

—John Peterson, The Miracle Seven

"Those seven exercises that are John McSweeney's creation accomplish an extraordinary amount of benefit that is far beyond other forms exercise. They strengthen and stretch virtually every muscle while promoting youthful elasticity and blood flow. I believe the Tiger Moves and the many other exercises of the same type in Living Strength will make it possible for everyone to remain incredibly youthful as will be obvious by the way they move and the youthful silhouette they cast."

—John Peterson,
    Transformetrics Forums

THE 12 EXERCISES FOR OVERALL STRENGTH

The following 12 SMR exercises start with your head (the Neck Roll) and move through your feet (the Calf Raise), strengthening your entire body. While each exercise focuses on one general area, they all work multiple muscle groups, giving you multi-joint functional training.

By the time you finish an SMR workout, you should feel warm (even sweaty) and a little tired.

"This routine consists of twelve exercises, and each one is vital in that it targets different muscle groups."

—John Peterson

Your whole body should feel stretched out and exercised. You should not feel sore or injured but rather you should have a sense of soaring energy.

DÉJÀ VU: I'VE SEEN THIS EXERCISE BEFORE

You'll notice that a few of these exercises—the Six-Way Neck Movement, the Knee Bend, for example—also appeared in the range-of-motion dynamic stretches in Chapter 11. That's not a mistake.

You'll see calf raises and knee bends again when I talk about circuit-training and body-weight exercises because both of those moves are also body-weight resistance moves.

So what's the difference here? What makes a calf raise dynamic stretch different from a calf raise SMR?

The difference is visualized tension. When you do a calf raise as a dynamic stretch, you're just performing the motion, gently engaging the muscles to get them warm. When you do the calf raise as an SMR, you will add tension by "thinking into" the muscles and tensing them as you perform the motion, increasing the effort so that you can build strength in the muscle.

If you're starting with low muscle mass, SMRs can help you get ready for body-weight exercises. Knee bends are precursors to full squats—as you practice SMR knee bends, you're building muscles around your joints that will help you when you start doing the deeper knee bends of squats. (When you squat, you should never go below 90 degrees.)

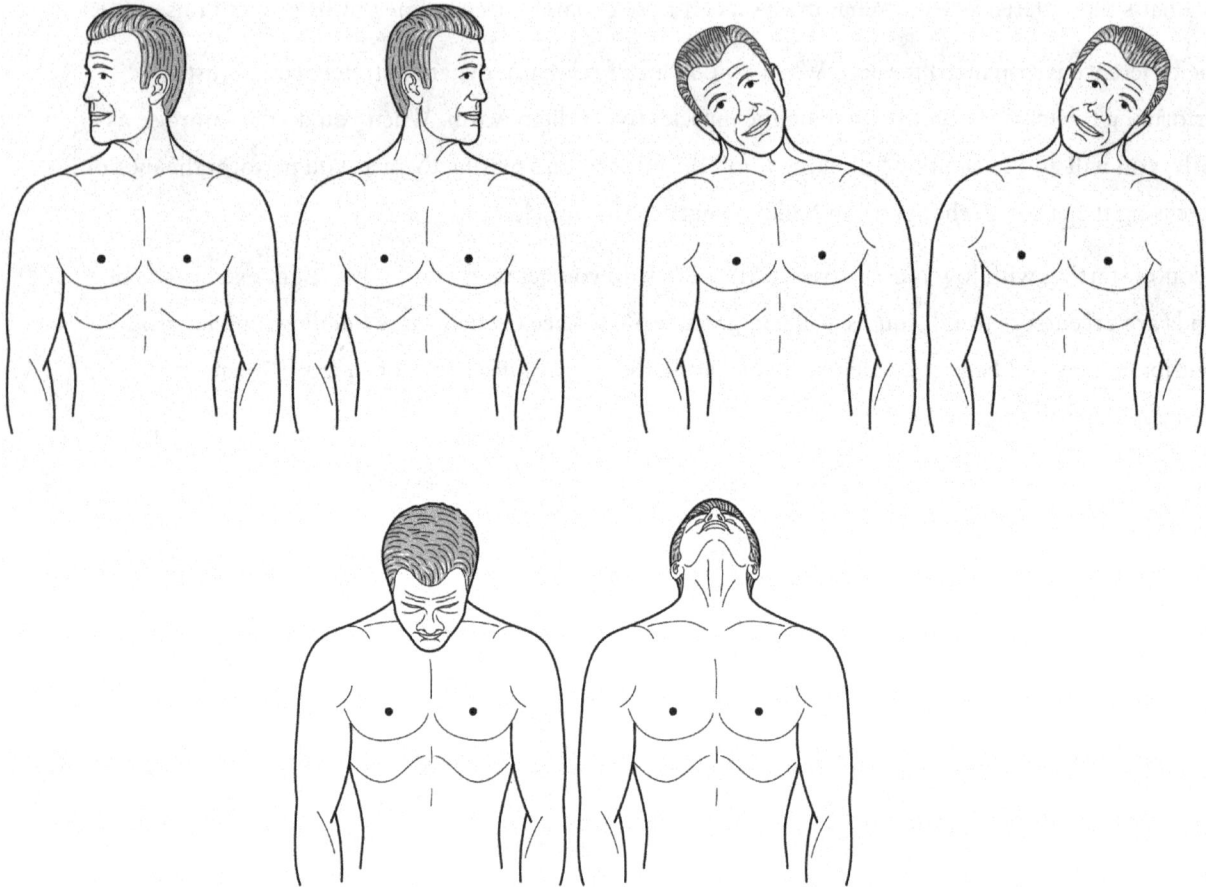

1. Stand with your feet shoulder-width apart, your head forward, and relax your arms. Tighten the muscles of your neck with light tension to begin. Keep the tension as you move your head.

2. Turn your head to the left as far as you comfortably can, release the tension for a moment (less than a second) and turn it to the right. Repeat for your number of repetitions.

3. When you finish step 2, return to the starting position of step 1. Tilt your head to the left, bringing your ear toward your shoulder. Release the tension for a moment and tilt it to the right. Repeat for your number of repetitions.

4. When you finish step 3, return to the starting position of step 1. Tilt your head forward, bringing your chin toward your chest. Release the tension for a moment and tilt your head backward, looking toward the ceiling.

5. Repeat for your number of repetitions.

As I noted earlier, the key phrase is "As far as comfortable." If you feel discomfort, use less tension and/or don't stretch as far.

VARIATION: SIX-WAY NECK MOVEMENT WITH DYNAMIC SELF-RESISTANCE (DSR)

When I do the Six-way Neck Movement, I like to use my hands to add a little extra resistance. I do this three times a week, a couple of sets for each position.

Side to Side, Turning: Turn your head as far as you can to the right. Put the heel of your left hand on the left side of your head, in front of your ear in line with your forehead. With your left hand resisting, turn your head to the left as far as you can. Repeat ten times.

Reverse the position of your head and your hand—beginning with your head turned to the left and using the right hand to resist—and repeat ten times.

Side to Side, Tilting: Put your left hand above your left ear on the side of your head. Bring your right ear as close as you can to your right shoulder. While resisting with your left hand, bring your left ear as close to your left shoulder as you can. Repeat ten times.

Reverse the position of your head and your hand—beginning with your left ear at your left shoulder and using the right hand to resist—and repeat ten times.

Forward and Back: Put the heels of your hands in the middle of your forehead. Bend your head back, then bend your head forward while resisting with your hands. Do that ten times.

While your chin is touching your chest, put your hands on the back of your head (opposite your forehead). Move your head back while resisting with your hands. Start off with gentle resistance, and as your neck gets stronger, increase the resistance of your hands.

Reps: Light tension—10; Moderate tension—8; Heavy tension—6.

Sets: Light tension—3; Moderate tension—2-3; Heavy tension—2.

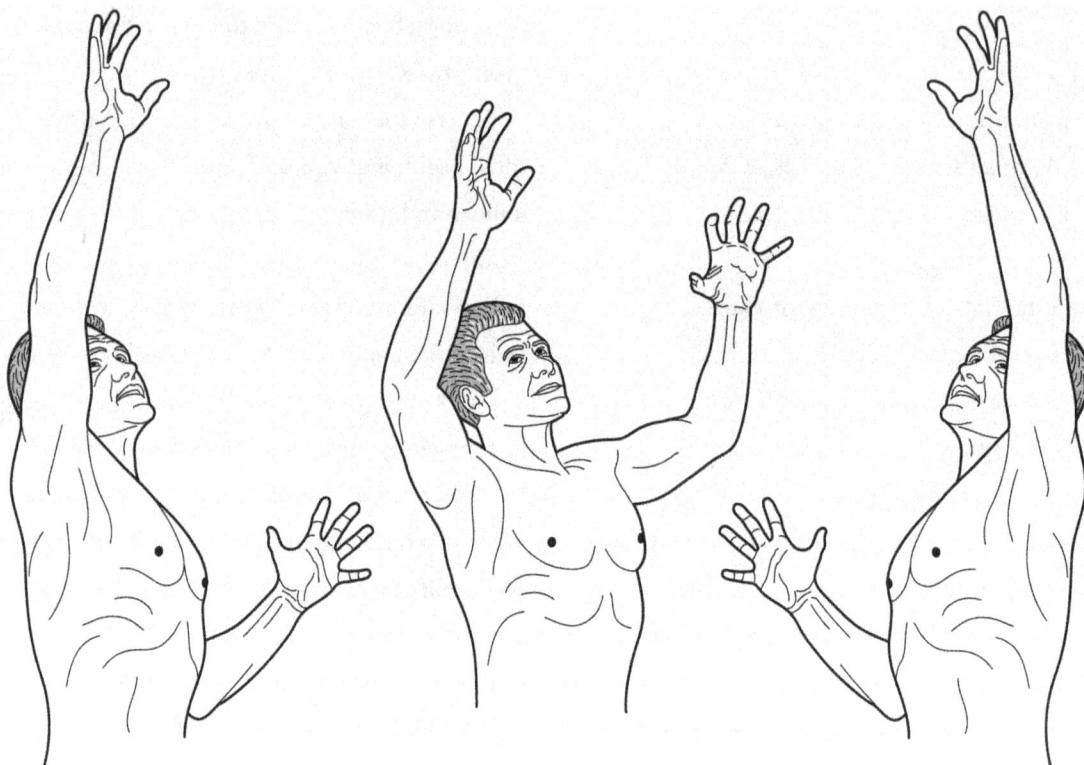

1. Stand with your feet shoulder-width apart and your chin tilted up slightly (you can look up or look at your mirror). Hold your hands in front of you at shoulder height with your elbows bent—this is a tiger move, so keep your "paws" up like you're about to pounce.
2. Tense your muscles, lightly at first, and reach your right arm upward (you can let your left arm drop a little as the diagram shows). Imagine that you're moving through the exercise with the brakes on. Reach up as high as you can, maintaining tension, and then return to the starting position.

3. Release the tension for a moment, then repeat the motion with the left arm.
4. Do your number of repetitions for each arm.

Try it:

You can leave your hands open or, for an extra forearm workout, clench your fists.

Reps: Light tension—10; Moderate tension—8; Heavy tension—6.

Sets: Light tension—3; Moderate tension—2-3; Heavy tension—2.

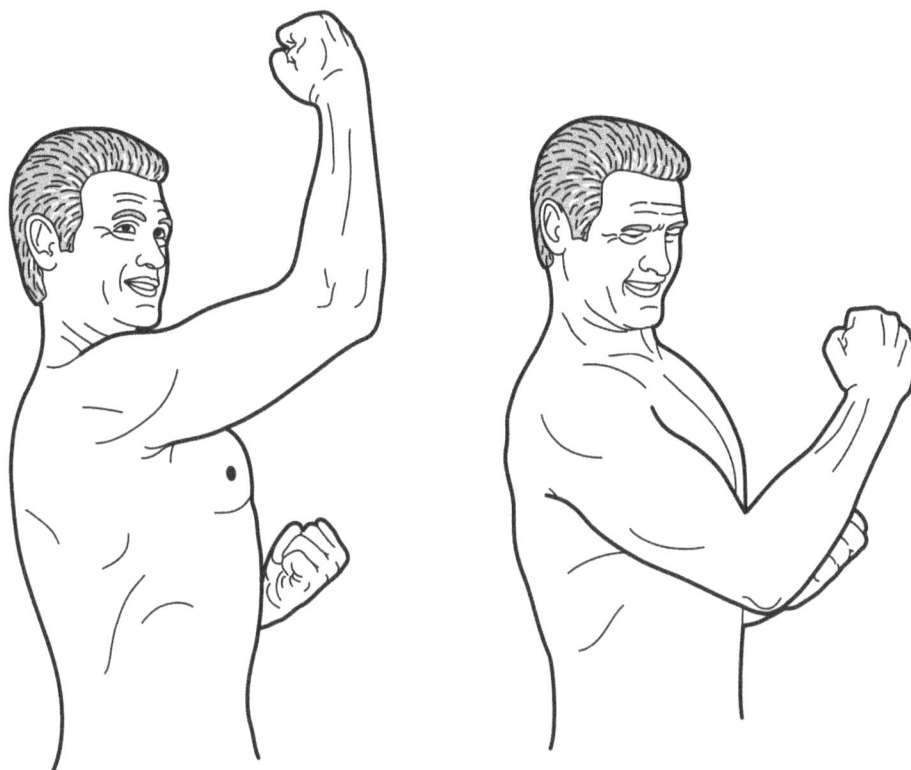

1. Stand with your feet shoulder-width apart. Bend your elbows and make fists with your hands. Make sure your palms face you.

2. Raise your right hand above your head (as shown in the diagram) and imagine that you're grabbing a handle just above your head. Flex your muscles lightly and pull your arm down, imagining that you're pulling against a heavy weight. Move your hand along the midline of your body (face, sternum, navel) as you bring it down.

3. As you pull your right arm down, bring your left arm up with tension. Raise your left arm up to your imaginary handle, relax your flexed muscles for a moment, and then grab the handle with your left hand and pull down with tension.

4. Do your number of repetitions for each arm.

Reps: Light tension—10-12; Moderate tension—8-10; Heavy tension—6-8.

Sets: Light tension—3; Moderate tension—2-3; Heavy tension—2.

Watch your form: Keep your hand moving along the midline of your body so that you engage the muscles in your shoulders and back. If you keep your hand in front of your shoulder, you'll work different muscles. That's a good exercise too, but make sure you do this exercise as shown to get the benefits for your core.

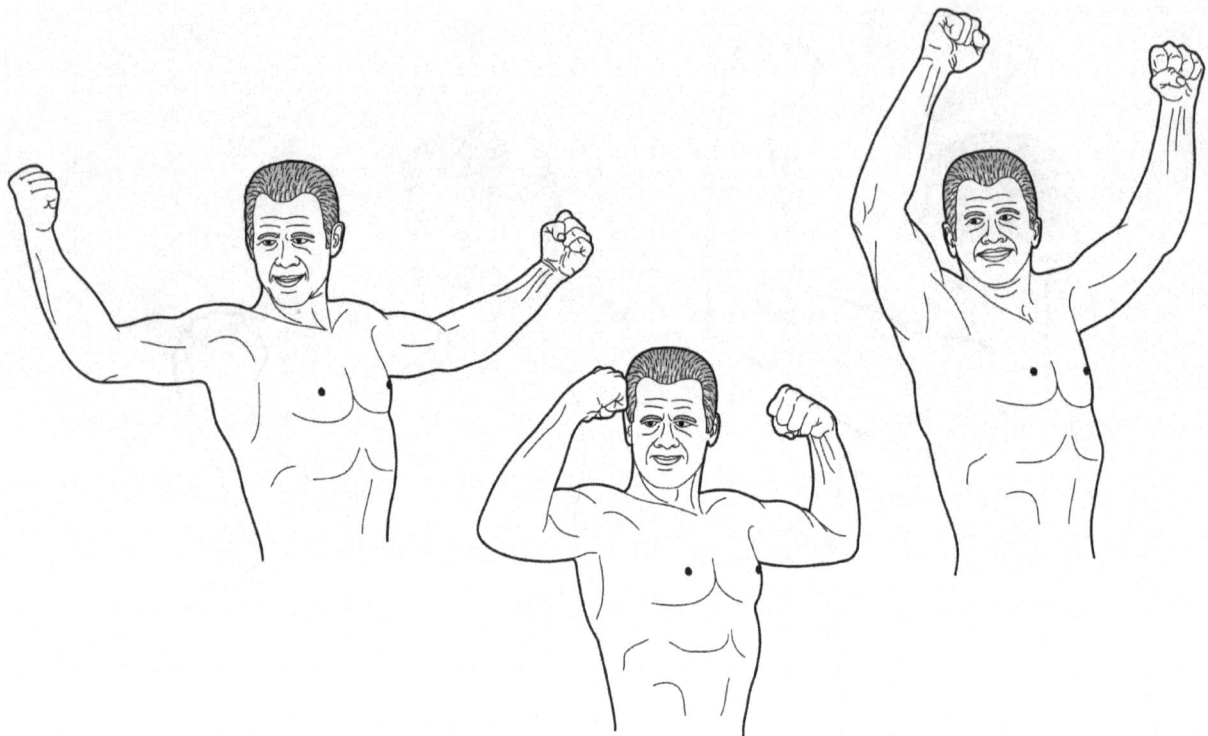

1. Stand with your feet shoulder-width apart. Extend your arms to the side with your hands in fists, palms facing up.
2. Tense your muscles and then bend your elbows, bringing your arms toward your shoulders as shown in the diagram.
3. When your hands get close to your shoulders, rotate your palms forward and extend your arms overhead as shown. Maintain tension through the whole movement.
4. When your arms are fully extended over your head, release tension for a moment (less than a second), then tense again and reverse the movement, bringing your hands back to your shoulders, then out to the side and back to the starting position, with tension.
5. Release tension for a moment and then repeat the exercise.
6. Do your number of repetitions.

"A big component of the Atlas system included what I call Dynamic Self-Resistance exercises (DSR). These exercises are a first cousin to the DVR exercises, which were also a part of the Atlas system, and allow you to contract with maximal force as you use one limb or muscle group to resist another."

— John Peterson,
   The Miracle Seven

Reps: Light tension—10-12; Moderate tension—8-10; Heavy tension—6-8.

Sets: Light tension—3; Moderate tension—2-3; Heavy tension—2.

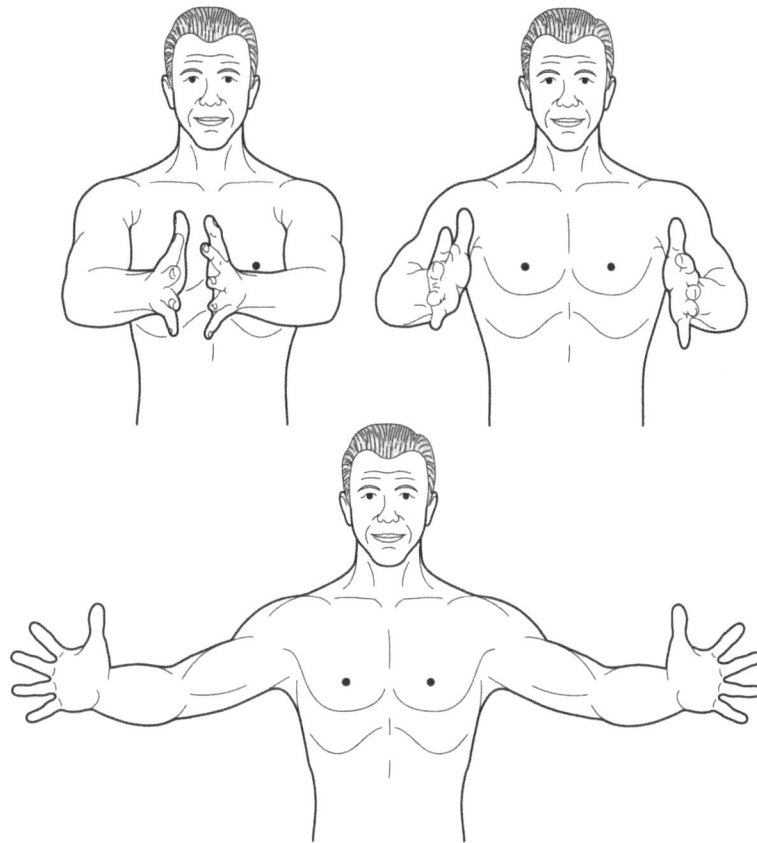

1. Stand with your left foot about one step in front of your right foot. Extend your arms in front of you with your palms facing each other, as shown in the diagram.
2. Tense your muscles and slowly open your arms, contracting your back muscles, until your arms are open at your sides. Hold this position for one full second.
3. Release tension for a moment, then tense your muscles and slowly bring your hands together again, contracting your chest as well as your arms and shoulders. Keep a slight bend in your elbows.
4. Release tension for a moment and then repeat the exercise.
5. Do your number of repetitions.

"[Tiger Moves] require no gym and no equipment and can be done anywhere and anytime. They are far superior to weights [or] machines … and I'm living proof of their effectiveness."

— John McSweeney

(as told to John Peterson)

Reps: Light tension—10-12; Moderate tension—8-10; Heavy tension—6-8.

Sets: Light tension—3; Moderate tension—2-3; Heavy tension—2.

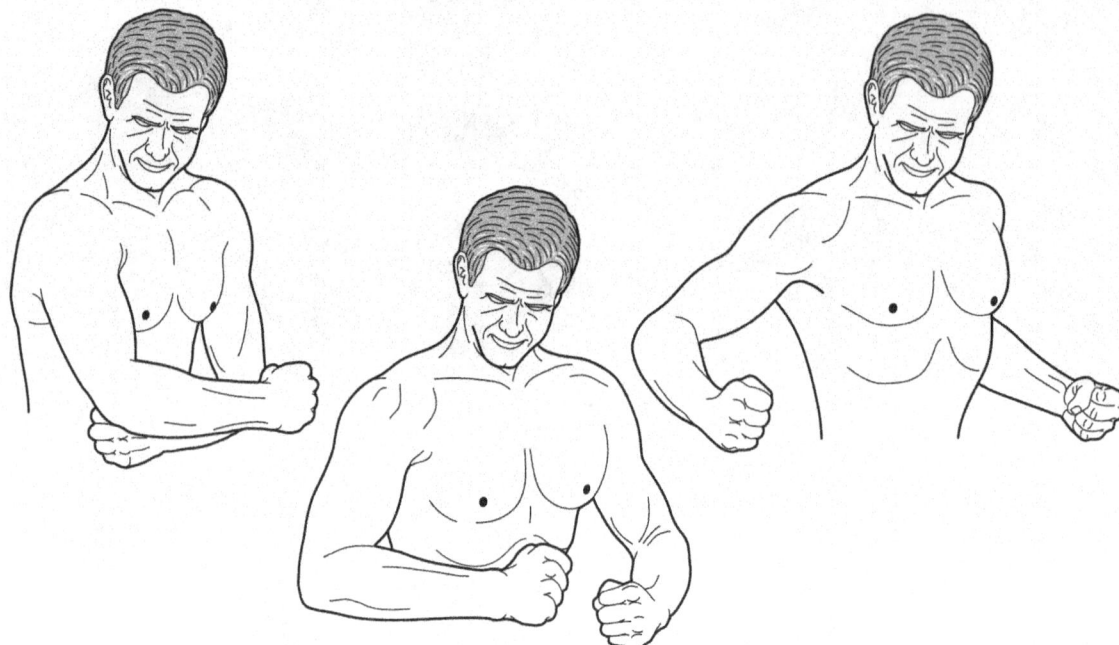

1. Stand with your left foot about one step in front of your right foot. Bend your elbows, make fists with your hands, and cross your left forearm above your right forearm as shown in the diagram. Contract your chest and stomach slightly and let your shoulders roll forward.
2. Tense your muscles and slowly open your arms, shoulders, and chest, contracting your back muscles so that your shoulders roll back as shown. Imagine that you're trying to pull something apart. Hold this position for one full second.
3. Release tension for a moment, then tense your muscles and slowly roll your shoulders forward again, this time crossing your right forearm above your left forearm.
4. Release tension for a moment and then repeat the exercise, switching your forearms with each contraction. Keep your forearms parallel to the ground throughout the exercise.
5. Do your number of repetitions. (You don't need to do your number of reps for each arm—if you do 10 reps, do 5 with the right forearm above and 5 with the left forearm above.)

"Once you have mastered the movements you can apply greater tension. Your sets and repetitions will then change to [include varied levels of tension]."

— John Peterson,
   Pushing Yourself to Power

Reps: Light tension—10-12; Moderate tension—8-10; Heavy tension—6-8.

Sets: Light tension—3; Moderate tension—2-3; Heavy tension—2.

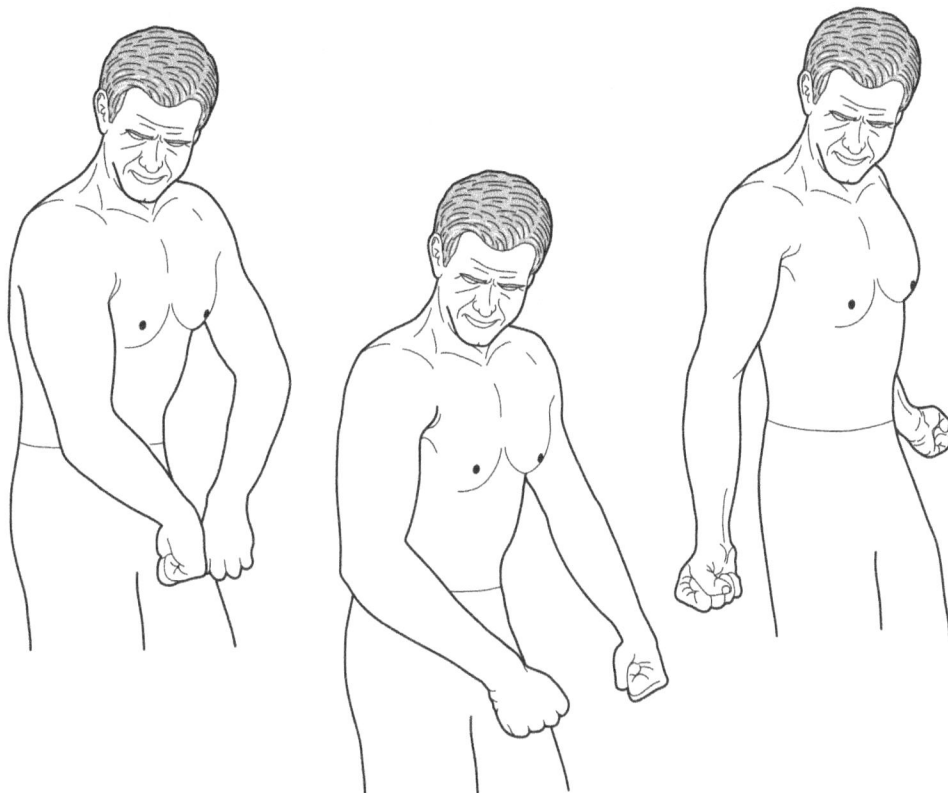

1. Stand with your left foot about one step in front of your right foot. Hold your arms in front of your body, make fists with your hands, and turn your wrists so that the backs of your hands almost touch. Keep your arms low and close to your body. (Ladies, if you need to bend your elbows a little or keep your arms a little farther apart to accommodate your chest, that's fine.)
2. Tense your chest, arms, and shoulders, then slowly rotate your arms until your palms face forward as shown. Flex your back and arm muscles and hold this position for a full second.
3. Release tension for a moment, then tense your muscles and slowly rotate your arms back to the starting position.
4. Release tension for a moment and then repeat the exercise.
5. Do your number of repetitions.

"If you are currently among the large numbers of people who have been injured through exercise, Tiger Moves can go a long way to helping you achieve dynamic, pain-free mobility."

—John Peterson,

The Miracle Seven

Reps: Light tension—10-12; Moderate tension—8-10; Heavy tension—6-8.

Sets: Light tension—3; Moderate tension—2-3; Heavy tension—2.

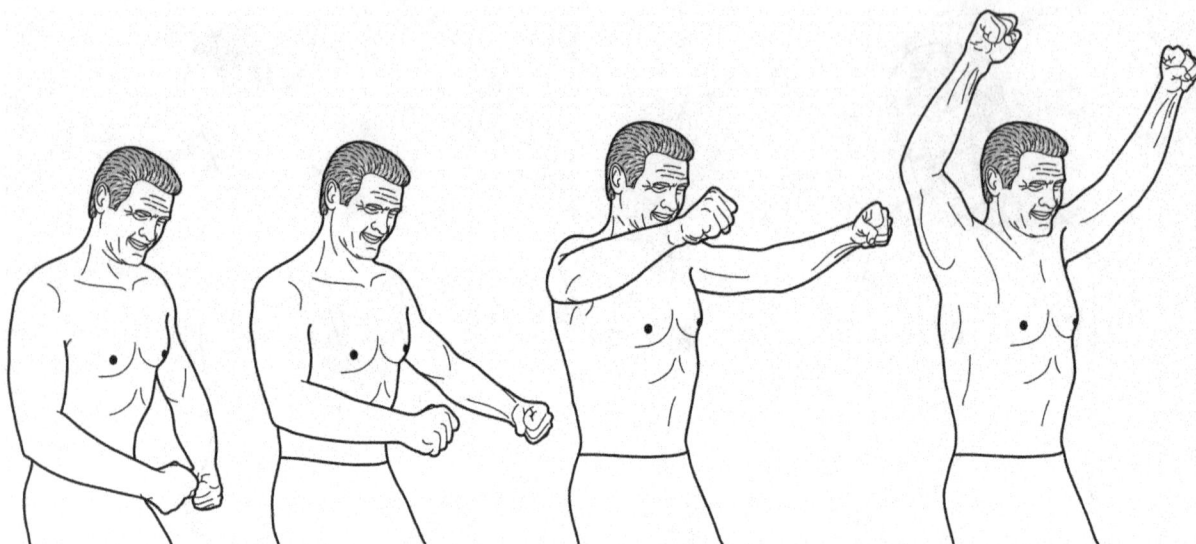

1. Stand with your feet shoulder-width apart. Extend your arms in front of you at about hip level, as shown in the diagram, and make fists with your hands.
2. Tense your muscles and slowly raise your arms upward until they are straight above your head, as shown. Keep your elbows slightly bent throughout the movement so that you're almost closing a circle when you bring your hands up.
3. Release tension for a moment, then tense your muscles and slowly lower your arms to the starting position. Don't drop your arms—maintain tension as you lower them.
4. Release tension for a moment and then repeat the exercise.
5. Do your number of repetitions.

"Many exercise systems can harm the body and hasten the aging process ... The late running guru Dr. George Sheehan wrote that 'if you want to know what you will look like in 20 years, just look in the mirror after having run a marathon.'"

—John Peterson,
Pushing Yourself to Power

Reps: Light tension—10-12; Moderate tension—8-10; Heavy tension—6-8.

Sets: Light tension—3; Moderate tension—2-3; Heavy tension—2.

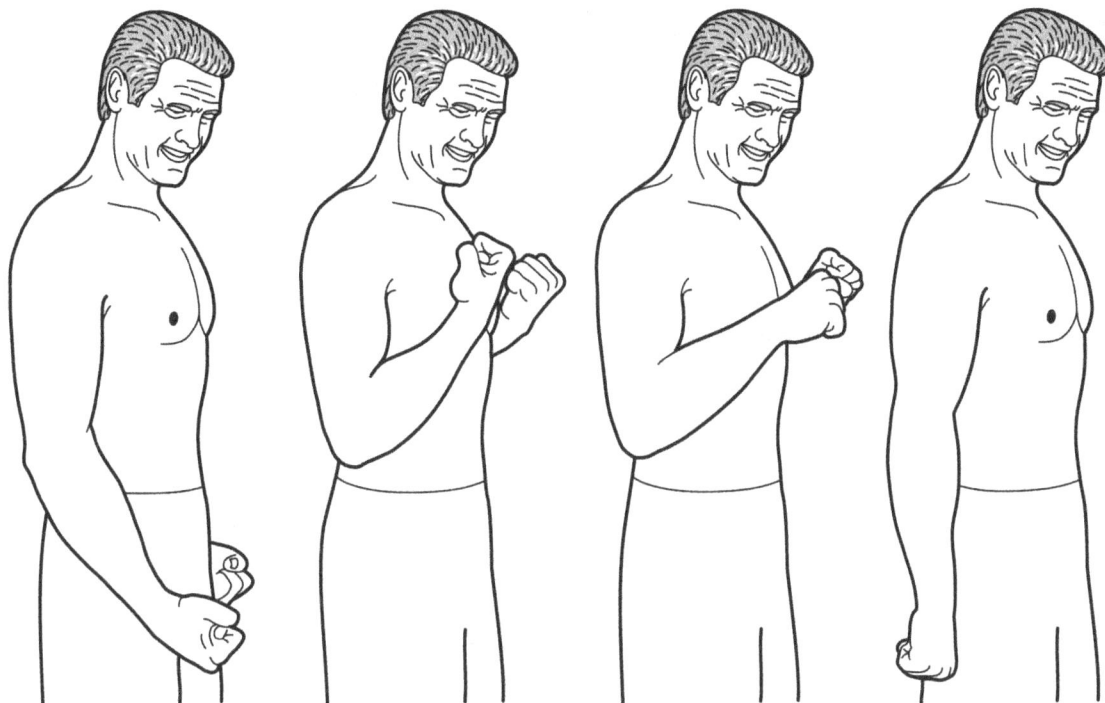

1. Stand with your feet shoulder-width apart. Keep your hands at your sides, make fists with your hands, and turn your hands so that your palms face forward.
2. Tense your muscles and slowly bend your elbows, bringing your hands up toward your shoulders. (Your palms will now face you.) Imagine that you are lifting a heavy weight in your hands as you do so.
3. Release tension for a moment, then tense your muscles and rotate your wrists so that your palms face forward and away from your body. Slowly straighten your elbows until your hands are back at your sides. (Your palms will now face backward.)
4. Release tension for a moment, then rotate your palms forward and repeat the exercise.
5. Do your number of repetitions.

Reps: Light tension—10-12; Moderate tension—8-10; Heavy tension—6-8.

Sets: Light tension—3; Moderate tension—2-3; Heavy tension—2.

Note: Read these instructions fully before you begin the exercise.

In Farmer Burns's version of this exercise, you hold your breath while trying to force the air out. It's very challenging and can leave you quite dizzy. In this version, you're going to let a little air escape, but slowly and with great control, making the "sss" sound as you exhale.

Standing variation:

Stand with your feet shoulder-width apart, shoulders relaxed, and arms hanging at your sides. Make sure you remember to curve your hips forward as you pull in and contract your stomach. Do this exercise near a wall so that you can catch yourself if you get dizzy.

Other variations: Give yourself an extra pump of energy by clenching your fists as you contract. For an extremely strong pump, tighten every muscle in your body as you contract.

1. Lie on your back with your knees bent. Inhale through nose as deeply as you can, letting your belly rise first and then your chest.
2. As you exhale pull your stomach in—try to touch your belly button to your spine. Your pelvis will naturally start to tilt your hipbones to the mat—increase the benefit by tightening your abdominals. You'll create a powerful scooping action with your abdomen (and your back will love it).
3. As you exhale, contract your throat and mouth; your mouth should be slightly open and your teeth lightly closed. Make the "sss" sound until you exhale all the air. Exhale for as long as possible—5 seconds is a good start, but you can gradually increase the time. Try to empty your lungs completely by contracting your abdominal muscles deeper and deeper.
4. Repeat for a total of 12 breaths, taking as long as you need to complete them. Keep your abdomen tight and rigid and your hips curved toward your chest until you have completed 12 breaths.

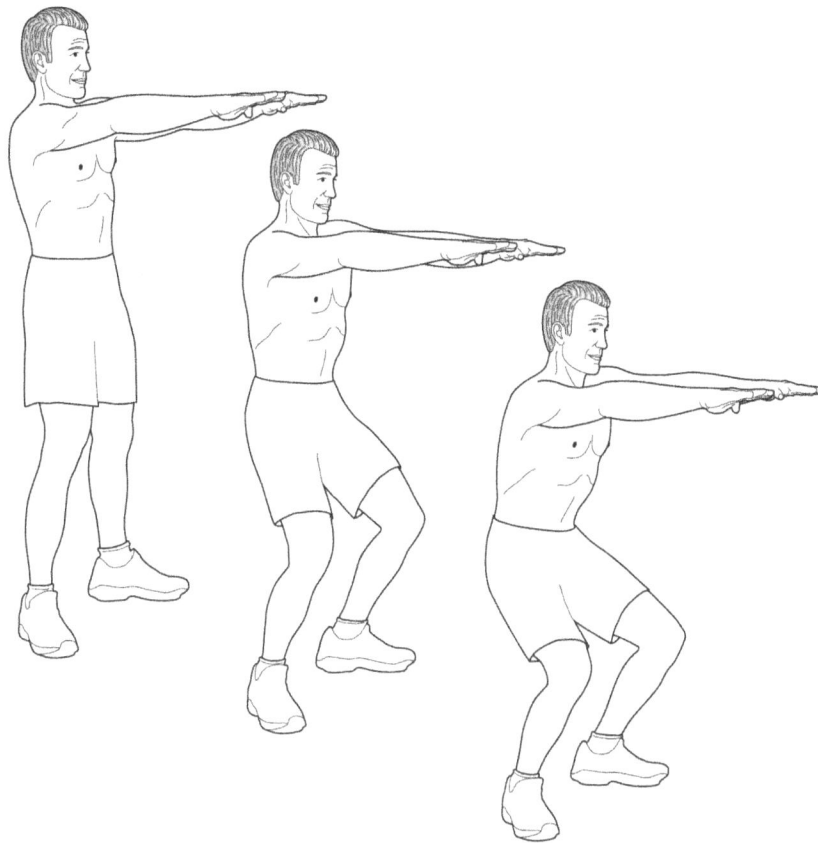

1. Stand with your feet close together and rotate your legs so that your feet are angled slightly outward, as shown in the diagram. Hold your arms in front of you or to the sides for balance.
2. Tense your muscles and slowly bend your knees, lowering yourself as far as you comfortably can, but don't go past 90 degrees. Imagine that you're holding a heavy weight on your shoulders as you bend your knees.
3. Release tension for a moment then tense your muscles and slowly straighten your legs, returning to your starting position.
4. Release tension for a moment and then repeat.
5. Do your number of repetitions.

When you're doing knee bends as an SMR, make sure to apply tension rather than relying solely on your body weight for resistance. In fact, by "thinking into" and contracting the muscles around your knee, you will build up protective muscle around that joint because you're moving carefully and mindfully. You never want to drop your body weight (or any other kind of weight) on your joints without control.

Do you want a bigger challenge? Try doing it one leg at a time.

Reps: Light tension—10-12; Moderate tension—8-10; Heavy tension—6-8.

Sets: Light tension—3; Moderate tension—2-3; Heavy tension—2.

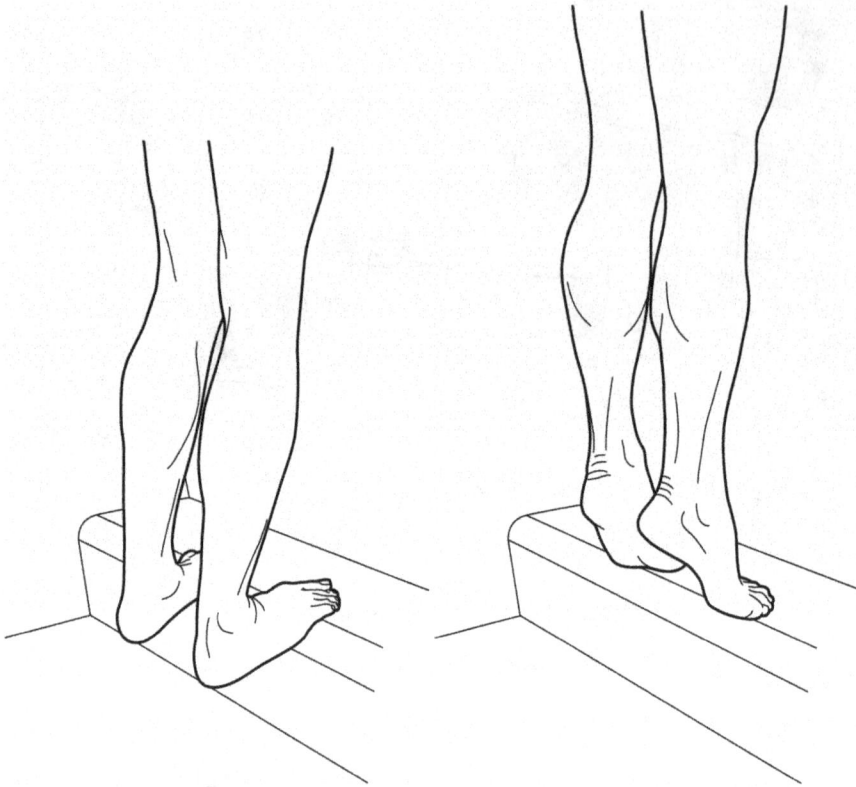

1. Find a stair, a thick block, or a heavy piece of wood that will support your weight and won't slip out from under you. Stand on that object with your toes on it and your heels off. Place your feet about shoulder-width apart, or whatever distance allows you to maintain your balance.
2. Tense your muscles and slowly lower your heels as far as you comfortably can, then slowly raise yourself up onto your toes as high as you can.
3. Release tension for a moment, then slowly lower yourself down as far as you comfortably can.
4. Release tension for a moment and then repeat the exercise.
5. Do your number of repetitions.

"Translate these gentle yet powerful movements to an exercise system and you energize the body and fight the aging process by increasing blood flow through even the smallest capillaries, especially those located in the facial skin."

—John Peterson,
    Pushing Yourself to Power

Reps: Light tension—10-12; Moderate tension—8-10; Heavy tension—6-8.

Sets: Light tension—3; Moderate tension—2-3; Heavy tension—2.

MORE SMRS — THE POSSIBILITIES ARE ENDLESS

There you have it. These 12 exercises can deliver whole-body strength to you without causing you pain or injury. If you love them, you will never need to do any other kind of strength training in your life. And if you really love them, you can do more.

I have done dozens of different SMRs since I started performing them ten years ago. I have made up my own—exercises that fit the way I move in my life that help me strengthen my body to get the results I need.

Any movement can be an SMR if you apply tension during the action. Think about what your body does when you reaching for something on a high shelf or across the table. Turn that into an SMR exercise by doing the motion under tension during your exercise session, performing several reps and sets. Be creative and use your own movements and ranges of motion to develop your personal SMRs.

"Perhaps most significantly, though, strength training causes self-esteem, body image, and confidence to soar—and the value of those changes can't be overstated."

— Metzl
The Exercise Cure

When you become aware of the way your body moves in space, you will figure out what it requires for functional fitness. You will discover what you need to do to make it stronger. Just listen to your body.

CHAPTER 14

CALISTHENICS CIRCUIT FOR AGELESS STRENGTH AND FITNESS

■ ■ ■

Your strength-training choices are endless, and that's great news. As an Ageless Boomer, you're going to be doing strength training for the rest of your life, and it's going to be a long life. If you don't feel like doing the same exercise all the time, you can change up every single workout. What's the bottom line? Keep it interesting and exercise several times a week.

STRENGTH TRAINING:
MORE OPTIONS

"Rod," you might ask, "if SMRs are so great, why do you have another strength training chapter?" Good question. I have three answers.

One, some people find that SMRs take some getting used to. They have a hard time visualizing a non-existent weight and creating the tension of one muscle working against another. If you're one of these people, that's OK. If you keep at it, you will get it, and a mirror will help.

However, that doesn't mean you can skip strength training. If you're in doubt about it, please go back and read the first few pages of Chapter 13. Strength training is critical for your lifelong health and function, especially as you get older, and especially for you ladies. Aerobic exercise alone isn't the answer, as Jordan Metzl, M.D., explains in *The Exercise Cure*:

> Starting 20 years ago … research began pouring in about how strength training could provide different benefits that may be equally—if not more—important than those derived from aerobic training. As it turned out, strength work afforded exercisers many of the same benefits that came from cardio work: heart and lungs got stronger, blood pressure dropped, glucose metabolism improved. At the same time, strength training elicited changes not typically associated with aerobic exercise: more muscle mass; more strength and mobility; denser, stronger bones; better body composition.

The bottom line: If you want to be an Ageless Boomer, you **must** strength-train 3-4 times per week.

Remember, *functional fitness* is your goal. You want to keep your body strong, limber, and vital for whatever daily activities you choose. The exercises in this chapter are all multi-joint motions that train your body for real life.

Two, as you start building up your muscles and strength with SMRs (or if you're already pretty fit when you start this program), you may find that you want to add a level of challenge to your workouts. The exercise circuits in this chapter will give you a host of ways to increase your strength and musculature. They complement and augment your SMR routines. (You can get along with just SMRs for the rest of your life, but adding calisthenics is good, and I do them. It's not necessary, but it's still productive, and it can help you get to the next level.)

Don't be intimidated by the word "challenge." The exercises in these circuits range from easy to difficult, but all of the difficult exercises, from push-ups to pull-ups, have variations that will allow you to start where your body strength is now and progress as far as you're willing to go. Do you think that you can do a full push-up? Maybe not today, but if you follow this program, you will. Do you think that you can do a push-up against a wall? Absolutely you can.

Three, you may want variety. If you become an Ageless Boomer, you'll be doing strength training for decades to come. You don't want to get bored—exercise should be **interesting**! And you don't want your body to get too accustomed to one range of movement. To build strong muscle and joint tissue, you need to continually challenge yourself. You can increase the difficulty of the exercise by slowing down the speed at which you perform the movement, or challenging yourself with the intensity of your sets; you can also try different exercises that work the same muscle from a different angle.

So there you go: I just want you to have options. And keep in mind that you don't have to choose between SMRs and a calisthenics circuit—I mix the two together all the time (and I'll tell you how). The two approaches work together beautifully, and the options are endless!

CIRCUITS GIVE YOU RESULTS QUICKLY

The exercise circuits here are just a small group of different exercises that work your entire body. If you've spent any time in a gym, you've probably run across the idea that you should only strength-train one area of your body on any given day. You may also have been told that you should either strength-train or do cardio. Neither of those things is true, as Metzl explains in *The Exercise Cure*:

> "I don't think programs that divvy up the body like dotted lines on a butcher's pattern—arms one day, chest the next, and so on—are a very good use of your time. These programs require you to do a high volume of exercise for one part of the body in a single day and are designed solely to bulk up the muscles. This is great if you're a body-builder but that's … not what we're going after here."

Metzl (who is both a doctor and an Ironman triathlete) also explains that it's a backward idea to think that cardio and strength training can't go together. In both types of exercise, you're getting your heart beating and your blood pumping, so they naturally support one another.

A whole-body exercise circuit is a great way to achieve overall strength and fitness in a short amount of time. Some circuit workouts have you perform the same exercises over and over again, but the Ageless Boomer circuits are a flexible menu that lets you choose different exercises each time you do them. It's more fun and better for you (although doing the same set of exercises for 4-6 weeks is fine).

The Ageless Boomer circuit workout makes it easy and fun to get a full body workout. To begin, you choose one exercise from each of five categories:

- Push
- Pull
- Hip Extension
- Core
- Cardio

Next, you do one set of each exercise. That's one circuit. Then you do a second circuit: you can use the same exercises as your first circuit or you can choose different exercises, as long as you pick one exercise from each category. You do one set of each exercise, finishing your second circuit. Finally you do a third circuit, either repeating a previous circuit's exercises or choosing new exercises.

Your circuits might look like this on one day:

	Push	Pull	Hip Ext.	Core	Cardio
1	Push Ups	Doorknob Rows	Wall Squats	Flutter Kicks	Jumping Jacks
2	Push Ups	Doorknob Rows	Wall Squats	Flutter Kicks	Jumping Jacks
3	Push Ups	Doorknob Rows	Wall Squats	Flutter Kicks	Jumping Jacks

But on another day, they might look like this:

	Push	Pull	Hip Ext.	Core	Cardio
1	Push Ups	Doorknob Rows	Wall Squats	Flutter Kicks	Jumping Jacks
2	Cross Punches	Pull Ups	Lunges	Leg Outs	Rebounding
3	Chair Dips	Ledge Curls	Side Lunges	Planks	Power Walking

It's like a salad bar—you get to pick out the exercises you want to do and build a full-body workout with them.

"But Rod," you ask, "how many repetitions do I do of each exercise in a set?" It depends on the exercise, and it depends on you. Later in this chapter I'll explain how you figure out the number of reps that are best for you and you alone.

You do need to follow a few rules:

- Choose one exercise from each category for each circuit
- Don't skip any categories
- Do at least three full circuits

Beyond those rules, you can create any circuits you want and go for it.

FUNDAMENTALS
OF HEALTHY CALISTHENICS

If the word "calisthenics" reminds you of the high school gym teacher you couldn't stand, please take a deep breath and let that thought go now. I'm not here to criticize you and blow a loud, annoying whistle, but I am going to coach you through a few basic principles.

As you know from reading my story at the beginning of this book, I've been athletic from the time I could walk. From climbing trees to climbing ropes in gymnastics, I loved to move and test the abilities of my body. Calisthenics—classic, time-tested exercises—were a big partof my experience, and I loved doing them. But that's not true for everybody, and it may not be true for you.

If you hated calisthenics as a kid (and maybe you still hate them), I'm willing to bet it was because you were force-fed a one-size-fits-all program for every kid in the school. It didn't matter whether you could keep up, and if you couldn't, you were probably embarrassed in front of everyone. In the years since, maybe you visited gyms or classes where the trainers and instructors took the same one-size-fits-all approach, and that made you hate calisthenics even more.

That was then, this is now. I'm not going to tell you to drop and give me twenty. I'm telling you to listen to your body, start where you are, and then slowly and steadily build your strength. You are **not** too weak. You are **not** too old. You can do this.

The rest of this section will give you some guidelines for safe and effective exercise.

"Variety is the spice of life. Forget about doing the same sets and exercises day in and day out, maybe hitting the same treadmill every day, like a gerbil trapped in a wheel. And there's no need to change clothes, pack a gym bag, drive, park, find a locker, find an open machine … then, after a long, boring workout, do the whole process in reverse."

— Mark Lauren, former special ops exercise instructor and author, You Are Your Own Gym

PRECAUTIONS: TALK TO YOUR DOCTOR, LISTEN TO YOUR BODY

As always, before you begin any exercise program, talk to your health care professional to make sure it's safe for you. This precaution is especially important if you've had any kind of cardiovascular disease or joint injury/replacement.

Once you've gotten the green light from your doctor, make sure to listen to your body when you're exercising. Warm, working muscles are good; pain is bad. An elevated heart rate is good; a racing heartbeat is bad. Getting a little sweaty is good; getting overheated, flushed, and dizzy is bad. If any of those things happen, stop, drink some water, and reset. Dial down the difficulty. Pay attention to your body's cues to make sure your exercise is healthy and safe.

Every type of exercise requires you to warm up. In general, if you use the Range of Motion exercises in Chapter 11, you will be warm and ready to start a strength-building circuit.

If you would like to warm up a little bit more, you can use SMRs at light tension to work on certain areas. For example, if you're going to do push-ups as your push exercise, you might want to do a set of High Reach SMRs to get your shoulders extra warm and loose. Remember, if you're doing SMRs as a warm up, just use light to moderate tension.

FORM AND POSTURE

Correct form in an exercise is very important—it helps you prevent injury and get the most from your exercise. It can also be really hard to get right when you're working on your own. You don't get the best view of your own body from inside your own head, so you need to use tools to make sure you're doing an exercise correctly.

First, you have to see what proper form looks like, so you need a model, e.g., the pictures in this book or a video online. A push up is a push up is a push up, so it doesn't matter whether you watch me do one, or John Peterson, or Mark Lauren—as long as the person knows what he or she is doing, you can use that person as a model.

Second, you have to be able to watch yourself. The easiest tool for this task is a mirror. Whenever possible, exercise in front of a full-length mirror in snug-fitting or minimal clothing.

Range of Motion Exercises:

Six-way Neck Movement

Neck Circle

Shoulder Roll

Arm Circle

Maximum Amplitude Arm Circle

Y Arm Movement

T Arm Movement

W Arm Movement

L Arm Movement

I Arm Movement

Wrist Rotation

Torso Twist

Torso Rotation

Forward Bend

Hip Rotation

Knee Bend

Knee Rotation

Ankle Rotation

Heel Raise

Some exercises, however, can be hard to do while

looking in a mirror. A push up, for example, requires you to keep your body straight from shoulders to heels, even if you're doing it against a wall. To look in a mirror to check your form, you have to turn your head to the side while you're doing the exercise, which isn't easy when you're engaging your shoulders in the push up. An alternative is to have another person check your form and tell you what to correct. If you don't have someone who can check your form, you can try using a video camera (a lot of us have them on our phones now) to record yourself and then review your form.

Eventually, if you learn how to do the exercise with correct form, you'll be able to feel when your form is incorrect and you'll be able to correct yourself without looking. Thus it's all the more important to learn your form correctly from the beginning.

The same considerations apply to posture. When you have good posture, you reduce your risk of injury, you look younger, and you look thinner. As I noted in the last chapter, good posture means that your spine is elongated so that you're not swaybacked. Tuck in your bottom and tighten your abdomen so that you're lengthening your spine rather than compressing it. Keep your head lifted, your neck long, and your shoulders back.

Q: DO I NEED SPECIAL EQUIPMENT?

A: No. You can do almost all of these exercises without any equipment at all. The rest you can do with household items and furniture.

One exception is a chinning bar. If you're going to do chin-ups and pull-ups, you will need a stable bar that you can attach to your home's structure, usually a doorway. Many chinning bars can be placed in a doorway without causing damage to the structure.

MODIFYING THE DIFFICULTY

Traditional calisthenics like push-ups, pull-ups, and chin-ups can be tremendously difficult, and that scares away many people. They've never had a chance to learn that all these exercises have easier versions that help you build your way up to those full versions.

In some cases, they've had bad information. The "girl" push-up, as many people called it, where you perform a push-up with your knees on the floor instead of your toes, isn't that much easier than a full push-up, and it's not a good way to train yourself for a full push-up. I'm going to teach you a much better way.

IT'S A MATTER OF PHYSICS

The body-weight exercises in this chapter use your weight as a source of resistance so that you can build muscle. In most cases, you're resisting the force of gravity on your body. That's what your weight is, actually—the amount of gravity the earth exerts upon you. (That's why astronauts weigh less on the moon; you could do some fun calisthenics up there, including a one-finger pull-up!)

So if you want to change the amount of weight you're trying to move, you have to use some simple physics.

Take push-ups, for example. When you start doing them, you're going to stand with your palms flat against a wall and your feet an arm's length away from the wall. You will lean your body into the wall, bending your elbows, until your chest touches the wall. Then you will straighten your arms, pushing back to your start position. That's a perfect push-up, but it used a fraction of the force of a full push-up. Why?

Because you changed the angle of your body in relation to gravity. When you stand, your feet are still holding most of your weight. When you do a full push-up on the floor, a huge proportion of your weight has shifted from your feet to your arms. Your legs, instead of holding your weight, are stabilizing you as your arms, shoulders, and chest do most of the work.

"Unless you work at it for a long time, the visible changes you get from aerobic training are fairly subtle: You're a little leaner, a little more toned. But most people who begin regular strength training—and work hard at it—see some pretty substantial improvements in how they look after just a few weeks."

—Metzl,
The Exercise Cure

If you haven't done a push-up since high school, it might take several months or more to go from a wall push-up to a full push-up. And that's fine! You're going to be doing this exercise for the rest of your life. Give yourself time to do it right. Like Laurence Morehouse said, for a beginner, one push-up does more than an advanced person doing 100 push-ups because you're working just as hard. As long as you're working hard enough, it's getting the job done.

As you get stronger and stronger with your push-ups, you will change the angle of your body when you do them. To change the angle, you keep finding lower and lower places for your hands—from wall to counter, from counter to table, from table to chair, from chair to floor. You will slowly and steadily put more of your weight on your upper body.

The same force of gravity applies to pull-ups and chin-ups. You're not going to start doing pull-ups like a Navy SEAL. You're going to start doing them while standing on a chair. You'll pull yourself up, but your legs will do most of the work, pushing your weight. As you get stronger, you'll let your arms take on more weight. When you're finally ready to lift your legs off the chair, you'll start from the top of the pull-up and lower yourself down, working to slow your descent. And when you're finally ready, you can do pull-ups without any support. It will take time, but Supine Pull-ups will help you get there as well.

CHOOSE YOUR OWN CHALLENGE

Not all the exercises in this chapter are as challenging as a pull-up—in fact, most of them aren't. Each exercise is rated from easy to hard with the following system:

Easy ◆

Medium ◆◆

Hard ◆◆◆

Exercises like the push-up, which can go from very easy to very hard, will have a range, like this: ◆ - ◆◆◆. When in doubt, start out easy. If you find yourself breezing through it, try a harder version for your next set.

REPETITIONS

So you know the basics of a circuit now: a Push, a Pull, a Hip Extension, a Core, and a Cardio. One set of one exercise from each category equals a circuit. But how many repetitions equal one set?

Like everything else in this chapter, the number of reps in your sets depends on your current level of fitness. In order to determine how many reps you should do, you need to start off with a test.

SELF-TEST: DETERMINE YOUR MAXIMUM

Choose your exercise. Make sure you read the instructions and know how to perform it properly. Now, perform that exercise with as close to perfect form as possible and repeat. When your form is less than perfect, stop. Write down the number of repetitions you performed (there's a place after each exercise where you can write it down). This number is your maximum. (Don't worry if the number is low right now—it will increase as you get stronger, and you will most certainly get stronger.)

BREAK IT DOWN: DETERMINE YOUR NUMBER OF REPS

Now you decide how hard to push yourself. You can do 25 percent (one-quarter) of your maximum, 50 percent (half) of your maximum, or 75 percent (three-quarters) of your maximum.

What's the right number for you today? Listen to your body and determine it for yourself. If you're in doubt, start with 25 percent. If that feels easy, increase to 30 percent for the next set. If your max number falls in between the numbers in the chart, you can calculate each percentage by multiplying your max by 0.25, 0.5, and 0.75. If your max number is 12, then

12 x 0.25=3,

12 x 0.5=6, and 12 x 0.75=9, so your reps would be 3, 6, and 9.

For timed exercises like the plank, multiply your max time in seconds by 0.25, 0.5, and 0.75.

"Don't ever think, 'I'll wait and see if I have time [to exercise],' or 'I'll try to squeeze it in later.' That'll never happen. Make a date with yourself. Then hold yourself accountable. The great thing is that this set time is whenever works best for your schedule."

—Lauren,
Body by You

For example, if you did 10 Counter Push-ups in your test set, then 25 percent would be 2.5, so you can do 2 to 3 Counter Push-ups in a light set. **Do not** do your maximum again after the test set—pushing yourself to the physical limit on a regular basis will overtax your muscles and your central nervous system.

You can also take a bell curve approach—start with 25 percent on Monday, increase to 50 percent on Tuesday or Wednesday, increase again to 75 percent on Thursday, back down to 50 percent on Friday or Saturday, and 25 percent on Sunday. (You don't have to train every day, but you can if you choose to.) Or you can ramp up steadily during the week, starting at 25 percent on Monday and increasing to 75 percent by Friday or Saturday. Never do two hard days in a row.

The following chart breaks down the different sets based on your percentages. (Don't try to figure out what 2.5 push-ups look like—just choose to do 2 or 3.)

Max	25%	50%	75%	Max	25%	50%	75%
5	1.25	2.5	3.75	40	10	20	30
10	2.5	5	7.5	45	11.25	22.5	33.75
15	3.75	7.5	11.25	50	12.5	25	37.5
20	5	10	15	55	13.75	27.5	41.25
25	6.25	12.5	18.75	60	15	30	45
30	7.5	15	22.5	65	16.25	32.5	48.75
35	8.75	17.5	26.25	And so on …			

SELF-TEST AGAIN BECAUSE YOU'RE GETTING STRONGER

Every few weeks (every week, if you're improving quickly), perform a self-test. You will get stronger when you perform these exercises consistently, so your maximum reps will be moving up weekly to monthly. Keep checking and updating your number as you gain strength.

Circuit training keeps you moving, making the most of your time. You don't need to pause and rest in between sets because you're changing between different muscle groups, so you're not overworking.

If you need to rest to catch your breath, don't sit down. You want "active rest" that keeps you moving and warm between sets. You can walk around, bounce on the rebounder, dynamic stretch, do light-tension SMRs, or simply take deep breaths during recovery. You can certainly take a walk to your water bottle—make sure you stay hydrated!

INDEX OF EXERCISES

Burpee

Calf Raise

Chair Dip

Chair Squat

Chin up

Cross Punch

Doorknob Row

Farmer Burns Stomach Flattener

Flutter Kick

Good Morning

Isometric Curl

Jumping Jacks

Leg Curl

Leg-Out

Leg Raise

Liederman Chest Press

Lunge

Mountain Climber

Pelvic Tilt

Plank

Pull up

Push up

Rocking Horse

Self-Resistance Curl

Side Lunge

Sit Back

Straight Punch

Standing Side Leg Lift

Step-Up

Supine Pull-up

Wall Squat

| "MENU" OF EXERCISES

Push	Pull	Hip Ext.	Core	Cardio
Push up	Pull up	Chair Squat	Good Morning	Burpee
Cross Punch	Chin up	Lunge	Flutter Kick	Jumping Jacks
Straight Punch	Doorknob Row	Standing Side Leg Lift	Farmer Burns Stomach Flattener	Mountain Climber
Liederman Chest Press	Isometric Curl	Leg Curl	Leg-Out	Rebounding
Chair Dip	Self-Resistance Curl	Wall Squat	Rocking Horse	Walking
	Supine Pull-up	Step-Up	Leg Raise	Stair
		Side Lunge	Pelvic Tilt	
		Calf Raise	Plank	
			Sit Back	

1 Push

1 Pull

1 Hip Extension

1 Core

+ 1 Cardio

1 Circuit

| PUSH EXERCISES

Push exercises are exactly what they sound like—movements that require you to push against some resistance. The resistance comes from gravity (as in the push-up), or from yourself (as in the Liederman Chest Press).

These Push exercises emphasize the chest, shoulders, and arms, but they also work your core, and in some cases also work your legs. You will feel significant effort in your trapezius muscles (the muscles between your neck and shoulders), deltoids (shoulder) muscles, triceps (the back of your upper arms), and pectorals (the muscles of the chest).

This section includes the following Push exercises:

- Push-up
- Cross Punch
- Straight Punch
- Liederman Chest Press
- Chair Dip

The push-up is the king of all exercises. It has been celebrated by people from Charles Atlas to Herschel Walker. In his book *Death, Taxes, and Push-ups*, Ted Skup, a fellow Boomer, describes doing 1,000 push-ups a day as his only exercise. I don't recommend that approach for most people, but it's a good demonstration of their effectiveness.

Push-ups work every part of your body—chest, shoulders, arms, core, even legs. You have to use all your major muscle groups to stabilize yourself and keep everything tight while you raise and lower yourself. They're absolutely amazing.

"No other exercise …works the upper body musculature as synergistically including chest, shoulders, arms, upper/lower back, and abs as well as the push-up."

— *John Peterson and Rod Fisher,*
Ultimate Push-ups for the Awesome Physique

And yes, a full push-up can be really hard. Unless you're an athlete, a fitness enthusiast, or been in the military, you probably never developed enough upper body strength to do a full push-up. That's why I'm describing a range of push-ups to build your strength.

"Development of the chest was the first priority of both Earle Liederman and Charles Atlas. The reason is simple: It's not possible to develop your chest without simultaneously developing your arms, shoulders, and upper back."

— *John Peterson, fitness expert and author,*
Pushing Yourself to Power

Laurence Morehouse explained this transition in *Total Fitness in 30 Minutes a Week*: Start by pushing away from the wall, then move to a counter, sink or chest of drawers. "From the counter or sink or chest of drawers, move next to a table … From the table, move to a chair or bench. From the chair or bench, move to the floor."

WALL PUSH-UP

To quote Morehouse, "Stand a little beyond arm's reach from a wall. Put your hands against the wall at the height of your shoulders. Lean forward until your chest comes near the wall. Then push away until you're back in the starting position. If that's too hard, step in closer." Keep your body straight and solid from your head to your heels, just as you would for a push-up on the floor. To make the exercise a little harder, move your feet back from the wall a little. The farther back you go, the more challenging it will get.

Max Reps: _____

25% _____   50% _____   75% _____

COUNTER PUSH-UP

Put your hands against a counter, sink, dresser, or any other stable object that "lowers the height of your hands below the height of your shoulders," as Morehouse says. Lean forward on your hands, elbows out, until your chest lightly brushes the object. Then push back to the starting position.

Max Reps: _____

25% _____   50% _____   75% _____

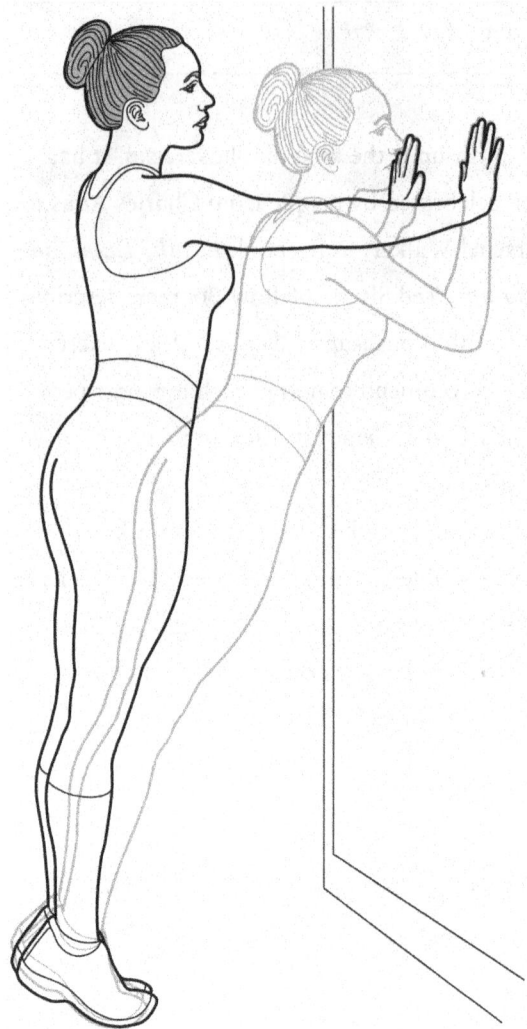

"Throughout the entire movement, your body should be in a straight line. From your heels to your neck, nothing should be bent. Be especially certain not to let your pelvis drop toward the ground, or let your butt stick up in the air at all. Weak form means a weak core. Keep your midsection tight!"

—Lauren,

You Are Your Own Gym

TABLE PUSH-UP

Find a table that is about waist-height. At this stage, your body will lean at about 45 degrees. Place your hands on the edge of the table and lower your body until your chest lightly brushes the table, then push back up.

Max Reps: _____

25% _____   50% _____   75% _____

CHAIR PUSH-UP

You're really starting to work hard now! Put your hands on two stable chairs, a bench, even a sturdy coffee table. It should be about knee-height. Lower yourself down until your chest lightly brushes the surface, then push yourself back up.

Max Reps: _____

25% _____   50% _____   75% _____

"Keep your butt tucked under, with your buttocks/glutes contracted tightly, your thighs together contracted hard, and your abdominals tight. This will make your push-ups look crisp and keep your body in a straight line from your shoulders to your heels, while it protects your lower back from sagging and hurting."

— Peterson and Fisher,
   Ultimate Push-ups for the Awesome Physique

NEGATIVE PUSH-UP (ALMOST THERE!)

You might need one more stepping stone to get yourself to a full push-up. If that's the case, try negative push-ups first. "Negative" means the less-strenuous part of the exercise; in the case of push-ups, that's the part where you lower yourself down.

Place your hands on the floor, straighten out your legs and body, and put the rest of your weight on your flexed toes. (You can work on holding this position—it's a version of the plank—to build up your strength.) The slower you go, the greater the effectiveness.

Slowly bend your elbows and lower yourself down to the floor. Return to the starting position by kneeling and repeat.

Max Reps: _____

25% _____   50% _____   75% _____

FULL PUSH-UP

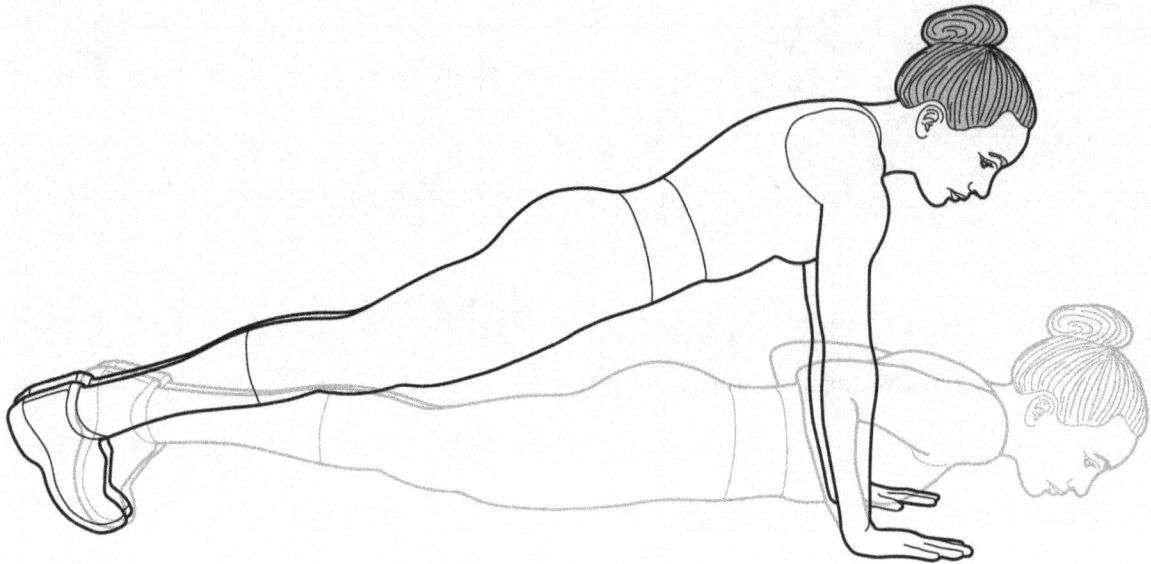

1. Get on the floor in a plank position with your arms straight, hands directly under your shoulders, and your body in one straight line from your shoulders to your heels. Rest your weight on the palms of your hands and the balls of your feet.
2. Bend your arms and lower your body toward the floor until your chest lightly brushes the floor.

3. Push upward, engaging your arms, chest, and back, until your arms are straight (but your elbows are not locked). Tighten your abdominals and legs to keep your body straight. Repeat the exercise.

Do your number of repetitions.

Max Reps: _____ 25% _____ 50% _____ 75% _____

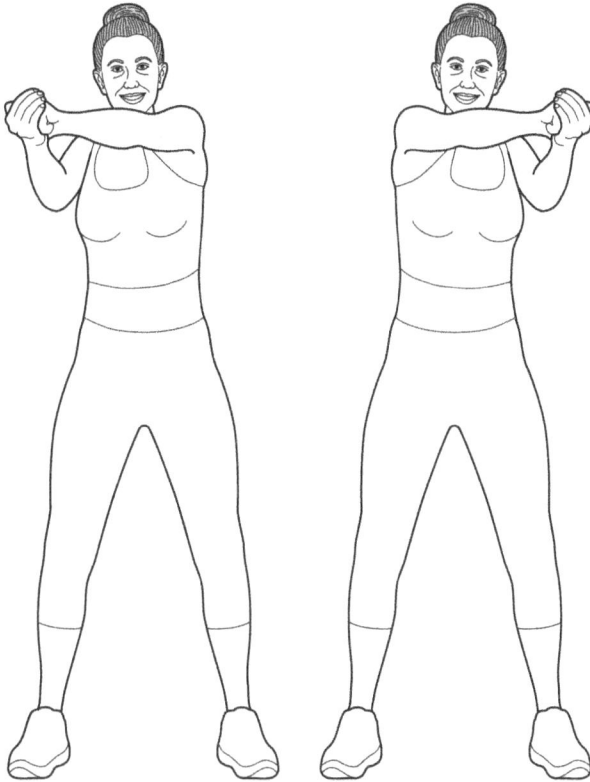

I recommend Monday, Wednesday, Friday, or Tuesday, Thursday, Saturday, etc.

1. Stand with your feet shoulder-width apart. Bend your elbow and pull your right hand up a little higher than your waist. Make a fist as if you were about to punch someone. Place your left hand over your right fist.
2. Tense your left arm and press against your right fist as if you were trying to stop your punch. At the same time, press your right fist forward, down, and across your body. Press forward until your right arm is fully extended; your right fist should be slightly below or even with your left hip (see illustration, above).

3. Slowly reverse the movement, making sure you maintain resistance by pushing your hands against one another, and repeat.

Do your number of repetitions with your right arm, then do the same number with your left arm.

Max Reps: _____ 25% _____ 50% _____ 75% _____

1. Stand with your feet shoulder-width apart. Bend your elbow and pull your right hand up just above your waist. Make a fist as if you were about to punch someone. Place your left hand over your right fist.
2. Tense your left arm and press against your right fist as if you were trying to stop your punch. At the same time, press your right fist forward until your right arm is fully extended. Continue resisting with your left hand; the farther forward the right arm goes the harder it will be to resist, but continue applying as much resistance as you can.
3. Slowly reverse the movement, making sure you maintain resistance by pushing your hands against one another, and repeat.

Do your number of repetitions with your right arm, then do the same number with your left arm.

Variation: You can vary the angle of this exercise; instead of going straight out, go up at a 45-degree angle, or do it as an overhead press straight up toward the ceiling.

"These exercises are just as beneficial for women as they are for men. In both cases the body starts to take on the lithe, highly defined, beautifully sculpted contours of a well-trained gymnast or martial artist. Following these exercises you can literally develop your body to its peak of natural perfection without ever worrying about becoming massively overdeveloped."

—John Peterson and Wendy Pett,
The Miracle Seven

Max Reps: _____ 25% _____ 50% _____ 75% _____

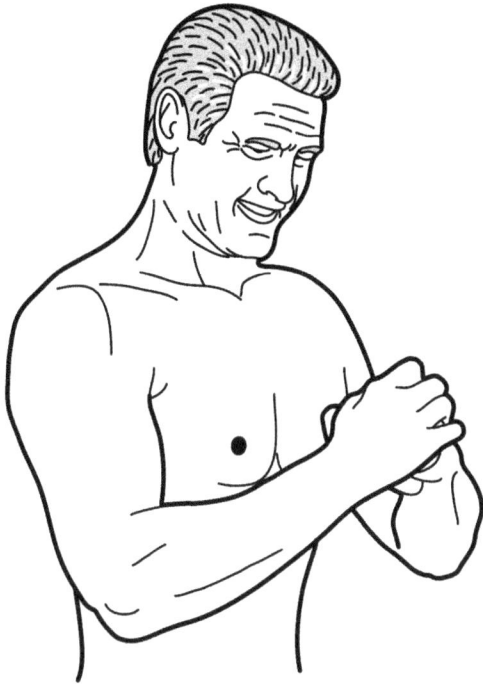

"The harder you resist in this exercise, the more benefit you will get out of it. This exercise will outline your pectoral muscles better than any other movement, as it hits them direct."

— Earle Liederman,
early 20th century strongman and fitness teacher

This exercise is great to do on the rebounder because it engages your upper body along with your legs. You can also do it anywhere, for example while you're standing in line.

1. Stand with your feet shoulder-width apart. Clasp your hands together, or put one fist into the opposite palm, bend your elbows, and hold your hands close to your chest with your elbows sticking out to the sides.

2. Push your hands against each other, creating resistance. Push a little harder with your right hand, moving your hands to the left. Keep your hands level with your chest as you move.

3. Go as far to the left as you can, then switch and push a little harder with your left hand, moving your hands to the right.

Repeat for your number of repetitions on each side.

Max Reps: _____ 25% _____ 50% _____ 75% _____

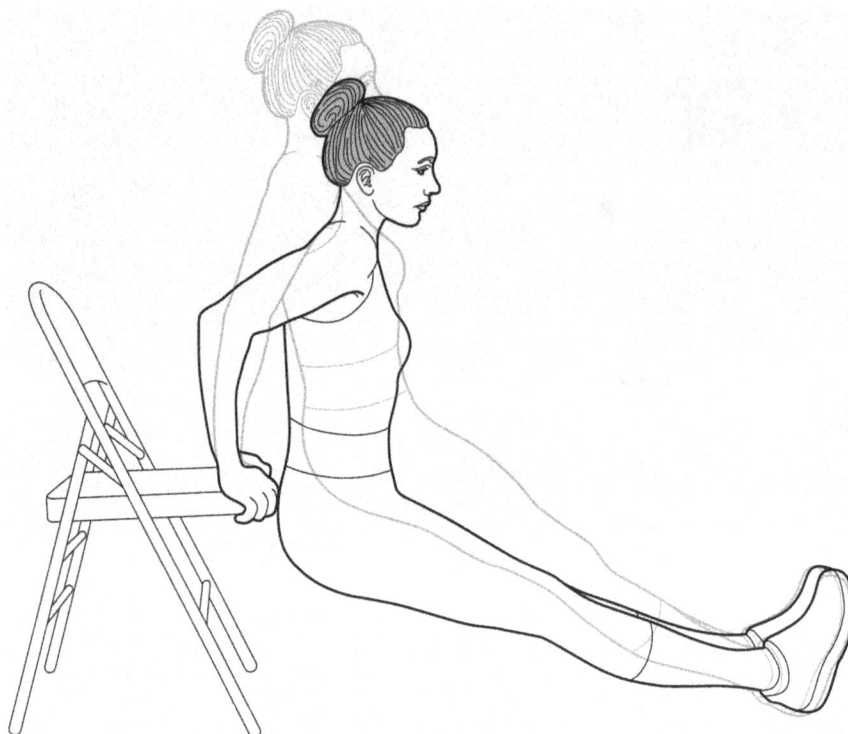

1. Find a stable chair or bench. Sit near the edge of the seat with your feet on the floor and your legs straight. Place your hands on the front edge of the seat with your palms down and your fingers curled around the edge for stability. You can have your knuckles face forward or to the side, whatever works best for you.
2. Slide your bottom forward and off the edge of the chair. Your arms are supporting some of your body weight. Keep the rest of your weight on your heels—don't lean forward onto your toes.
3. Bend your elbows and lower your body down as far as you can go. Work toward lowering yourself until your elbows bend to a 90-degree angle.
4. Push down and straighten your elbows. Keep your body in a straight line as you push to the top. Repeat.

Do your number of repetitions.

Think of this exercise like a reversed push-up—you keep your body straight and stable while your arms do the work. If you need to modify it to make it easier, you can bend your legs. The straighter your legs are, the harder it is. If your legs are bent, they're helping.

Max Reps: _____ 25% _____ 50% _____ 75% _____

254

| PULL EXERCISES

Pull exercises require you to pull something toward you against resistance. In the case of pull-ups, chin-ups, and others, that resistance is gravity; in the case of self-resistance curls, it's your own strength (you probably guessed that from the name).

Pull exercises complement Push exercises because they work all the muscle groups that Push exercises don't. You will feel significant effort in your latissimus dorsi muscles (the muscles of your back), biceps (the upper part of your upper arms), and forearms.

"All pulling movements work your entire back — lats, spinal erectors, rhomboids — as well as your biceps, forearms, rear deltoids, and core."

— Mark Lauren,
  Body by You

This section includes the following Pull exercises:

- Pull-up
- Chin-up
- Doorknob Row
- Isometric Curls
- Self-Resistance Curls
- Supine Pull-ups

"For some people, a major obstacle to working out alone is the lack of confidence to correctly and effectively strength train without an 'expert' telling them how to. In my experience … many gym trainers just throw random workouts together based on the handful of exercises they know and prefer."

— Lauren,
  Body by You

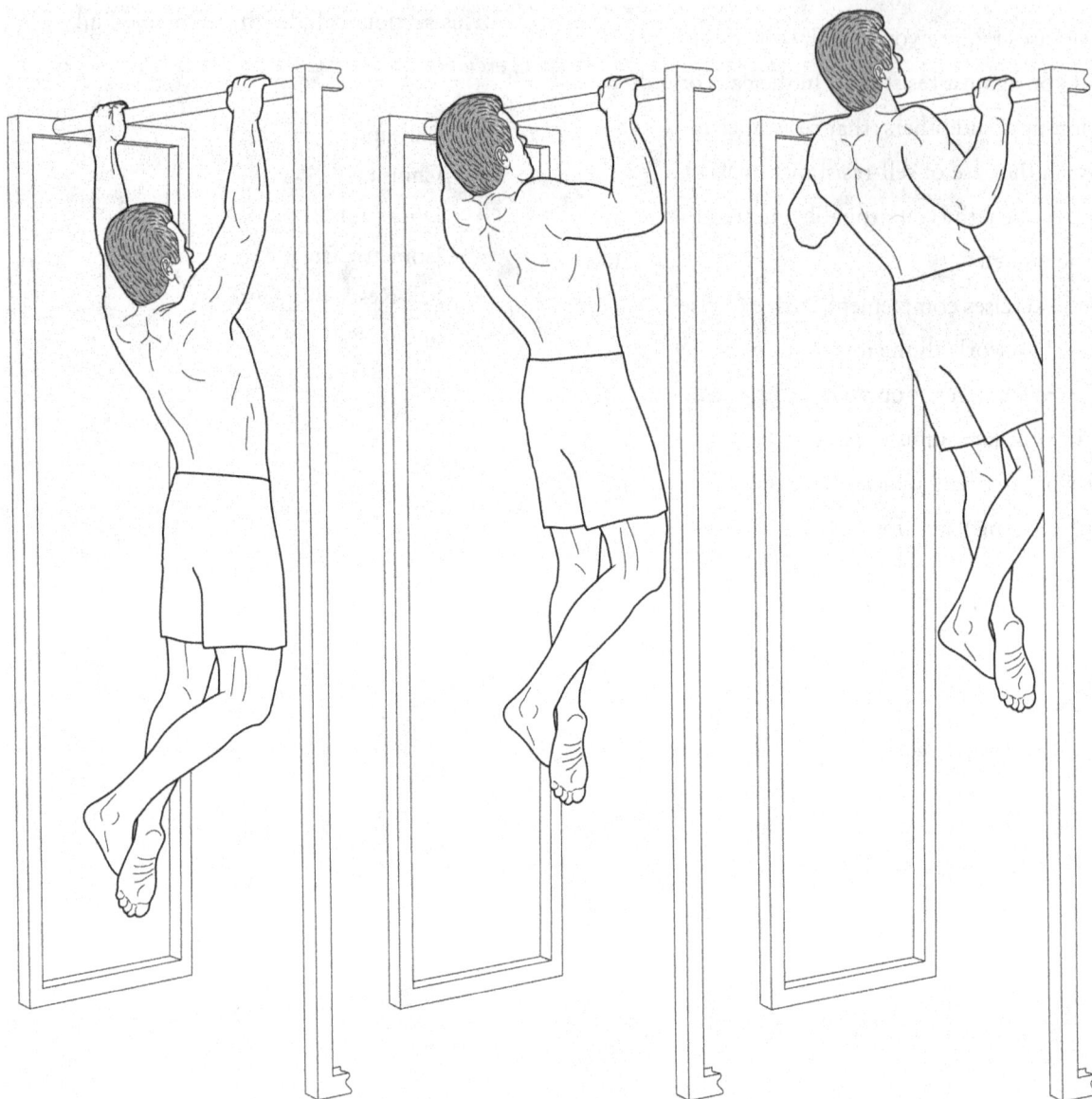

Full pull-ups are very difficult, but they are wonderful for strengthening your arms, back, chest, shoulders, and abs. It works every muscle from the waist up. To adjust the difficulty of your pull-up, use your legs. Place a stable chair or stool under your chinning bar. When you stand on the chair with your legs straight, your chin should be just above the bar.

1. Stand under your chinning bar, either on a stool or on the ground. Extend your arms out to your sides, then bend your elbows 90 degrees and point your forearms directly to the sky, like a football goalpost. Your hands should be slightly more than shoulder-width apart. Make sure your palms are facing **away** from you when you do pull-ups.

2. If you're on a chair or stool, your hands should already be nearly at the level of the bar, so grab hold. Bend your knees until your arms are straight. If you're on the ground, keep your hands the same distance apart as they are in the goalpost position, then reach up and grab the bar. Your hands should face **away** from you.

3. Pull your body up until your chin clears the bar. If you're using your legs, press up slowly, allowing your arms to take as much weight as they're ready to hold. Pull your elbows in close to your body as you approach the top. Pause at the top.

4. **Slowly** lower your body back down to your starting position. Do not simply drop your body—you could hurt your elbow and shoulder joints by suddenly putting that much stress on them. Always use control—you pick the speed, not gravity.

Do your number of repetitions.

"I have personally practiced various types of chins and dips and know from experience that they are great exercises for teaching your muscles to work together in groups, thus maximizing athletic fitness."

— Peterson,
   Pushing Yourself to Power

Max Reps: _____ 25% _____ 50% _____ 75% _____

Except for your grip, a chin-up is identical to a pull-up. The difference is that with a chin-up, your palms face toward you instead of away.

1. Stand under your chinning bar, either on a stool or on the ground. Extend your arms out to your sides, then bend your elbows 90 degrees and point your forearms directly to the sky, like a football goalpost. Your hands should be slightly more than shoulder-width apart. Make sure your palms are facing **toward** you when you do chin-ups.

2. If you're on a chair or stool, your hands should already be nearly at the level of the bar, so grab hold. Bend your knees until your arms are straight. If you're on the ground, keep your hands the same distance apart as they are in the goalpost position, then reach up and grab the bar. Your hands should be slightly more than shoulder-width apart. Your hands should face **toward** you.

3. Pull your body up until your chin clears the bar. If you're using your legs, press up slowly, allowing your arms to take as much weight as they're ready to hold. Pull your elbows in close to your body as you approach the top. Pause at the top with your chin over the bar.

4. Slowly lower your body back down to your starting position. Do not simply drop your body—you could hurt your joints by suddenly putting that much stress on them. Let your elbows be almost straight but not completely straight (applies to pull ups too). Maintain the tension and don't stress the joint.

Do your number of repetitions.

"Strength training has also been shown to be effective in easing depression, possibly because it enhances self-efficacy — or the feeling of having control over your environment."

—Metzl,
The Exercise Cure

Max Reps: _____ 25% _____ 50% _____ 75% _____

"First, added strength will allow you to perform better in life—a life that requires you to stand, lunge, bend, twist, and lift on a daily basis.

"Second, you will be strengthening not only your muscles, but also your bones. Dropping all animal protein from your diet in conjunction with strength training is a must for preventing osteoporosis.

"Isotonic exercise is any exercise where actual movement is required. Calisthenics, gymnastics, weightlifting, swimming and running are all examples of isotonic exercises."

— Peterson,
    Pushing Yourself to Power

"Third, as we age, our muscles atrophy at an accelerated rate in a process called sarcopenia. This weakening can be prevented and even reversed with consistent strength training.

"Finally, by consuming a calorie-light and nutrient-heavy plant-powered diet, complemented with a strength training program, you will give your body a beautiful one-two combination punch that will maximize weight loss in the healthiest and most effective manner."

—Rip Esselstyn, firefighter and triathlete, The Engine 2 Diet

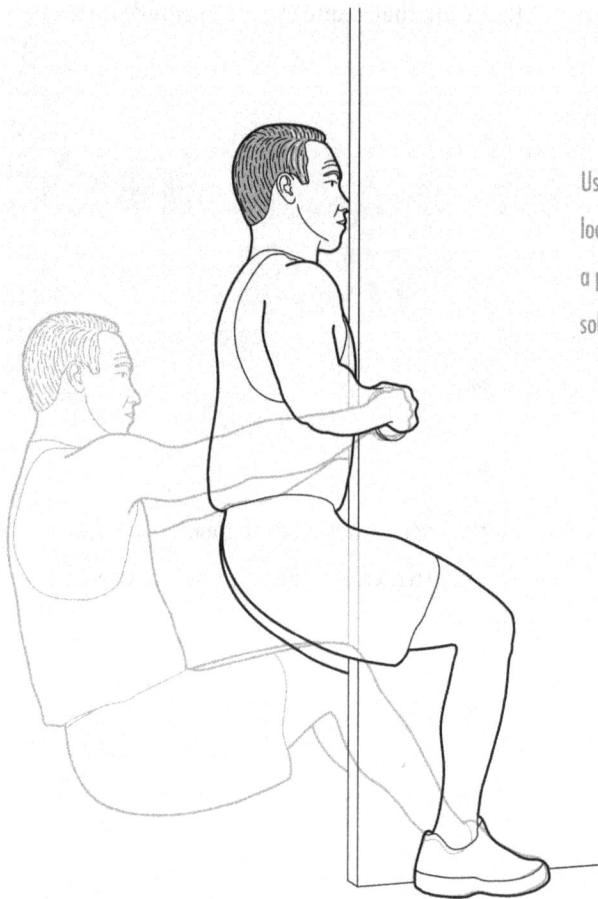

Use a small towel to make it easier to grip. If you're using a doorknob, loop the towel around each knob and then hold the ends. If you're using a post, wrap the towel around it once and hold the ends. It's a great solution if you have sweaty palms!

This exercise is a great way to work on your lats as well as your biceps. I used to do these when I was waiting for the bus as a teenager—instead of a doorknob, I'd wrap my hands around a lamppost. You can use a doorknob (make sure it's a strong door and doorknob!), or you can use a pole or post. Any vertical support that will support your weight as you lean back is fine.

1. Stand with your feet next to but not straddling the door. Make sure your feet won't slip—wear athletic shoes if necessary. Hold onto the knobs (or your towel—see sidebar). Bend your knees so that the door or post is between them.

2. Straighten your arms and lean back, keeping your back straight. Bend your knees until your thighs and your back make an L-shape. (You are going to maintain this L-shape through the whole exercise.)

3. Now comes the work. Pull yourself up toward the door or post by bending your arms and flexing the muscles in your back, but don't move anything else. Keep your back straight, making that L-shape with your thighs, and keep your toes down. Pull up until your chest lightly touches the door or post.

4. Go slowly back, letting yourself return to the position in step 2. Repeat the exercise.

Do your number of repetitions.

If you want to increase your level of difficulty, move your feet in so that your heels are right underneath the doorknobs. As you move your feet farther away from your hands, the exercise will get harder.

Max Reps: _____ 25% _____ 50% _____
75% _____

ISOMETRIC CURL ◆

Find a waist-high horizontal surface, like a shelf, railing, counter, or ledge, that's very heavy or very firmly affixed to your home's structure. You're going to put all your strength into lifting it upward, so make sure that it isn't going to move.

1. Stand in front of your ledge with your feet shoulder-width apart. Place your hands underneath the ledge, palms up; if you're using a railing, you can grip it with your palms up. Start with slightly bent arms.
2. Tense your arms and pull up as hard as you can against the immovable object. This is an isometric curl. If you don't have access to a ledge or rail, use your left hand over your right palm and push down with your left as you resist with your right, then reverse with your left arm. Exhale on the exertion.

3. Hold for 7-12 seconds, then slowly release the tension as you inhale. Your resistance will increase as you get stronger.

Do your number of repetitions.

Variation: Try this exercise with your elbows bent at different angles. Pick out three different angles—for example, elbows straight, elbows at 90 degrees, and elbows midway between 90 degrees and fully bent.

Max Reps: _____ 25% _____ 50% _____ 75% _____

261

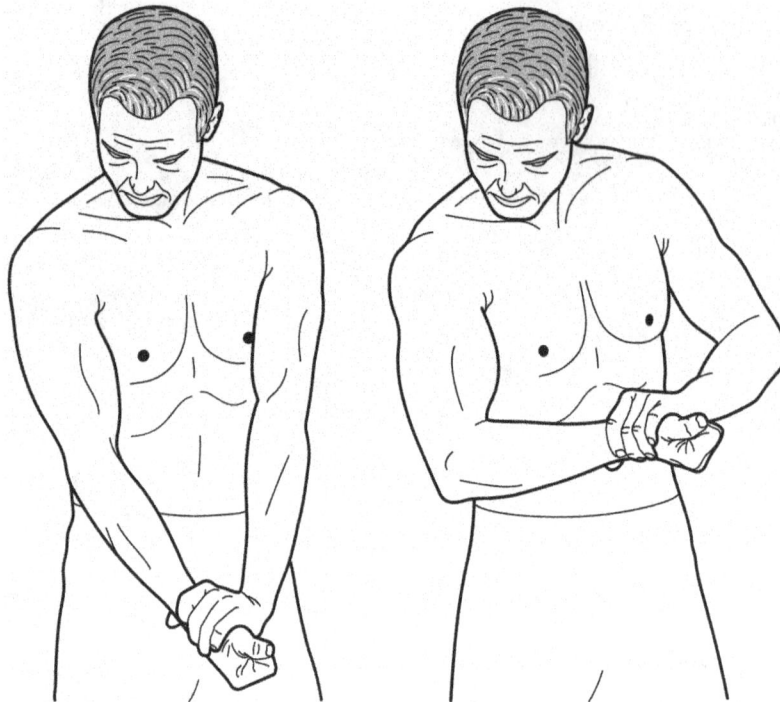

1. Stand with your feet shoulder-width apart. With your right arm at your sides, make a fist with your right hand, palm facing up, as shown above. Keep your right elbow close to your side. Place your left hand on your right hand or right wrist.
2. Press down with your left hand at the same time you start pulling your right hand up toward your shoulder.
3. Bring your right hand as close to your right shoulder as possible, then slowly reverse the movement. Repeat.

Do your number of repetitions with your right arm, then do the same number with your left arm.

Variation: You can do this curl with your palm facing down or in the neutral position with your thumb facing the ceiling (a thumb-up curl).

"I say it often: Strength controls pain. Exercise improves osteoarthritis symptoms by helping you lose weight so that the pressure on your joints is reduced, and by strengthening the muscles around the joints—so your bone surfaces absorb less pressure."

— Metzl,
The Exercise Cure

Max Reps: _____ 25% _____ 50% _____ 75% _____

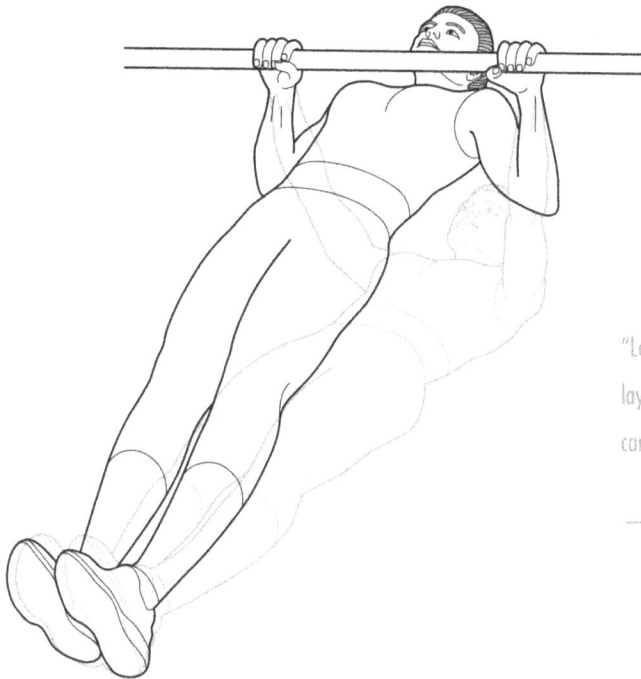

"Look around your home and be creative. I first started doing these by laying a sturdy broom across the tops of two tall stereo speakers. You can also use a mop or any pole that won't break."

—Lauren,

  You Are Your Own Gym

Before you begin, make yourself a pull-up bar that you can use while lying on the floor. You can place a broom handle across two chairs, two stools, or two tables of the same height. Ideally, the broom handle or pole will be just out of your arms' reach when you lie on your back underneath it. Make sure that this arrangement is stable enough to hold your weight. If the broom/pole slides around at all, place a towel under each end to keep it in position.

1. Lie on your back under your pull-up bar; position your chest directly under the bar. Grab the bar with your hands directly above your shoulders; make sure your palms face your feet.

2. Bend your arms and pull yourself up toward the bar; keep your body rigid from your shoulders to your ankles like you are doing an upside-down push up. Squeeze your shoulder blades together and keep pulling up until your chest touches the bar.
3. Slowly lower your body back to the floor—don't let your body drop quickly. Use the last part of the exercise to slowly stretch out your back and arms.

Do your number of repetitions.

Variations: You can reverse your grip with palms facing your head, or you can do them with a strap so you're your palms face each other.

Max Reps: _____ 25% _____ 50% _____ 75% _____

| HIP EXTENSION EXERCISES

Don't be fooled by the name of this category: hip extension exercises work every part your body from the waist down. That includes your glutes (your buttocks and hip flexors), your quads (the four muscle groups on the front of your thigh), your hamstrings (the long muscles on the back of your legs), the muscles of your calves, and the muscles of your ankles and feet.

Your legs have some of the hardest working muscles in your body—at least, I hope they do! If not, get up out of your chair. Sitting may feel relaxing, but it can be tough on your hips to keep them compressed in the same position for hours on end. These functional hip extension exercises can give you more strength, balance, and flexibility in your all-important legs.

Just so you know, one of the best hip extension exercises is probably already in your house: stairs. Climbing stairs works every muscle in your lower body, but especially your legs. And it's terrific cardio.

This section includes the following Hip Extension exercises:

- Chair Squat
- Lunge
- Standing Side Leg-Lift
- Leg Curl
- Wall Squat
- Step-Up
- Side Lunge
- Calf Raise

"Using machines makes you good at, well, using machines. Not much else.

"Our training must reflect the demands of the real world to be most effective. Bodyweight exercises teach us to function naturally, as a cohesive whole, as we do in everyday life.

"Don't waste your time becoming proficient at using fitness machines. Instead, become proficient at using the one thing that you are never without: your body."

—Lauren,
   Body by You

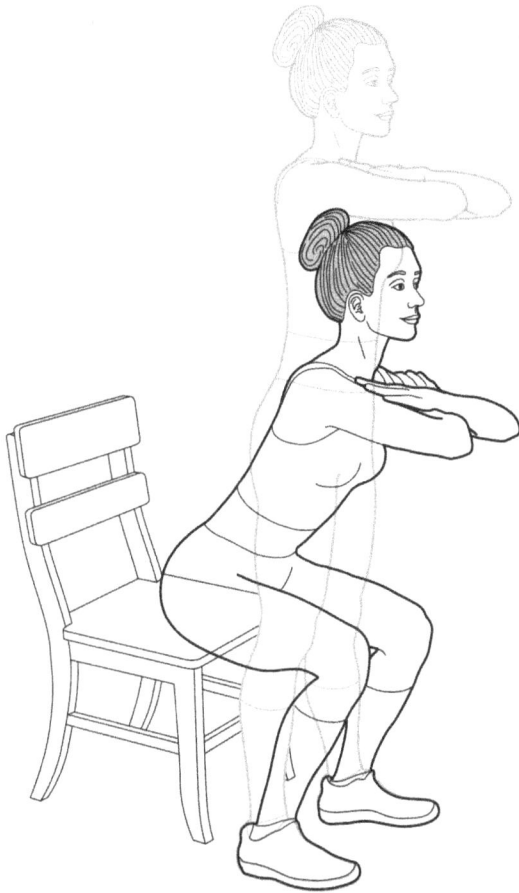

"The best way to prevent hip trouble, or to reduce minor hip pain? Get your butt moving — literally. The muscles of your buttocks play an enormous role in stabilizing and properly mobilizing your hip joint, as do the all-important core muscles. Fire them up and say good-bye to hip pain."

— Metzl,
The Exercise Cure

This exercise is very simple but very effective. When you begin, you can keep your feet close to the chair and allow your bottom to lightly touch the seat; to increase the difficulty, move your feet farther from the chair so that the back of your rear end touches the seat.

1. Stand in front of a chair with your feet shoulder-width apart.
2. Lower your bottom toward the chair as if you were going to sit down. Keep going until your bottom barely touches the seat.
3. Slowly straighten yourself back up to standing. Keep your weight over your heels, not your toes, for the whole movement.

Do your number of repetitions.

Max Reps: _____ 25% _____ 50% _____ 75% _____

Lunges are a classic, time-tested exercise, but you must take care of your knees when you perform them. **Make sure your front knee does not extend beyond your toes when you lower yourself down.** Most people should not let the knees bend more than 90 degrees.

If you need a little extra help with balance, perform these next to a wall or railing.

1. Stand with your feet close together, a little closer than shoulder-width apart. Put your hands on your hips or out to the side for balance.
2. Take a long step forward (about the length of your thigh), and bend your front knee as you move your weight onto your front leg. Keep your back foot in place and bend your back knee. Bend as far as you comfortably can—if both knees bend to 90 degrees, great; if not, stop before it hurts.
3. Push yourself back to standing by straightening your front leg. Keep your back and head straight throughout the movement.

Do your number of repetitions on each leg. You can switch from one leg to the other with each lunge or you can do one set for one leg, then one for the other leg.

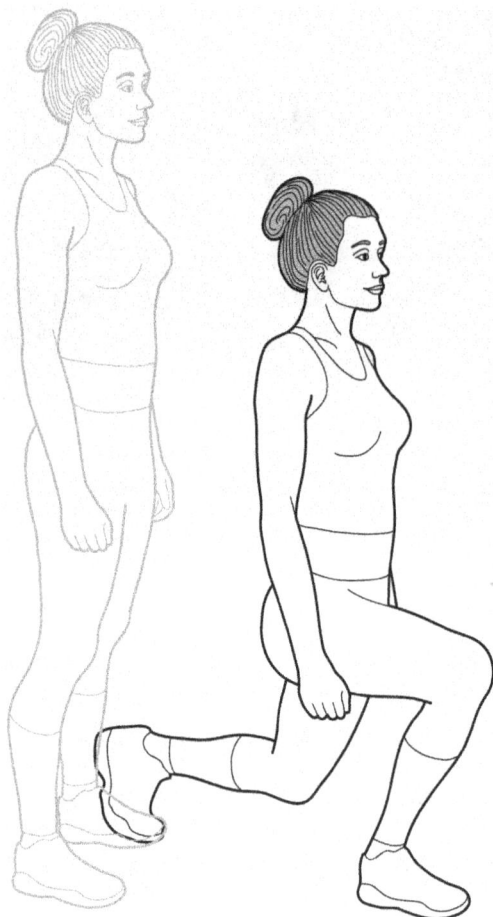

You can also start with your working leg forward. Instead of stepping forward and back each time, just keep one leg forward and bend your knees. Remember not to let your front knee go beyond your toes.

Max Reps: _____ 25% _____ 50% _____

75% _____

1. Stand with your feet hip-width apart; place your right hand on a wall, table, or desk for balance.
2. Shift your weight to your right foot and slowly lift your left leg out to the side. Keep your leg straight but don't lock your knees. Keep your foot flexed with your knee and toes pointed forward.
3. Raise your leg as far as you comfortably can; if you can get a 45-degree angle between your two legs, that's great. Hold your leg there for two seconds.
4. Slowly lower your leg back down.

Do your number of repetitions with the left leg, then the right.

Don't pop your hip up or stick your butt out: if your hip starts to lift up when you're raising your leg, stop. That's the highest you can go with good form.

Max Reps: _____ 25% _____ 50% _____ 75% _____

LEG CURL ◆ ◆

You can do these leg curls SMR-style for a greater challenge. Just perform the movement slowly at different levels of tension.

1. Stand with your feet hip-width apart; place your hands on a wall, table, or desk for balance.
2. Extend your left leg behind you and bend it as much as you comfortably can; your left hip will raise up a little, but keep both hips facing forward.
3. Bend your left knee and bring your heel toward your bottom. Bring it as close to your bottom as you comfortably can.
4. Hold and squeeze for three seconds.
5. Slowly lower your leg to the starting position.

Do your number of repetitions on the left leg, then the right.

"Your knee joint is like the middle child in a family of three: always taking the blame for everyone else's mistakes. When your knees hurt, it's often because of a problem in the joints above or below, rather than a problem in the knee itself: If your ankles and hips aren't adequately strong and flexible, your knee joints can suffer."

— Metzl,
The Exercise Cure

Max Reps: _____ 25% _____ 50% _____ 75% _____

For this exercise, wear a shirt that covers your back so that you can slide up and down the wall.

1. Stand with your feet shoulder-width apart and your back against a wall. Slide your feet forward one step. Keep your body from your hips to your shoulders against the wall.
2. Bend your knees and slide your upper body down the wall. Keep sliding down until your knees are bent at 90 degrees (or as far as you are comfortable). You should look like you're sitting in an invisible chair.

3. Straighten your legs and slide your body back to the starting position.

Do your number of repetitions.

You can also try holding this in place as if you're sitting on a non-existent chair. Start by trying to hold it for 5 seconds, and work up to 3 minutes or more.

If you're a skier, this exercise is a great way to prepare your body for ski season.

Max Reps: _____ 25% _____ 50% _____ 75% _____

Climbing stairs is one of the best exercises known to man. If you don't have a flight of stairs handy, you can do this exercise. Start with a low step (about 6-7 inches) and increase the height of the step to increase your challenge.

1. Stand in front of a step with your feet hip-width apart.
2. Place one foot on top of the step. Using your front leg (the one on the step), push yourself up until you're standing on the step
3. Slowly lower yourself back down. Try to keep your descent smooth to soften the impact on your ankles.

Do your number of repetitions for each leg.

Jordan Metzl recommends step-ups, along with several other exercises, for women experiencing menopause symptoms:

"A 2006 study found that middle-aged women who started an exercise program saw a marked reduction in symptoms after 12 months; in a control group of women who had no exercise at all, symptoms got worse."

—Metzl,
The Exercise Cure

Max Reps: _____ 25% _____ 50% _____ 75% _____

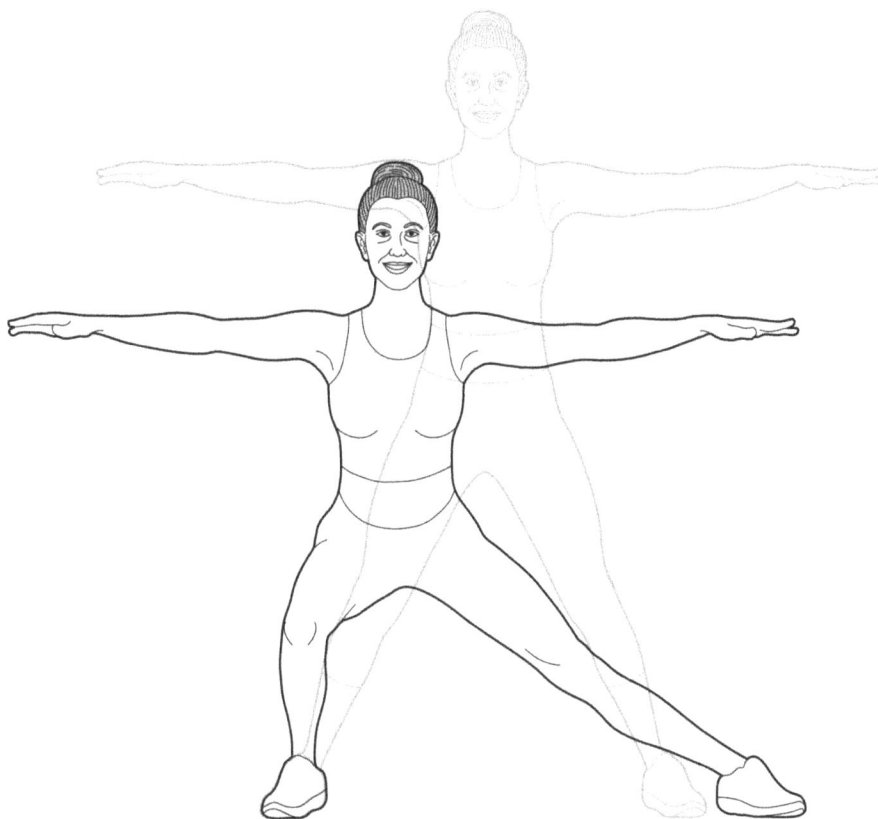

This exercise builds flexibility and strength in all your leg muscles. Make sure that when you bend your knee you do not let your knee go beyond your toes.

1. Stand with your feet hip-width apart and your arms out to the side for balance.
2. Step your left foot out wide to the side (how far depends on your flexibility). Bend your left knee, lowering your upper body. Keep your upper body upright and your right leg straight. You can let your bottom stick out a little as you bend your knee. Bend as far as you comfortably can, and **do not let your knee go beyond your toes.**

3. Slowly push against the floor and straighten your leg, returning to the starting position.

Do your number of repetitions on the left leg, then the right.

Start slow—keep your legs closer together and don't bend your knee as deeply as the diagram shows. Increase the range of the movement as you get stronger and more flexible.

Max Reps: _____ 25% _____ 50% _____ 75% _____

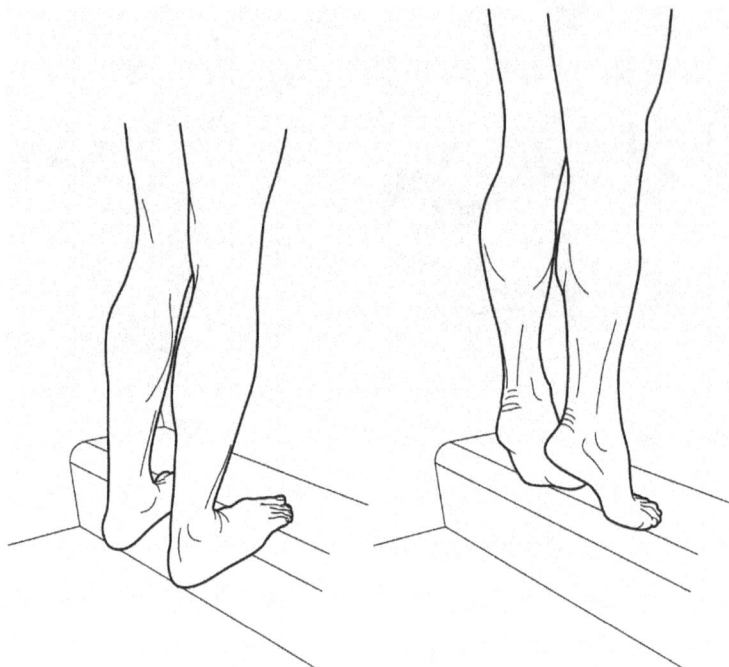

1. Find a stair, a thick block, or a heavy piece of wood that will support your weight and won't slip out from under you. Stand on that object with your toes on the object and your heels off the object. Place your feet about shoulder-width apart, or whatever distance allows you to maintain your balance.
2. Slowly lower your heels as far as you comfortably can, then slowly raise yourself up onto your toes as high as you can.
3. Slowly lower yourself down as far as you comfortably can. If you go past your stair, you're getting a great stretch in your calves and hamstrings, and Achilles tendon. But don't go too far down—you should not feel even slight discomfort. Some people prefer to use a book so that they have the floor as a safe stopping point.

Do your number of repetitions.

"Anything you do that is bad for your health is the equivalent of racking up huge amounts of debt … You'll pay for it tomorrow, or the next day, but make no mistake, whether you pay it off by sacrificing something valuable or find yourself choking on debt payments months or years from now, *you will pay.*"

—*Metzl,*

The Exercise Cure

Max Reps: _____ 25% _____ 50% _____ 75% _____

CORE EXERCISES

When people think about core exercise, too often they just focus on the abdominal muscles, but your core includes your entire trunk from your neck to your bottom. It includes your back as well as your abs. As you get older, maintaining a strong, balanced core is critical.

You'll notice that many core exercises involve moving your legs. Remember that they're not leg exercises—their goal is not to strengthen your legs, even though they will have that side effect. The goal is to strengthen and stabilize your core, so when you're doing Flutter Kicks or Leg-Outs, make sure to focus on your abdominals and back. You're using your core to hold and stabilize your legs, giving your lower abdominal muscles a great workout.

This section includes the following Core exercises:

- Good Morning
- Flutter Kick
- Plank
- Leg-out
- Rocking Horse
- Leg Raise
- Pelvic Tilt
- Farmer Burns Stomach Flattener
- Sit-back
- Seated Russian Twist

"Your core is just that: the center of your entire body. Its importance in form, function, and fashion cannot be overestimated. Ninety percent of backaches can be eliminated by strengthening your core muscles. In addition to making pain history, a strong core will let you ... carry your grandkids around ... instead of having them carry you around in a wheelchair."

—Lauren,
  You Are Your Own Gym

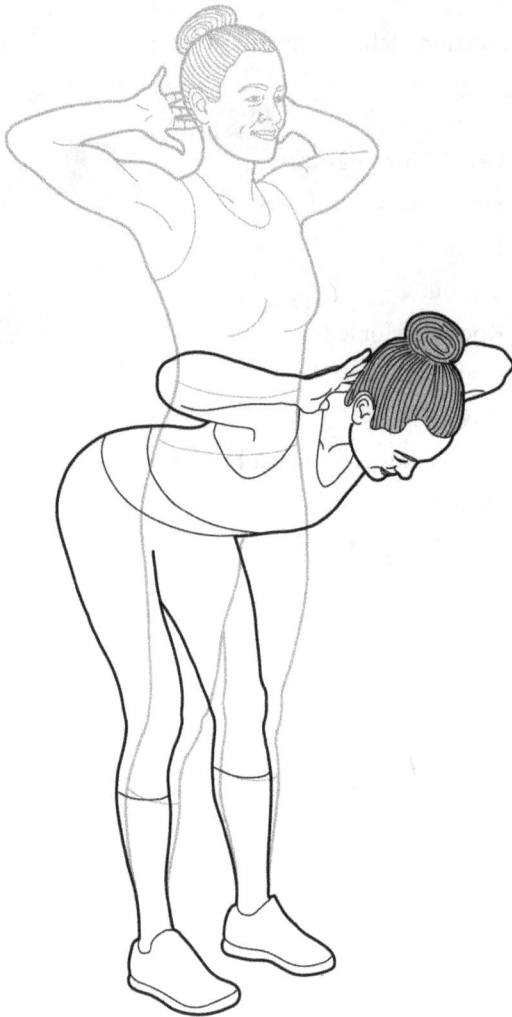

A "Good Morning" is similar to a forward bend dynamic stretch, but you're using the weight of your torso to strengthen your core.

1. Stand with your feet shoulder-width apart and your knees slightly bent; extend your arms out to the side for balance or place them behind your head for a little extra weight.
2. Bend forward at the waist, keeping the rest of your body still. Don't round your back—keep just as straight as it is when you're standing. Bend as far as you comfortably can—if your torso makes a 90-degree angle with your legs, that's great.
3. Slowly straighten back up to starting position.

Do your number of repetitions.

"The most important exercise you can do for your lower back is to get up out of your chair as often as you can: Sitting weakens the muscles that surround your spine and leaves you vulnerable to injury."

—Metzl,
The Exercise Cure

Max Reps: _____ 25% _____ 50% _____ 75% _____

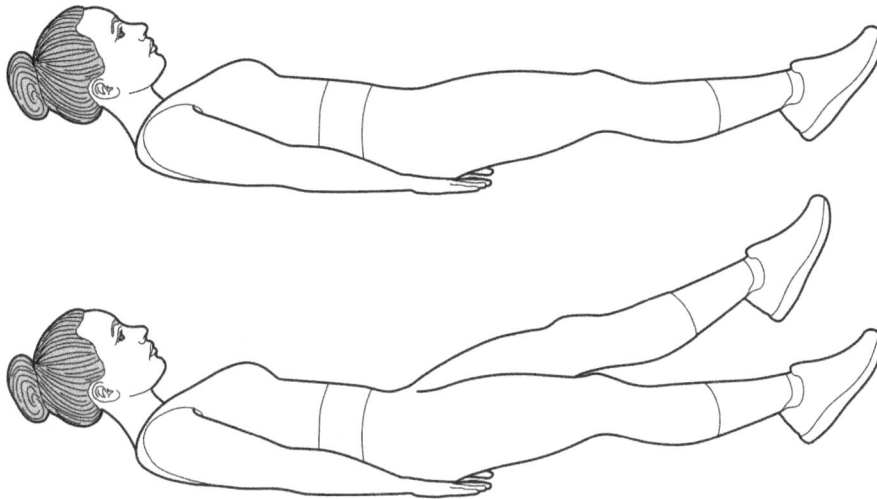

1. Lie on your back on a firm surface. Place your hands under your bottom and raise your head, looking toward your belly. Keep your entire back flat to the floor (tilt your pelvis to flatten the back fully).
2. Raise your legs off the floor until they form a 90-degree angle with your torso. Slowly lower them until you cannot keep your back flat on the floor. The lower you go, the harder you'll work, but you need to keep your back flat.
3. Keeping both legs straight, raise one leg, then lower it. As you lower one leg, raise the other. Continue these small straight-leg kicks—the "flutter" in Flutter Kicks. You can go fast or slow as long as you keep your back flat on the floor.

Continue for your amount of time (e.g., if your max is 60 seconds, 25 percent is 15 seconds).

Max Reps: _____ 25% _____ 50% _____ 75% _____

"After about age thirty, natural bone growth ceases, and steady bone loss begins in various parts of the body. If you don't act to delay or stop this bone loss, you're likely to end up with a fragile bone structure by the time you reach your later years.

"Fortunately, you can begin to act against this deterioration at any age, and one of the best strategies is to include weight-bearing exercise in your fitness program."

—Kenneth Cooper, MD, and Tyler Cooper, MD,
Start Strong, Finish Strong

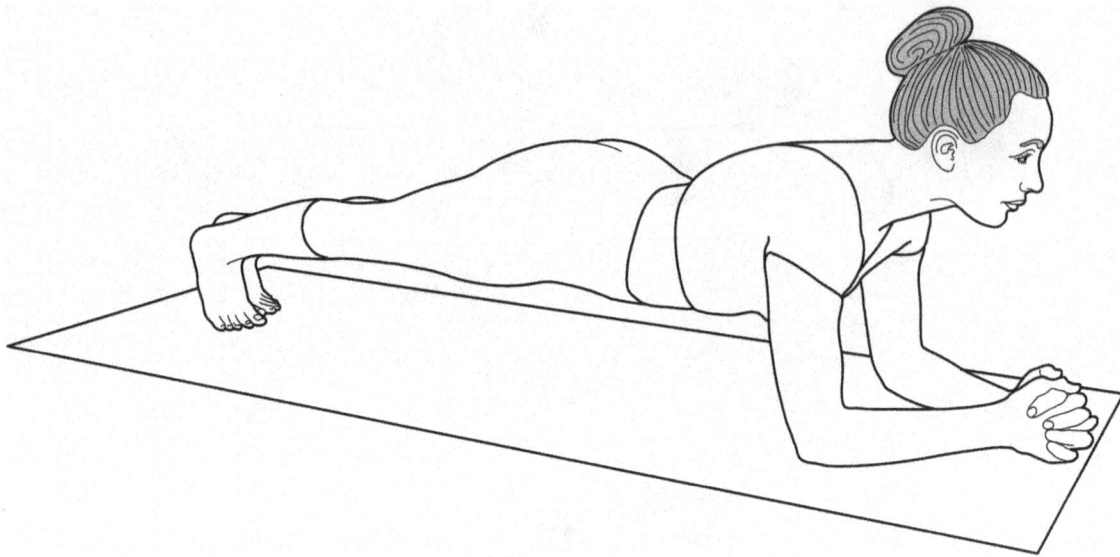

You can do a plank two ways—in push-up position with your arms straight, or in a bent-arm position. Both are great whole-body exercises.

1. Lie on your stomach on a firm surface. Lift your chest and rest your weight on your forearms, keeping them shoulder-width apart with elbows bent at 90 degrees.
2. Push your body up until all your weight rests on your forearms and your toes. Keep your body straight just as you would in a push-up.

Hold this position for your amount of time (e.g., if your max is 60 seconds, 25 percent is 15 seconds).

"Crunches are also what might be called a 'nonfunctional' exercise. Think about it: When you're standing, walking, and otherwise going about your life, your spine is elongated, a position that the abdominal muscles help support. The only time the abs shorten into a crunch-like position is when you're getting up off the floor or slumping on the couch — not something you need any more practice doing.

"I much prefer planks to crunches … planks are no-impact, and you can do them anywhere."

— Metzl,
   The Exercise Cure

Max Reps: _____ 25% _____ 50% _____ 75% _____

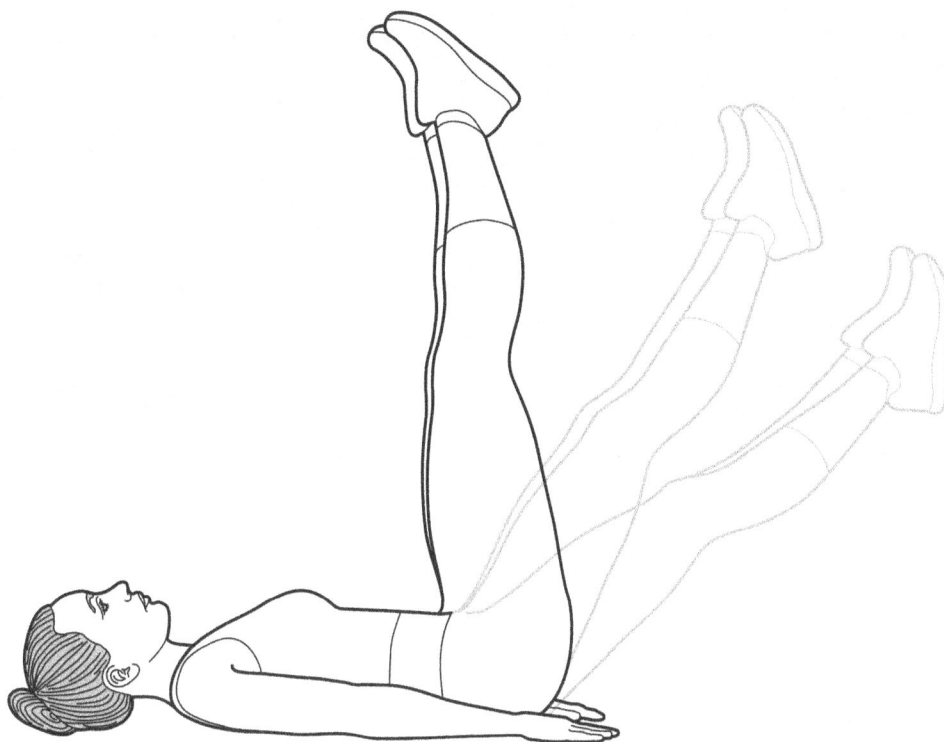

1. Lie on your back on a firm surface with your legs straight together and your hands flat under your bottom. Keep your lower back flat on the floor.
2. Raise your legs off the floor until they form a 90-degree angle with your torso. Slowly lower them until you cannot keep your back flat on the floor. The lower you go, the harder you'll work, but you need to keep your back flat. This is your start position.
3. Bend your knees and bring your legs in toward your chest, then straighten them out and return to your start position.

Do your number of repetitions.

Max Reps: _____ 25% _____ 50% _____ 75% _____

"Exercise, combined with weight loss, may relieve arthritis: Researchers at Wake Forest University studied 316 men and women, age 60 and older, who were suffering from osteoarthritis (wear-and-tear arthritis) of the knee. They found that a weight-loss diet, combined with exercise (including moderate walking sessions) had a greater effect on pain than did diet alone."

—Cooper and Cooper,
    Start Strong, Finish Strong

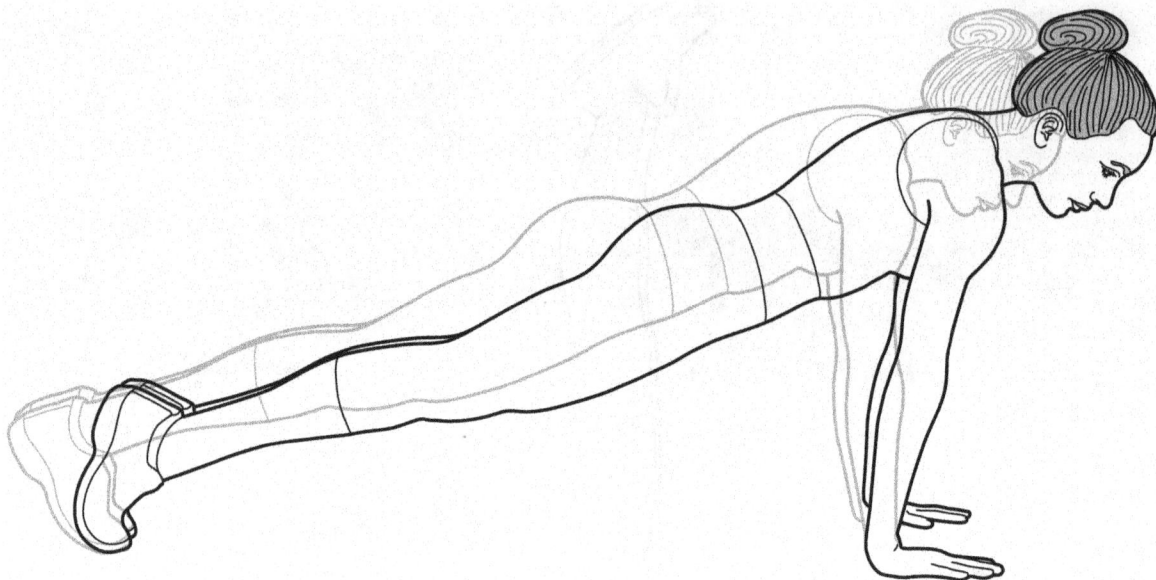

This exercise builds balance through your core, but it does put significant pressure on the wrists. Use the adaptation in the sidebar if you need to.

1. Place your hands on the floor and get into push-up position. Make sure your hands are directly below your shoulders. Keep your body straight.
2. Using your toes, push your body forward, letting your wrists bend beyond 90 degrees. Go as far as you comfortably can—6-10 inches is great.

3. Slowly return to your starting position.

Do your number of repetitions.

If your wrists hurt when you perform this exercise, you can place a small rolled towel or washcloth under each hand (just make sure your fingertips touch the floor so you don't slip). If you have push-up handles, you can use them to make your wrists more comfortable.

Max Reps: _____ 25% _____ 50% _____ 75% _____

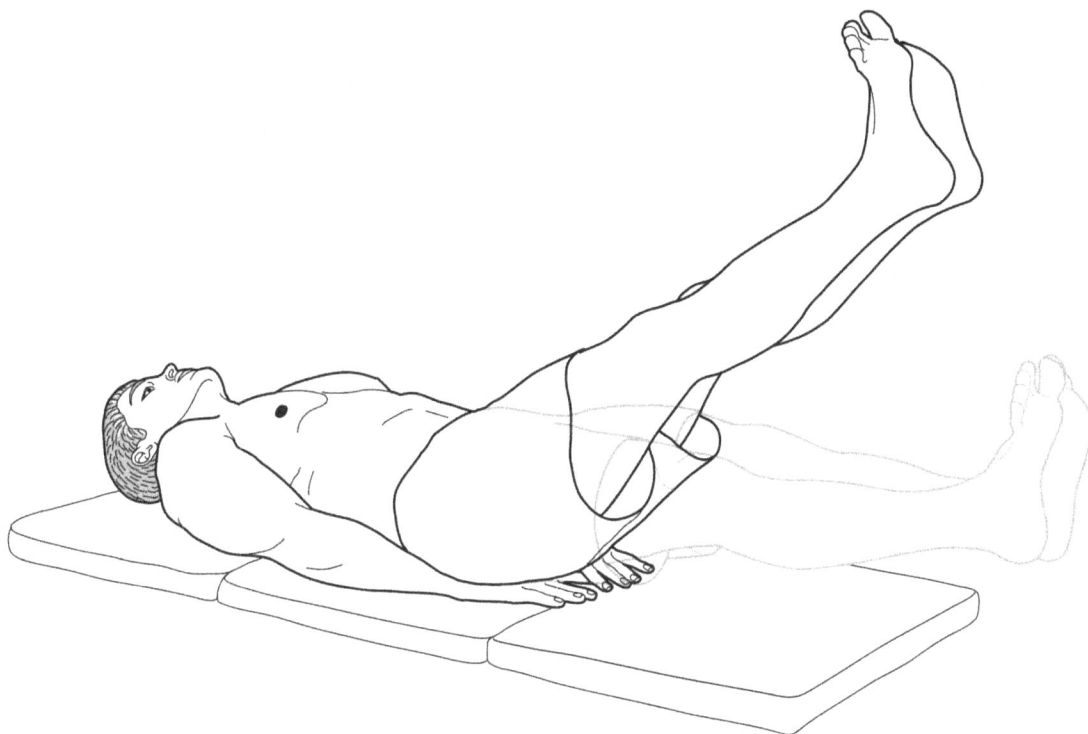

1. Lie on your back on a firm surface with your legs straight together and your hands flat under your bottom. Keep your lower back flat on the floor.
2. Raise your legs off the floor until they form a 90-degree angle with your torso. Slowly lower them until you cannot keep your back flat on the floor. The lower you go, the harder you'll work, but you need to keep your back flat. This is your start position.
3. Keep your legs straight and raise your feet up to 90 degrees, then lower them to your start position.

Do your number of repetitions.

"I look at daily exercise [including walking] as a healthy addiction. We have so many obesity-related health issues that are not treated until after they happen. Hypertension and diabetes are preventable with daily exercise. Exercise is medicine, preventive medicine, and it needs to be a daily ritual just like brushing your teeth."

— Metzl,
The Exercise Cure

Max Reps: _____ 25% _____ 50% _____ 75% _____

In the 1970s, I had a back injury that just wouldn't heal, so I signed up for a course called "The Y's Way to a Healthy Back" at the YMCA. The course had been created for President John F. Kennedy by his doctor, Hans Krauss. Krauss's approach strengthened the abdominals to the point where they became a brace for the back.

This exercise was a cornerstone of his treatment, and it did wonders for my back. It's so easy anyone can do it, no matter your age or level of ability.

1. Lie on your back on the floor with your knees bent. Keep your back flat against the floor.
2. Tighten your abdominal muscles and tilt your pelvis up slightly. Hold for up to 10 seconds while exhaling, keeping your abs flexed.

Do your number of repetitions.

Dr. Krauss was a remarkable example of healthy aging. In his eighties, he could do 10 full-range pull-ups.

Max Reps: _____ 25% _____ 50% _____ 75% _____

Note: Read these instructions fully before you begin the exercise.

1. Lie on your back with your knees bent. Inhale through nose as deeply as you can, letting your belly rise first and then your chest.

2. As you exhale pull your stomach in—try to touch your belly button to your spine. Your pelvis will naturally start to tilt your hipbones to the floor—increase that motion by tightening your buttocks. You'll create a powerful scooping action with your abdomen (and your back will love it).

3. As you exhale, let air hiss out through your lips and teeth. Make an "sss" sound until you exhale all the air. Exhale for as long as possible—5 seconds is a good start, but you can gradually increase the time. Try to empty your lungs completely by contracting your abdominal muscles deeper and deeper.

4. Repeat for a total of 12 breaths, taking as long as you need to complete them. Keep your abdomen flexed tight and rigid and your hips curved toward your chest until you have completed 12 breaths.

Standing variation:

Stand with your feet shoulder-width apart, shoulders relaxed, and arms hanging at your sides. Make sure you remember to curve your hips forward as you pull your stomach in. Do this exercise near a wall so that you can catch yourself if you get dizzy.

Other variations: Give yourself an extra pump of energy by clenching your fists as you contract. For an extremely strong pump, tighten every muscle in your body as you contract.

Max Reps: _____ 25% _____ 50% _____ 75% _____

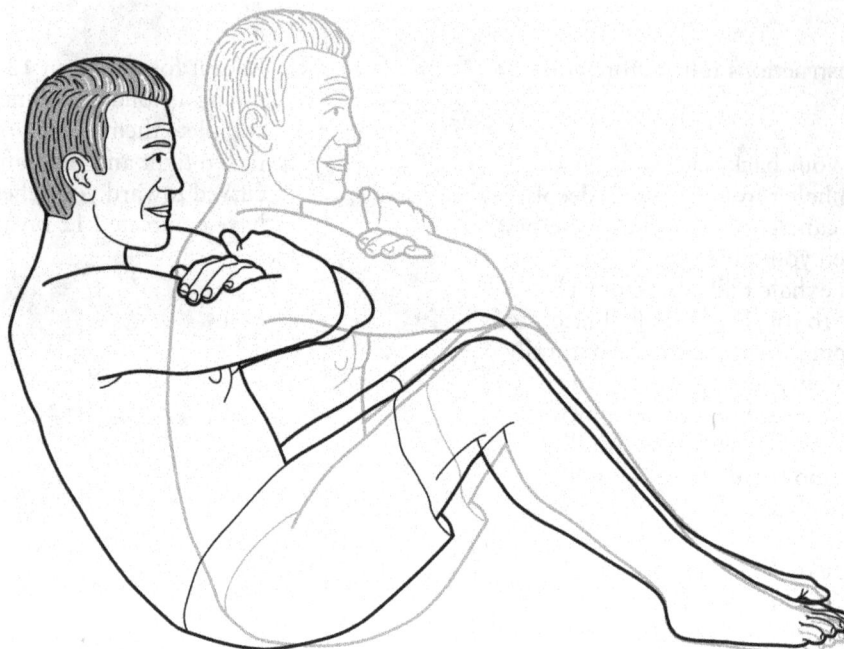

"In the sitback, it's almost impossible to move backward without involving the abdominal muscles … You'll feel them harden as they come into action, and soften as they relax."

—Laurence Morehouse,

  Total Fitness in 30 Minutes a Week

Back in the 1970s, Laurence Morehouse developed the sitback as an alternative to the sit-up or crunch. His research at the time told him sit-ups and crunches were ineffective, and modern research has since proved him right. His sitback continues to be a terrific core exercise.

1. Sit on the floor with your knees bent. To start, you can anchor your feet under a heavy piece of furniture, but as your abs get stronger, you won't need to anchor your feet. Bring your chest as close to your knees as it will go. Place your hands on your belly so that you can feel your muscles.

2. Slowly lean your upper body backward until you feel your abdominal muscles begin to tighten. Start slow: lean back a few inches and then return to your starting position. If that's easy (and you don't feel your muscles engage), lean back a little farther on your next sitback. Keep going until you find the spot where your abdominals are working but not exhausted. Morehouse explains, "As your condition improves, your point of moderate effort will drop farther and farther backward. Eventually, your shoulder blades will lightly brush the floor."

3. Hold this position for your amount of time (e.g., if your max is 60 seconds, 25 percent is 15 seconds). "Start with a degree of effort that enables you to hold the position for 15 to 20 seconds. The last few seconds the belly muscles will begin to quiver. Work up to a full 20 second sitback before quivering commences, then try a deeper sitback."

No More Crunches!

"Recently, in large part thanks to the work of spine biomechanics expert Dr. Stuart McGill, crunches have been shown to be detrimental to spine health. According to McGill, there may be no quicker way to herniate a disk than to flex the spine forward over and over again, as in the crunch exercise."

— Metzl,
The Exercise Cure

Max Reps: _____ 25% _____ 50% _____ 75% _____

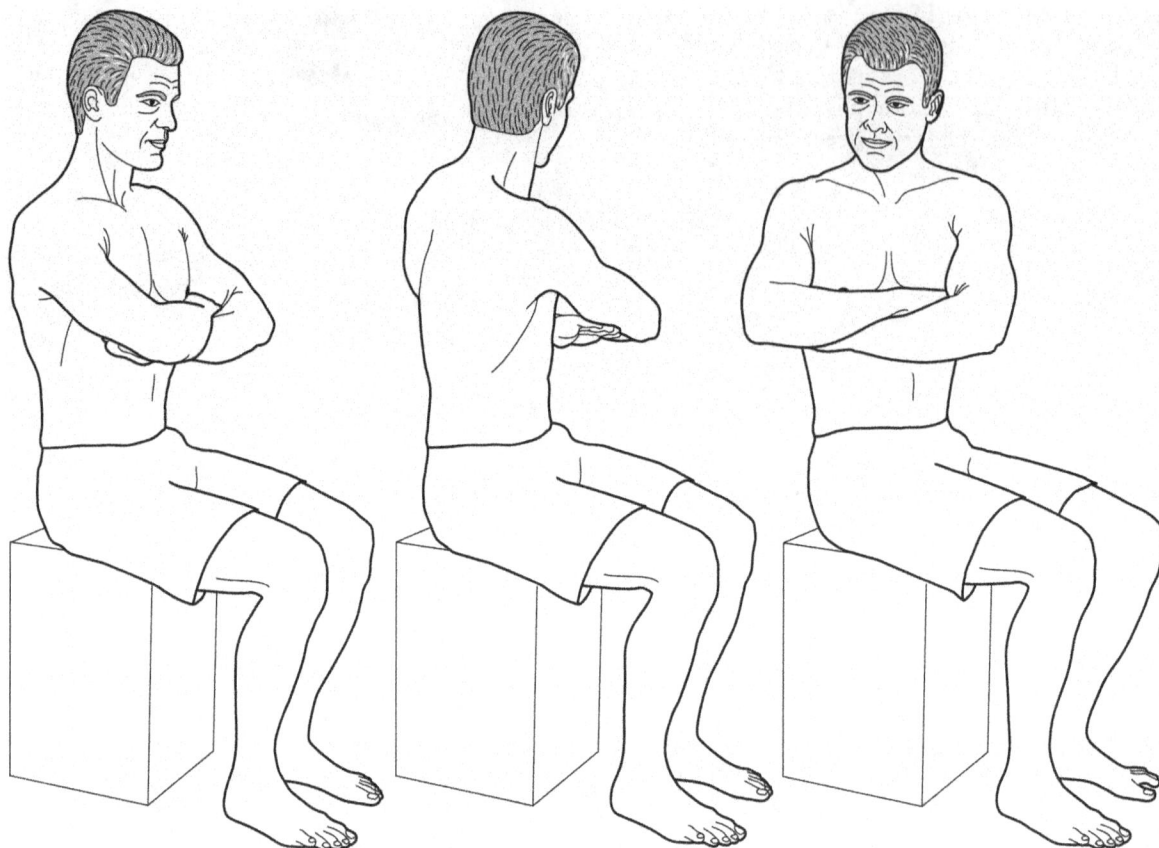

This very easy, very simple exercise will help develop flexibility and mobility in your core.

1. Sit on a chair or stool, fold your arms in front of you, and face straight ahead. Place your feet about shoulder-width apart on the floor.
2. Twist your upper body as far to the left as you comfortably can. Move slowly and smoothly—don't jerk your body.
3. Twist your upper body as far to the right as you comfortably can. Keep the movement slow and smooth.

Do your number of repetitions.

"Different people have different flexibility needs. But the majority of people these days need stretches that will *undo* the tightness and tension that result from lots of sitting."

—*Metzl,*
The Exercise Cure

Max Reps: _____ 25% _____ 50% _____ 75% _____

CARDIO EXERCISES

As I pointed out earlier in this chapter, all the exercises in these circuits raise your heart rate. When you insert cardio into the mix, you give your heart an extra boost, maximizing the work you're doing.

As Metzl explains, "[Hybrid] strength training workouts will ... affect your heart and lungs, and feel a little more like cardio workouts ... Every workout, to a certain degree, will help you build muscle, improve your cardiovascular system, *and* help you burn fat. That's one-stop shopping and incredibly time-efficient."

If time-efficiency is critical for you, you don't need to walk or rebound on a day when you do circuit training because you're doing cardio. Keep in mind that the benefits of walking and rebounding go beyond basic cardio exercise, though. You may not want to skip them and miss out on those benefits.

You can also use rebounding or walking as your Cardio exercise in the circuit—see my notes at the end of this section.

This section includes the following Cardio exercises:

- Burpee
- Jumping Jacks
- Mountain Climber

"But what's the secret to starting — and sticking with — [a fitness] program? The absolutely essential first task is to identify a personal passion or conviction that will motivate you profoundly — a hot button that will spark an inner drive to enable you to maintain your body and mind in the best shape possible."

— Cooper and Cooper,
Start Strong, Finish Strong

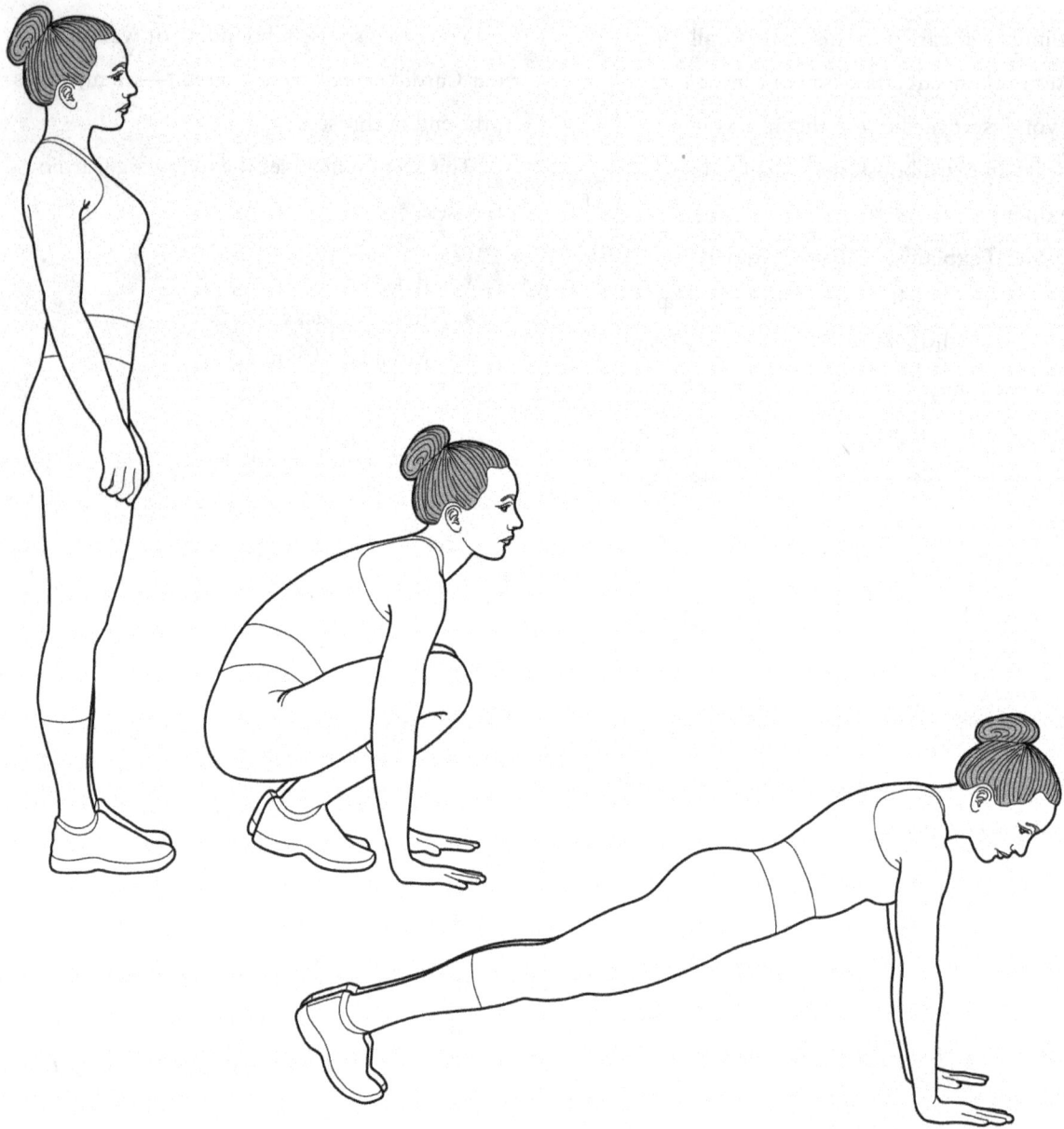

Burpees are tough, so don't push yourself to try
these until you're already doing full push-ups.

1. Start in a standing position and drop into a squat position (as if you're sitting back into a chair) with your hands on the ground.
2. Bring your palms to the floor and extend your feet back in one quick motion to assume the front plank position.
3. Return to the squat position in one quick motion.
4. Return to an upright standing position.

Do your number of repetitions.

"All exercise should be progressive: You should be trying to get stronger, faster, more flexible, more enduring, pretty much all the time, for your whole life. But it rarely works out that way: Instead, we tend to get comfortable doing a certain number of reps ... and we settle for 'good enough.' Then, over time, the 'good enough' bar tends to backslide ... and our fitness starts to fade.

"The solution? Keep it progressive."

—Metzl,
The Exercise Cure

Max Reps: _____ 25% _____ 50% _____ 75% _____

JUMPING JACKS ◆

You've seen this exercise before—it's an oldie but a goodie.

1. Stand with your feet hip-width apart and your arms at your sides.
2. Jump up and land with your feet apart. At the same time, raise your arms and touch your hands together above your head.
3. Jump again and return to the start position.

Do your number of repetitions.

"Regardless of your age, it's important to remain keenly aware that the Great Downward Curve of Life is always lurking in the background— and that you must do all you can to counter those threats that have the power to prevent you from [maintaining optimal health]."

— Cooper and Cooper,
Start Strong, Finish Strong

Max Reps: _____ 25% _____ 50% _____ 75% _____

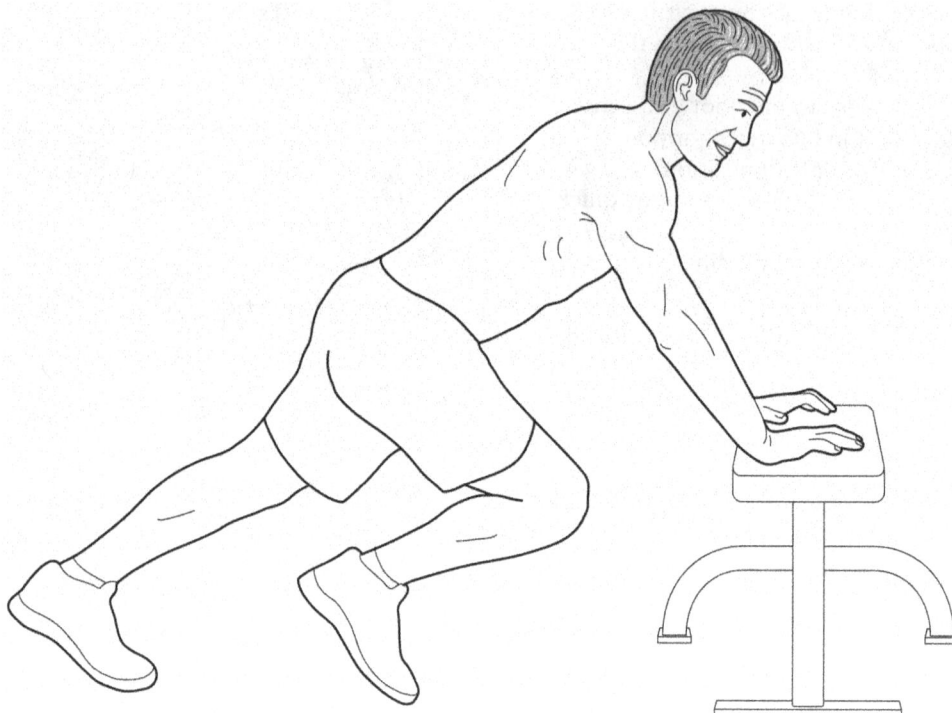

You can adjust the difficulty of Mountain Climbers the same way you adjust a push-up: if you're ready for the full effect, place your hands on the floor. If you need to take things more slowly, raise your hands to a chair or table. You're moving your knees forward, so you can't really do them against a wall, but even leaning on a table will make these a lot easier.

1. Place your hands on the floor, a chair, a table, or a counter. Straighten out your body as if you were going to do a push-up. (If your hands are on the floor, it's OK for your bottom to stick up a little as you move your legs). Take a big step forward with one leg. The front leg should be bent and the back leg should be straight.

2. With a very low jump, switch your legs so that the front leg is extended back and the back leg is bent in front.
3. Continue switching your legs.

Continue "climbing" for your amount of time (e.g., if your max is 60 seconds, 25 percent is 15 seconds).

"Pretend you are less than one hundred feet from the top of Mount Everest. This is your last push to the top!"

— Esselstyn,
    The Engine 2 Diet

Max time: _____ 25% _____ 50% _____ 75% _____

Be creative with your cardio. If it gets your heart rate up, it fits the bill. Try several minutes of energetic dancing (no slow dances in your circuit). Hop on your rebounder and do some Twist Bounces. Or do your Jumping Jacks on the rebounder for an extra boost.

"May we all exercise for the next 100 years ... and beyond."

— Metzl,

The Exercise Cure

Walking can work for cardio, but make sure you are raising your heart rate. You may need to walk fast or walk up a hill. If you're moving around your house or your neighborhood during your circuit, you can walk up and down a flight of stairs for your cardio—it's a fantastic exercise. (And you're strengthening your legs at the same time as you're working your cardiovascular system).

If you're lucky enough to work out near a pool, you can swim a few laps as your cardio. If you're working with the most basic situations, you can jump rope or jog in place (although jogging on the rebounder is much easier on your joints).

Keep it safe, keep it interesting, and keep it fun. If your exercise has those three qualities, you'll have no problem exercising for the rest of your long life.

T.J.'S STORY: FROM BUSTED-UP AT 33 TO HEALTHY AND BUILT FOR YEARS TO COME

The following story comes from T. J. Walsh, a young man in his 30s who pursued weight-lifting with a passion until it hurt him so badly he couldn't do the other physical activities he loved. Using body-weight exercise and some good advice from John Peterson, he healed his injuries, became pain-free, and developed the lean body he really wanted. He also happens to be my son-in-law, so you'll see that I play a part in his story, too.

Growing up, I was always told I had to lift weights in order to "get built" and develop a sculpted, heavily muscled physique. Heavy weights. In fact, the heavier the better. Over the years, I followed the advice about nearly every bodybuilding scenario presented in the health and fitness magazines to the letter. None of it, however, worked as promised in the magazines, not even close. But I persisted because I didn't know

There was no way I could keep up with this 62-year-old man, no matter how hard I tried, and I was barely in my 30s. I was thinking, Doesn't this guy ever get tired? He's been talking, laughing, joking, and having a great time, and I can barely get a breath to answer him.

any better. Eventually I injured my back weight-lifting, and the pain crippled my ability to engage in some of the activities I loved.

Yet, in spite of the constant pain, the fact was that I had put on a lot of muscle as a result of using heavy weights—didn't that mean it worked? That was my mind-set when my father-in-law, Rod Fisher, told me, "T. J., I found a way that you can build and sculpt your muscles just the way you want and get rid of your pain simultaneously. It worked for me, and I know it can work for you." The moment he said those words, the red flags immediately went up. The old "If something sounds too good to be true, it usually is" scenario was kicking in loud and clear.

Nevertheless, here I was, constantly wracked in pain, looking at a man in his 60s whom I considered to be in phenomenal shape, bursting with energy, with a lean, sculpted build that most guys half his age can't achieve. And the man is 100 percent pain free! As I looked at Rod, I recalled a winter family vacation we had all taken to Park City, Utah, not too long before. One morning, Rod said, "T. J., let's go snowshoeing." I agreed. I knew it would be a great workout, but I didn't realize what a reality check it would be. On the ascent of a double black diamond peak, it wasn't long before I fell a good 50 yards behind and was immediately humbled. Bottom line: there was no way I could keep up with this 60-something, no matter how hard I tried, and I was barely in my 30s. I was thinking, Doesn't this guy ever get tired? He's been talking, laughing, joking, and having a great time, and I can barely get a breath to answer him.

Reminding myself of that day, I let go of what I thought was right. I figured, if I can get to where he is, it's worth a shot. Rod really had found the secret of pain-free strength and fitness, and I wanted to know it.

Rod introduced me to John Peterson's book *Pushing Yourself to Power*. He said, "This was the exercise system I used to heal my shoulder, T.J. Just read it and see if what he says makes sense to you." So I did. It took a while for me to believe it, but I was so interested that I arranged to meet John, who lives in Minneapolis, in June 2009.

When I first saw him, it was hard to believe that a 57-year-old guy was in such unbelievable shape. Then again, it was my father-in-law who started me on this, so seeing another man, older than myself, who was in the shape I wanted to be in, reassured me that I was on the right path to finding an exercise program that really works. At that moment, I still wasn't fully convinced, but I really wanted to get away from the pain in my lower back that kept me from snowboarding, golfing, and running—my favorite activities. I'm only 33 years old, and I was afraid I'd have this pain for the rest of my life. So I decided to give it a serious try.

It's been 22 months since I started using John's training system. My workouts now consist of body-weight exercises alone. When I met John, I was going to the chiropractor three times a week. Now I may go once every three weeks. I'm stronger and leaner than I've ever been, and I feel absolutely amazing. I have a new confidence, and I truly owe it all to Rod and John.

T.J.'s story shows that no matter what your age, you can benefit from adopting a healthy approach to exercise, which includes safe strength-training.

CHAPTER 15

REBOUNDING — LOW IMPACT ON YOUR JOINTS, HIGH IMPACT ON YOUR HEALTH

■ ■ ■

Rebounding is easy on you and easy on your body, so
you will be able to stick with it. Put a bounce in your
step with this efficient, effective, and fun whole-body
exercise. Get ready to look good and feel better.

JUMP FOR JOY AND HEALTH—
START REBOUNDING TODAY

Walking, SMRs, and calisthenics are highly beneficial forms of exercise that will give your body a complete workout. I love doing all of them, and I believe you will too. Why, then, do I like to rebound too? And why do I recommend it to you?

By this point in the book you've already seen how much I love rebounding as a form of cardio and as an aid to detoxification. But I haven't really had a chance to explain all the things that make rebounding terrific, so that's what I'll do in this chapter.

"Rebounding is the closest thing to the Fountain of Youth that science has discovered. We found that jumping on good equipment is effective in improving the symptoms of over 80 percent of the patients reporting to our rehabilitation lab."

—James White, Ph.D.
Jump for Joy

FIND THE FUN

First of all, rebounding feels great, and I don't just mean it makes you feel great when you finish, which is true of all good exercise. I mean it feels great while you're doing it. It's very easy and very fun. It makes you feel like a kid.

I exercised as a kid, but I didn't think of it as exercise—it was just fun. There wasn't a day that went by that I didn't spend hours climbing trees. Kids play, and that's their exercise.

As adults, we "work out," we make it work. We schedule exercise into our days. Can we change that perception that exercise is always work? I think we can, and I think it's something we need to do. Part of being an Ageless Boomer is being young at heart, and rebounding can help you get that feeling.

Think about what happens when a baby stands up in the crib for the first time. They start bouncing on their legs. It's natural and fun. Rebounding can take us back to our childhoods where vertical movement was fun, invigorating, and healthy. Grownups lose that childlike quality, and sometimes we need to get it back, especially when it comes to being active.

REBOUNDING IS EASY AND EFFECTIVE

You know you need exercise to live a long and healthy life, but have you started yet? I hope after reading my other chapters you have, but maybe you're still reluctant to start. Maybe you're worried about aggravating old injuries or getting new ones. Sometimes it's hard to know what to do to work out or what workout gear to buy. Perhaps a medical condition has kept you from working out.

If any of these reasons has held you back, rebound exercise is an excellent place to begin. As

always, check with your health care professional before starting an exercise program. But when

you've got the go-ahead, get yourself a quality rebounder.

Rebound exercise is a whole-body exercise suited for everyone, regardless of their ages and present levels of fitness. In Karol Kuhn Truman's book *Looking Good Feeling Great* she writes, "If you can walk, you can rebound." Author Linda Brooks wrote several books on rebounding and was still promoting—and practicing—rebounding in her eighties. It's ideal for people of **any** age, those recuperating from injuries, or those hampered by preexisting conditions.

WHAT IS REBOUNDING?

"Rebound exercise" or "rebounding" is bouncing on a rebounder, which resembles a small trampoline. It involves bouncing up and down and landing on one or both legs. You can control the intensity of your workout by including shoulder, arm, hand, trunk, and leg movements.

The term "rebound" means springing back after an impact, which aptly describes the liberating weightless sensation you experience at the zenith of your bounce directly after feeling the weight of gravity at the lowest point of your bounce. Even though you experience a strong force of gravity on your way down, you don't have to worry about impact when you use a high-quality rebounder because the springs soften and redistribute the force of the bounce.

The force—literally—behind the benefits of rebounding is gravity. Al Carter, rebounding pioneer, says:

> Rebounding efficiently uses the vertical forces of acceleration and deceleration to produce internal loading by directly opposing the gravitational pull. This develops more biomechanical work with less energy expended. Less oxygen is used and less demand is placed on the heart while stimulating the whole body.

In layman's terms, this means that as you bounce on a trampoline or a rebounder, gravity works on you a little differently. At the bottom of your bounce, the forces of acceleration and deceleration (your up and down movement) combine with the natural force of gravity to make your body experience an increase in gravity (g-force or g's). At the top of your bounce, you experience a decrease in gravity. That's why it feels so good—you get that "butterflies in the stomach" sensation of lightened g-forces.

Why does gravity make such a difference? Because you're experiencing more weight on your body, and what's more, you're experiencing that weight change on **every cell** of your body. If you walk, you work your heart and lungs and pump more blood through your entire system, and that's great. You load your body weight onto your bones and muscles, which helps build bone density and muscle strength, and that's great. But the net effect of that exercise on each cell of your body is pretty minimal. It's necessary and beneficial, but it isn't as comprehensive.

REBOUNDING PIONEER

Al Carter was a wrestler and gymnast who toured as part of the "Gymnastics Fantastics" trampoline show in the early 1970s. His children eventually became performers in the show, and the way trampolining seemed to benefit them sparked his interest in the health benefits of the sport. In 1977 he published *Rebound to Better Health*, and in the nearly forty years since he has brought rebounding to the attention of the world. His company, ReboundAIR, makes one of the best rebounders on the market. He trained Dave Hall, founder of Cellercise (whose company makes the Cellerciser, another of the best rebounders on the market). Al Carter made rebounding the global phenomenon it is today.

When you rebound, you flex your muscles over 100 times per minute with more weight than you get in any other workout (because of gravity). You work every muscle during the course of one bounce. You get all the weight-bearing benefits and aerobic benefits of exercise. And, at the same time, you put weight on every cell in your body.

That unique process means that rebounding offers you a host of benefits:

- Increases balance and coordination
- Helps flush out the lymphatic system
- Lowers resting heart rate
- Speeds up metabolism
- Increases lung capacity
- Builds and tones all your muscles
- Improves digestion and elimination
- Allows for a deeper, more restful sleep
- Clears your mind and sharpens your mental skills
- Strengthens your immune system
- Helps with weight reduction
- Slows the aging process
- Strengthens your heart
- Reduces cholesterol and triglyceride levels
- Improves vision
- Oxygenates the whole body
- Reduces stress
- Reduces varicose veins by flushing the fluids that have accumulated in those veins
- Increases circulation
- Improves balance
- Clears sinuses
- Burns calories
- Reduces anxiety and depression
- Improves confidence

But what makes rebounding even better? It's safe and gentle. When your foot hits the ground when you run, for example, gravity is working on your whole body, but it's working extra hard on your joints, as I'll explain in this chapter. In

rebounding, the trampoline takes the force of your impact on the mat, spreads it out to the springs, and then sends the energy back to mat to propel you back upward. So instead of jarring your joints, you're bouncing them gently. They get a full workout without pain and damage.

Like all the exercises in this book, you get to

One of the best benefits is that you can do all this in your own home, on your own schedule. Your cells don't care if you're in a fancy gym or not. They respond to increased weight. You can rebound while watching a show, listening to music, chatting with friends and family, or even meditating.

control how easy or hard you want to work out on a rebounder. If you're a beginner, or injured, or frail, you can start rebounding right now (get your doctor's OK first). If you're a tough guy—or gal—don't dismiss rebounding as too easy for you (unless you like getting injured by your workouts) because you can work your butt off on a rebounder. I don't usually get very sweaty during a power walk, but after a hard workout on a rebounder, I'm soaked.

As rebounding expert Dave Hall explains, rebounding combines all kinds of exercise into one workout: aerobic, calisthenic, and more. Rebounding is the one form of exercise that will give you a total, complete body workout—it does what every other exercise does, and then some.

Why just stimulate specific muscles during exercise when—with even less effort—you can stimulate your entire body all the way down to your cells? Humans are composed of roughly 1 trillion cells, and during rebounding they flex around 100 times a minute—that's quite a workout!

Al Carter says, "Rebounding is a cellular exercise because it causes all of the cells of the body to physically adjust to what is perceived by them as more demanding internal environment."

If you want to lose weight, you can do it with diet and exercise. If you rebound, you'll lose weight, build muscle, strengthen bones, and do wonders for your immune system.

The resistance of the forces of acceleration, deceleration, and gravity make you stronger cell by cell, from the inside out. And no part of your body is left out—from your immune system to your bones to your non-physical energetic systems. This theory is supported by an observation recorded by NASA.

In space's zero gravity condition, astronauts have been recorded to lose as much as 15 percent of bone and muscle mass in just 14 days. This is because the weightless environment makes their cells think that they don't have to work as hard, so they just don't. Then, the principle of atrophy takes over: if you don't use something, you lose it. If you've ever been on bed rest, you have experienced this phenomenon firsthand.

Rebounding works the same way—except in reverse.

Imagine that you were sent to a planet that had three times the gravitational pull of the earth. Just to walk, your legs would be required to work three times harder and be three times stronger than on earth, yet your legs would still rise to the occasion. Similarly, in rebounding the resistance of the forces of acceleration, deceleration, and gravity work together to challenge your entire body and make it stronger, cell by cell.

Rebounding is amazing at getting your blood circulating and getting your body loose and flexible. You're not lifting weight away from your body—your own body's weight is adding the work. When you add work you become stronger. You exercise all the cells in your body, and if every cell is getting worked, then every body part and body function is being improved.

A report written by Craig McQueen, M.D., and A.W. Daniels, Ph.D., at the University of Utah compares the impact loads experienced during rebounding compared to running on a hardwood basketball floor. McQueen and Daniels concluded that rebounding diminished as much as 87.5 percent of the impact to feet, knees, and legs.

When you rebound, you burn calories more efficiently than you do in other forms of exercise. According to Dave Hall, rebounding burns calories ten times faster than walking, five times faster than swimming, and three times faster than running. Ken Cooper, MD, the founder of aerobics, has a system in which he gives point values to different types of exercise based on laboratory measurements. He gives 50 percent more points to rebounding than to power walking.

High-impact exercises such as running can create up to 15-20 G-Force on your feet, ankles, knees, and hips. That extreme force can cause cell rupture, internal hemorrhaging, and muscle tearing from the bone (known more commonly as shin splints).

Rebounding redistributes the force of impact, protecting your joints. A 1981 NASA study concluded that when rebounding, the lessened force is equalized throughout the body: "While jumping on a trampoline, the G-Force was almost the same at [the ankle, back, and forehead] and well below the rupture threshold of a normal healthy individual."

The reduced impact of rebounding makes it an excellent option for anyone with knee, hip, and ankle problems, but it also makes it one of the best long-term exercise options you can imagine. If you're going to be exercising for the rest of your life, and I hope you will, the smart choice is an exercise that gives you substantial physical benefits without substantial damage. Rebounding does exactly that.

Rebounding boosts your immune system, helping you bounce back more quickly from illnesses and even helping you avoid sicknesses altogether. It does this in two ways: it increases immune cell activity and it cleanses the lymphatic system.

INCREASES IMMUNE CELL ACTIVITY

Immune cells, also known as lymphocytes, are vital to your health because their job description involves neutralizing viruses, bacteria, and cancer cells. The more active immune cells become, the better they do their job. According to Carter, "Rebound exercise creates that high-G environment necessary to increase the strength and activity of individual lymphocytes. This increases the efficiency of the entire immune system both collectively and individually, cell by cell." If your cells are stronger and more active, you're making your immune system stronger, and you're much more resistant to any kind of disease.

Although it may seem hard to believe that gravity can make that big a difference for your immune cells, a study called "Human Lymphocyte Activation is Depressed at Low G and Enhanced at High G" provided some compelling evidence that it makes a big difference. The researchers tested astronauts after they spent time in the low-G atmosphere of space and found that their lymphocytes were 50 percent **less** active than the lymphocytes of a control group that stayed on earth. So less gravity meant less-active immune cells, but they didn't stop there. They took the astronauts' sluggish lymphocytes and spun them in a centrifuge for three days at 8 Gs of constant force. After the immune cells experienced those extra Gs they

became **twice** as active. So gravity makes a big difference for our immune systems.

CLEANSES THE LYMPHATIC SYSTEM

You have four times more lymph in your body than blood, yet this vital fluid is often overlooked. Lymph surrounds all the cells in your body, removes metabolic wastes, and circulates white blood cells—all vital activities essential to keep you healthy. Unlike the heart, which pumps blood, lymph fluid has no pump and is channeled in one upward direction through the body via lymph ducts that act as one-way valves.

The New England Journal of Medicine clearly states the problem inherent in this pumpless system:

> ...without adequate movement, the cells are left stewing in their own waste products and starving for nutrients, a situation that contributes to arthritis, cancer, and other degenerative diseases as well as aging. Vigorous exercise such as rebounding is reported to increase lymph flow by 15 to 30 times.

Dr. Morton Walker asserts in *Jumping for Health* that three dynamics are needed to boost lymph flow—muscular contraction from exercise and movement, gravitational pressure, and internal massage to the valves of the lymph ducts—and that rebounding reliably provides all three. Martial arts expert and personal trainer JB Berns agrees: "Rebound exercise is the only exercise which provides all three properties necessary to maintain and increase lymph flow."

Carter also believes that rebound exercise is the key to increase lymph flow—even up to 50-fold, depending on the intensity of the exercise you are practicing. Because of the one-directional nature of lymph flow, the vertical up-and-down movement of rebounding is extremely effective to forcefully flush the entire body down to the cellular level by moving the lymph fluid along the lymph vessels.

Dave Hall once said, "I don't know how you can get sick if you rebound." Rebounders consistently report a drastic reduction in sickness, and even those who do get sick experience sicknesses of far shorter durations than before they started rebounding. As you know from my own stories, I've barely been sick a day since I started living an Ageless Boomer lifestyle. I want the same to be true for you.

THE ELIMINATION MIRACLE

I once had the opportunity to accompany Al Carter to a presentation he gave at a senior living facility. He was letting them know about all the great things rebounding could do for their health, but the one benefit that got everybody's attention was easier eliminations.

It's true. If you get up in the morning and bounce on the rebounder for a few minutes, you'll need to head to the bathroom. If come back and bounce for a few more minutes, you'll need to go again. For some folks, that's the best thing a rebounder can do.

MINIMIZE RISKS FROM FALLS

For Boomers, a single accident may be one accident too many. As we become older and our bones become more brittle, any bumps and falls can have devastating consequences. The good news is that many accidents can be avoided simply with improved balance and coordination while stronger bones can lessen the impact of any tumbles. What's the solution? Rebounding!

Balance is controlled by the inner-ear organ, known as the vestibule. Rebounding improves balance by stimulating the vestibule, making it re-adjust to the gravitational pull 100 times per minute. You're engaging your sense of proprioception, the sense of your body's position in space. Your brain needs to know where every

"I keep my rebounder at the foot of my bed, and use it daily."

— Bob Hope

"If you see somebody jumping up and down on the second floor of the White House, that's me rebounding."

— President Ronald Reagan

part is moving and landing, and every time you jump, your brain is doing minute calculations to figure out how you land in order to maintain balance.

Improved coordination comes from time spent on the rebounder. If you worry about falling when you start rebounding, use a stabilizing bar (available for all the brands I recommend) at first. You'll find that your body quickly adapts to this new challenge and learns rhythm, timing, balance, and coordination.

Rebounding also increases bone density. Remember the astronauts who lost bone density in space? Carter says, "Increasing G-force, by rebounding, sends a message to the bone cells telling them the entire skeletal system needs to be mineralized, dense, and strong." This means that with stronger bones and improved coordination and balance, worry about debilitating falls will be a thing of the past.

GET THE BODY YOU'VE ALWAYS WANTED

Although it's a lot more important to be Ageless for health and vitality rather than for vanity, rebounding can do many things to help you feel better about the person you see in the mirror. According to Karol Kuhn Truman, rebounding slims the thighs, trims the hips, flattens the belly, tones the arms, and even (for ladies) firms the bustline. It does this by burning the unwanted fat deposits in your body while simultaneously toning and building muscle. Your muscles will become stronger, your fat will melt away, and the true shape of your body will start to emerge.

When you rebound, the benefits extend beyond your muscles to your skin cells, making them stronger and more supple. Your circulation is also improved, improving your complexion, and the fat deposits contributing to your wrinkles disappear. Then, the exercise tightens your skin. This results in a refined face with more resilient skin and a healthy glow.

"Rebound exercise does improve face, chin, neck, sagging skin, and complexion. I know because it's done exactly that for me, as well as for others I know: Sagging skin takes on new resilience and color, complexions just look healthier and more alive."

—Karol Kuhn Truman

With rebounding, you achieve all the established benefits of exercise—improved flexibility, better sleep, improved circulation, more efficient digestion, improved back and arthritis pain relief, strengthened heart, lowered blood pressure, improved eyesight, and increased IQ and memory, and many more. However, when rebounding, you achieve these benefits more efficiently and effectively than with other means of exercise.

As I stated before, unlike jogging, walking, bicycling, or weightlifting, rebounding is a whole-body exercise that strengthens the entire body at once. It's isotonic, isometric, callisthenic, and aerobic all in one. Rebounding is even more efficient than running. The NASA study on rebounding (see next page) concluded that rebounding produces improved conditioning, making it 68 percent more efficient than running on a treadmill. John Peterson used to be a marathon runner, but he stopped running when he discovered how much better rebounding is.

A study conducted at Ken Cooper's organization, the Institute of Aerobics Research in Dallas, Texas, compared subjects who were weight training with subjects who were weight training AND adding 30 seconds of rebounding in between each weight-lifting round. The study found that after just 12 weeks, the individuals who added rebounding to their weight-training circuits experienced as much as a 25 percent strength increase over those who only weight trained.

You can do the same: when you're doing SMR exercises, you can step onto your rebounder in between sets, bounce for a minute or so, and then begin another set. You can even do some of the upper-body exercises while on the rebounder, as long as you keep your feet in the right stance and keep your pace steady and slow.

The key factor driving this increase in strength may be because of mitochondria. Carter suggests that during rebounding, the mitochondria are replicated in every one of your cells. Mitochondria are known as "cellular power plants" because they supply energy to the cells. Carter adds that "the more mitochondria you have in the muscles you are using, the greater the endurance of those muscles." This power supply provides you with extra stores of energy to keep you going strong for the rest of the day, and you don't even have to break a sweat to start achieving the multitude of benefits rebounding provides.

THE NASA STUDY

I've mentioned this study several times in this chapter, and you may be wondering why NASA would study rebounding. The reason is gravity—astronauts have to endure unusual gravity conditions, and rebounding can offer certain benefits that other kinds of exercise can't provide.

The study itself was conducted through NASA by A. Bhattacharya, E.P. McCutcheon, E.Shvartz, and J.E. Greenleaf at the Biomechanical Research Division, NASA-Ames Research Center, in cooperation with the Wenner-Gren Research laboratory at the University of Kentucky. The results of the study were published in the *Journal of Applied Physiology* in 1980.

The researchers found that rebounding is more efficient than other tested forms of exercise (treadmill running) and that rebounding puts less stress on the joints than treadmill running.

CHOOSING THE RIGHT REBOUNDER

In 1981-1984, rebound exercise became extremely popular in the United States, but within a couple of years, the fad died out because of a mass import of poorly made foreign rebounders that flooded the U.S. market. Thus, the quality of rebounder will definitely make a difference. While options are available at every

price point, you will probably pay a few hundred dollars for a good rebounder. You can pay more for a rebounder that is worse, like some of the bungee-cord based models. You'll achieve the best results on a high-quality rebounder that is built for performance and tested for safety. A $30 model will not provide the same results as a high-quality rebounder and it may cause injury because it's too jarring.

The following are a few things to consider when selecting a rebounder:

- **Mat.** A quality rebounder uses a Permatron® mat, or equivalent, that will not distort or bend when you are bouncing, fully supporting your ankles, feet, and legs.
- **Springs.** Look for thick, heavy-duty springs that are thicker in the middle and tapered to the ends, giving a wide-bellied appearance.
- **Legs.** Higher quality models will have fold-down legs while cheaper versions will have legs that screw off.
- **Buoyancy.** Look for a rebounder that provides a soft and buoyant bounce with excellent lift that does not jar your back and knees.
- **Durability.** Choose a rebounder with quality parts that come with a warranty and are easy to replace.

302

- **Shape.** Over time, circular rebounders have proven to be the best, since they wear evenly.

Cellerciser and ReboundAir are the brands I recommend the most, although Needak is also good. Both Cellerciser and ReboundAir have an optional stabilizing bar to help with balance.

REBOUNDING WORKOUTS FROM MILD TO INTENSE

As you get started with your rebounding regimen, you can do as much or as little as you want. I have not included timing with the exercises because it's important to make the timing work for you. When I started I did two minutes a day and increased slowly from there. Any time from two minutes at set intervals throughout the day to 45-minute daily routines will work splendidly. Above all, listen to your body and progress at your own rate.

The techniques and routines discussed in this section are merely examples of movements to get you started as you progress from beginner, to intermediate, to advanced. Rebounding videos are widely available; Reboundair and Cellerciser come with videos.

You will find as you get bouncing that you will discover motions and movements that feel good to you. Feel free to get creative. Create your own workout. Dance on the rebounder.

TRY SHORT INTERVALS SEVERAL TIMES A DAY

You can start rebounding in multiple short doses throughout the day. Several short sessions are actually more effective than one long session. A great way to start is with the Health Bounce, where your heels don't leave the mat.

Linda Brooks suggests that if you've been sitting at your desk, go rebound once an hour for a few minutes. If you've been working for an hour and you want to be sharp again, go do the health bounce.

THE HEALTH BOUNCE

If you are just starting out, begin with a warm-up exercise called the Health Bounce. The

Health Bounce was developed by Al Carter and is ideal to start every session whether you are a beginner, intermediate, or expert.

1. Stand in the center of the rebounder mat with your feet about six inches apart. If you are unsure of your balance, hold the stabilizing bar.
2. Begin by bouncing on your toes by bending your knees and then straightening your legs. You do not need to let your feet leave the mat.
3. Continue bouncing for several minutes.

The Health Bounce should leave you with a tingling effect, which is a sure sign that you are cleansing your body and boosting your lymphatic system.

The following schedule is a good way to begin:

- Week 1: Health Bounce for 4 minutes; 4 to 5 times per day.
- Week 2: Health Bounce for 1 minute, jog for 2 minutes, Health Bounce for 1 minute; 5 times per day.

- Week 3: Health Bounce for 2 minutes, introduce the Strength Bounce (instructions in the next section), work up to 1 minute, jog for two minutes, Health Bounce for 2 minutes; 5 times per day.
- Week 4: Increase times across the board; continue repeating 5 times per day.

Once you get to 10 minutes, you can cut down on the number of times per day.

How fast should you go? At your own pace. I do the Health Bounce at 120 bounces per minute and the Strength Bounce at 100 bounces per minute. It's so consistent that I don't even need to time it any more. When I Health Bounce 120 times, a minute has passed.

Variation: You can try a Power Health Bounce where your heels leave the mat but your toes stay on the mat.

EASY DOES IT

When you are starting out, don't be afraid to use a stabilizing bar to hold on to if it will give you confidence in the beginning. You can increase the overall efficiency of the exercises by adding arm rotations, swings, or flaps. Truman also recommends putting your palms together and pushing to tone your arms and chest. Beginners do well with simple exercises punctuated with cool down intervals.

Boomers new to rebounding can try the following program:

1. Health Bounce
2. Walk in Place
3. Health Bounce
4. Twist Bounce or Jog in Place
5. Health Bounce

HIGH-KNEE WALK IN PLACE

The High-Knee Walk in Place is an ideal warm-up aerobic exercise to get your heart pumping. Do this for a couple of days before even starting the Health Bounce, just to get used to the feel of the mat.

1. Begin by walking in place on the mat.
2. Concentrate on lifting your knees up in front of you, one leg at a time.
3. Try leaning back slightly and keeping your back straight.

TWIST BOUNCE

The Twist Bounce is a fantastic exercise. It's ideal for Boomers with lower back problems because it targets and strengthens that area. It loosens the muscles in your back, increases blood flow to your spine, improves digestion, and massages your organs. Dave Hall attributes an inch of his height to this exercise.

1. Start bouncing, letting your feet leave the mat.
2. Twist your hips in the opposite direction of your shoulders and torso—when your torso and shoulders go right, turn your hips left. (Remember Chubby Checker and the Twist.)
3. Switch directions on the next bounce. Continue twisting, changing directions with each bounce.

If I wake up and can't sleep, I get on the rebounder, breathe deeply, and Health Bounce for 10 to 20 minutes. It's like a sleeping pill.

REBOUND JOG

1. Begin jogging in place.
2. Swing your right arm forward as your left knee rises.
3. Swing your left arm in front of you as your right knee rises.

4. Concentrate on breathing deeply.

Continue for as long as you like. You can regulate the speed of your jog depending on how hard you want to go.

SITTING BOUNCE

If you're frail, injured, or easily fatigued, you may find Sitting Bounces can be helpful.

1. Sit on the rebounder with your bottom in the middle of the mat and your feet on the floor. Rest your hands behind you on the far edge of the rebounder or on the mat at your sides.
2. Bounce, keeping your bottom on the mat.

Continue for as long as you like. If you want to make the Sitting Bounce more vigorous, place your hands behind you on the edge of the rebounder and lift your bottom off the mat as you bounce.

TAKE IT UP A NOTCH

Intermediate Boomers can incorporate elements from the beginning stage and build on them to take it up a notch. Instead of cooling down in intervals throughout the program, try warming up, reaching a peak, and then cooling down.

A sample program for intermediate rebounders is as follows:

1. Health Bounce
2. Rebound Jog
3. Kick Bounce, Twist Bounce, or Cross-overs
4. Rebound Jog
5. Health Bounce

KICK BOUNCE

The Kick Bounce really gets your lymphatic flow going. It can be executed while bouncing or while running or jogging.

1. Lean back on your heels.
2. Kick out straight with your left foot as you land solidly on your right foot.
3. Then do the opposite foot and leg on the next bounce.
4. Swing your arms opposite of your legs.
5. Try a variety of back kicks and side kicks.

CROSS-OVERS

Cross-overs will help you build coordination as you build strength.

1. Start your Rebound Jog or Run.

2. Touch your left elbow to your right knee as it comes up.

3. Touch your right elbow to your left knee as it comes up.
4. Repeat.

This is my favorite rebounding workout; although I do variations of this all the time, this is the basic workout. I love rebounding, and I've been doing it for a long time, so naturally I've developed some pretty vigorous workouts on the rebounder. This relatively short workout is one variation of many, but it should give you some ideas to create challenging rebounding workouts for yourself.

I start with a thorough warm up:

- Health Bounce (3 minutes). I start with my heels on the mat for the first minute. For the second and third minute, my heels leave the mat in a power health bounce.
- Slow Rebound Jog (3 minutes). I do it in the center of the Rebounder.
- Strength Bounce (1 minute).
- Twist Bounce (1 minute).
- Slalom Bounce (1 minute).
- Rebound Shuffle Bounce (1 minute).
- Jumping Jacks (2 minutes).
- Rebound Jog (1 minute). Active recovery.

Be careful not to go too wide with your Jumping Jacks, especially if you have long legs. Keep your feet on the mat!

Once I'm warmed up, I start doing intervals, which can include a whole bunch of different exercises. This is one variation:

- High-knee sprint (1 minute)
- Rebound Jog (1 minute)
- High-knee sprint again (1 minute)
- Rebound Jog (1 minute)
- High-knee sprint (1 minute)
- Rebound Jog (1 minute)
- High-knee sprint (1 minute)
- Rebound Jog (1 minute)
- High-knee sprint (1 minute)
- Rebound Jog (1 minute)

For you, your intervals could be one minute each or they could be five seconds each. If you're starting out, you can do shorter intervals of the hard stuff and longer intervals of the easy stuff, e.g., 10 seconds of hard, 50 seconds of easy.

Want a quick, heart-speeding workout?
Try the Four-Minute Workout:

Health Bounce
(1 minute), Strength Bounce (1 minute),
High Knee Sprint (1 minute)
Health Bounce
(1 minute)

You can also play with the number of interval sets you do. If I'm in a rush, I might do one interval set; if I'm not in a rush, I'll do five interval sets. Then I do more aerobic bounces, reversing the order I used the first time:

- Jumping Jacks (2 minutes)
- Rebound Shuffle Bounce (1 minute)
- Slalom Bounce (1 minute)
- Twist Bounce (1 minute)
- Strength Bounce (1 minute)

I cool down by reversing the warm-up exercises:

- Slow Rebound Jog (3 minutes)
- Health Bounce (3 minutes)

Minus the warm-up and cool down, the whole workout takes about 32 minutes.

"The single most important form of exercise in existence is the full body Isometric Contraction along with mastering Isometric Contraction for every muscle group ... The next most important form of exercise that one can possibly do, in my mind, in order to tie it all together and maintain and enhance strength, balance, speed (reaction time), coordination, muscular/cardio endurance, and aesthetics is R-E-B-O-U-N-D-I-N-G for 10 minutes each day."

— John Peterson,
    in his Transformetrics forums,
    on the subject of staying young

HIGH-KNEE SPRINTS

This is one tough exercise, I can tell you. Take the Rebound Jog to the next level by sprinting as quickly as you can comfortably and safely. This exercise works your cardiovascular system to peak efficiency.

1. Rapidly run as quickly as you can.
2. Lift your knees to waist level, one at a time.
3. Swing your right arm forward as your left knee rises to help you gain momentum.
4. Swing your left arm in front of you as your right knee rises.
5. Concentrate on breathing deeply.

Start by sprinting for 5 to 10 seconds and work up to sprinting for one minute.

THE STRENGTH BOUNCE

In the Strength Bounce, you're leaving the mat with both feet. Every bounce where your feet leave the mat is strength time. High jumps increase the G Force your body feels and resultantly strengthen every cell in your body. For more G Force and more strength, simply bounce higher; the higher you jump, the more effort you're putting in. Don't do it until you're sure of your balance, then have fun with it. Your balance will improve steadily by jumping on the rebounder.

1. Allow both feet to simultaneously leave the mat.
2. Bend and straighten your knees as your jump builds.
3. Swing your arms up and down with your bounce to help you gain momentum.
4. Jump as high as you can safely.

Make sure to consciously tighten your core as you jump. You can add variety to the High Jump by landing with one foot in front of the other and vice versa on the next jump

SLALOM BOUNCE

Imagine you're headed down a mountain on skis as you do this. Increase your challenge by jumping higher.

1. Bend your elbows and hold your forearms parallel to the ground.
2. Jump with both feet and turn your body to the right.
3. Jump with both feet and turn your body to the left.

"If you're having a bad day, try this: Jump up and down, wiggle around, you're going to feel better."

— Dr. Stuart Brown

REBOUND SHUFFLE BOUNCE

This move should look like cross-country skiing: you switch your arms and legs with each jump.

1. Stand on the rebounder with your right arm forward and your left leg forward.

2. Jump and switch the position of your feet and arms: the left arm comes forward and the right goes back as the right leg comes forward and the left leg goes back.
3. Keep jumping, switching legs with each jump.

CELLULITE BUSTER

Dave Hall says many women swear by this move as a way to burn off cellulite. No matter what state your legs are in, this exercise will get them burning. It's like a football player drill—you run fast with very small steps.

1. Stand on the rebounder with your legs about shoulder-width apart and knees slightly bent.
2. Start by moving your feet up and down in small steps, but they don't need to leave the mat.
3. Speed up and lift your feet off the mat. As Hall says, "Within about 20 seconds, I guarantee your thighs will be burning."

CREATE YOUR OWN REBOUNDING MOVES

While you're rebounding, you can augment the workout with different exercise techniques. You can target certain muscle groups by changing the position of your body while still working the whole body. For example, you can kick your legs out to the side, to the front, to the back. (Use a stabilizing bar if you kick out to the front.) By leaning forward and kicking backward you're strengthening your lower back and butt. By leaning back and kicking forward you're strengthening your quads and core. In addition, you're working your core as you maintain your balance.

SPRING INTO ACTION

Are you ready to get results with minimum effort, risk, or injury? Sound too good to be true? The only way to find out is to get started, and I dare you not to smile in delight as you do. Rebounding makes me feel like a kid jumping on my bed without my mother yelling at me to stop.

Don't be dissuaded by the misperception that exercise has to be hard to be effective. It is because rebounding is easy and fun, that you will be able to stick with it. In the end, you will look better and feel better, and the health benefits you experience will speak for themselves. So get yourself a rebounder, take off your shoes and socks, and get jumping. What do you have to lose, besides troubling health ailments and a little extra around the middle?

CHAPTER 16

MEDITATION AND BREATHWORK—PUSH-UPS AND STRESS MANAGEMENT FOR YOUR MIND

■ ■ ■

Breathing and meditation techniques are exercises that can help you reduce anxiety, sleep better, and live longer. And all you have to do is breathe your way to an Ageless version of you.

DON'T SKIP
THIS CHAPTER!

Meditation has a bad rep among a lot of Americans, especially people in our generation, who think of it as "hippy-dippy nonsense," even those Boomers who were hippies once themselves. You might be ready to skip past these exercises because you think they're silly or invalid. If so, you would be very, very wrong.

"Nothing's going to solve all of your problems, but meditation can change the relationship between you and that voice in your head which is responsible for most of the things you're probably most embarrassed about in your life."

— Dan Harris,
  author of 10 Percent Happier

Dan Harris, author of *10 Percent Happier*, once doubted the benefits of meditation, calling it "uniquely ridiculous." Harris had been the victim of a panic attack while reading the news in front of millions of television viewers. When his boss, Peter Jennings, assigned him to investigate religion and self-help, he became acquainted with the idea of "the voice in your head" that we all possess, the internal critic and instigator that often leads us to bad decisions. He recognized himself in that description, knowing that voice had led him to abuse drugs, which in turn triggered his panic attack.

He found that Buddhists had a suggestion to deal with that voice: meditate. At first, he scoffed, but as he investigated meditation, he found extensive scientific evidence to support it. "There's an enormous amount of science that says meditation is simple brain exercise that can have an extraordinary impact on your brain and your body. It can lower your blood pressure, boost your immune system, and literally rewire key parts of your brain that have to do with self-awareness, compassion, and stress," Harris said in an interview with bigthink.com.

Simple brain exercise. That's all.

"Meditation is the only intentional, systematic human activity which at bottom is about not trying to improve yourself or get anywhere else, but simply to realize where you already are."

— Jon Kabat-Zinn,
  Wherever You Go, There You Are

If you're tempted to discount meditation because of its connection to many world religions, then just think of it as exercise. For millions of people, meditation is much more than exercise, but for our purposes as Ageless Boomers, the important takeaway is that your health will improve if you incorporate meditation and breathwork as part of your exercise regimen.

STRESS IS
A KILLER

Stress is a significant factor in our lives today. Many Boomers are still working full-time jobs and dreaming of a seemingly unreachable retirement, while balancing the stresses of home life, adapting to new technologies, and constantly trying to do more in less time. Others may be retired and planning vacations but are still managing care-giving responsibilities and creating overload by trying to do too much too fast. The very technologies that are supposed to be making our lives easier are actually creating their own demands—we are at the mercy of e-mail, voicemail, texts, Facebook, Twitter, and more. As if that kind of mental anxiety isn't enough, there are also environmental factors such as pollution, aging bodies, digestive stress, and sleep deprivation. The bottom line is that no matter how hard we try, it's impossible to escape all stress.

More than 80 percent of Boomers said they feel moderate to high levels of stress related to the care or support they provide to their children, spouses, and/or parents, according to a 2014 research study conducted by The Hartford Financial Services Group and CornPsych.

We pay dearly when we fail to manage this stress over the long term. Stress triggers the release of the fight-or-flight stress hormones adrenaline, noradrenaline, and cortisol that increase heart rate and send increased blood to the muscles to prepare the body for battle—battle that generally never really happens, leaving us with an overcharge of hormones. According to leading neural-immune scientist Dr. Esther Sternberg, chronic exposure to these hormones elevates the risk of stroke and heart attack, suppresses the immune system, impairs cognition, decreases thyroid function, and drives the accumulation of abdominal fat. And the mind is not unaffected. Recent studies conducted in Argentina and Sweden found significant links between stress and mental diseases such as dementia. To top it all off, stress also disturbs our sleep, starting a grueling cycle of exhaustion, inefficiency, more stress, and less sleep.

While it's impossible to escape all stress, if you can reduce your stress levels, you will enjoy great health benefits over the long term. You can successfully reduce stress by learning and applying the healthy, simple, and effective practices to manage your stress levels discussed in this chapter.

MANAGE YOUR STRESS LEVELS

Stress is constant, so you need to practice stress management daily and consistently. Sometimes we think we're managing stress by drinking more coffee, getting more done, or sleeping less, but these practices ultimately charge a steep price. Good stress management practices feel great, so you'll look forward to doing them.

"We live longer than our forefathers; but we suffer more from a thousand artificial anxieties and cares. They fatigued only the muscles; we exhaust the finer strength of the nerves."

— Edward George Bulwer-Lytton

The first step to managing stress is to make yourself a priority. No matter how many responsibilities clamor for your time and attention, you have to take responsibility for yourself as well. When you make yourself a priority, you can make time for stress-reducing practices. Those practices include exercise (an incredibly good stress-buster), spending time with loved ones, and spending time outside in the sun and enjoying nature. I'll get into more detail about all these practices later in this chapter.

The second step toward managing your stress levels is to figure out which types of stress you can eliminate and which you can't. If you can reduce the overload on your mind and body in just a few ways, you will feel the benefits both in the short term and over the long term. Some of the stressors you need to eliminate will be unique to you: you might decide that serving on a particular committee is one stress too many. Other stressors are common to almost everyone: you can reduce the stress of exhaustion by getting better sleep (see Chapter 8), and you can reduce digestive stress by changing your diet (see Chapters 4, 5, 6, and 10).

GROW YOUR ENERGY BANK ACCOUNT

Think about your body as an energy bank account. That energy replenishes regularly, but different conditions affect the amount and speed at which your energy returns. You can increase "returns" two ways: by focusing on increasing the amount of energy you create or by decreasing the amount of energy you use. Ideally, you'd do a combination of both.

Exercise, for example, costs energy, but it's a worthwhile investment. It strengthens your entire body, which will enable you to expend less energy in the future, both when you exercise and in your daily life. You give up energy now to have more later. At the same time, exercise increases your overall energy reserves, giving you more energy—mental and physical—with which to tackle the tasks that demand your attention.

Exercise is also terrific at reducing stress, and it's nature's greatest tranquilizer, improving your sleep quality.

Likewise, spending time with loved ones and friends requires planning and energy, but it pays huge dividends in terms of reducing stress. Positive social contact not only improves your mood, it also increases longevity, improves mental function, staves off dementia, and reduces stress hormones.

Investing in exercise, spending time with friends, and getting adequate sleep can all increase your energy supply. Other practices, such as minimizing digestive stress (the amount of energy that gets diverted to digestion) can reduce energy depletion. Combine these different variables and you have a lot more energy in the bank.

Minimizing digestive stress is actually one of the best things you can do to reduce your overall stress level. As an example of how managing dietary stress can help, think about how you feel when you are tired, stressed, or anxious. Do you reach for a healthy snack or a sugary treat? We often crave something sweet, such as a chocolate bar or a cookie, but that's not what nature had in mind when it gave us a sweet tooth. What our sweet craving is trying to tell us is to reach for some fruit, which will give us a burst of vitamins and minerals, some hydration, and a sugar boost regulated by the fiber in the fruit so that we don't have an insulin spike and crash. Depending on the fruit we choose, it will also trigger a release of serotonin or dopamine, which will make us feel good. The problem with the cookie is that it provides too much refined sugar, a digestive overload, a crash, and no nutrition. The body doesn't recognize it since it's a processed food, which creates acidity in the body. So we end up cycling right back to being fatigued and stressed. The point? Reach for an apple next time you feel tired.

As Brendan Brazier explains, digestive stress can combine with other sources of stress into a toxic cocktail: "Combining the destructive nature of a largely refined-food diet with other common stressors to continue to the point at which they are chronic paves the way for many ailments—high blood pressure, blood sugar control problems, and elevated blood fats such as cholesterol among them."

But what about managing the inevitable stress that you can't eliminate? While you can't remove all sources of stress in your life, you can take steps to reduce its impact on your body. By relaxing your body, you can lower the amount of cortisol released into your body and brain. So what are the best ways to relax your body? I've got two simple and surprisingly powerful techniques. The first is to change your breathing patterns. The second is called "progressive muscle relaxation." If you practice these, you will discover new untapped reservoirs of energy and calm within yourself. And that newfound calm may very well change your life. It certainly changed mine.

CHANGE YOUR BREATHING, CHANGE YOUR LIFE

Yogi Ramacharaka once said, "Life is but a series of breaths." Breath is life. Without it we die. Breathing is obviously something we all do, but few of us give it much thought. However, it turns out that altering our breathing is a very powerful way to reduce our anxiety. Farmer Burns, a world champion "catch-as-catch-can" wrestler in the early 20th century, said, "Deep breathing alone can make a weak man strong and a sick man well." In addition to reducing stress levels, improving oxygen intake has myriad additional health benefits, including improving immune systems, lowering blood pressure, improving cell repair, removing toxins, helping to alkalize the body, driving the growth of grey matter in our brains, helping organs function better, aiding with more efficient digestion, and contributing to general mental and physical well-being. NASA reveals that astronauts are given 100 percent oxygen while on missions to promote clear minds, reduce stress, boost energy levels, and foster good health.

It is vital to ensure ample oxygen delivery down to our cells. Lack of oxygen has been revealed to be associated with cancer and all manner of diseases. Dr. W. Spencer Way related in the *Journal of the American Association of Physicians*, "Insufficient oxygen means insufficient biological energy that can result in anything from mild fatigue to life-threatening disease. The link between insufficient oxygen and disease has now been firmly established." Nobel Prize winner Dr. Otto Warburg, Director of the Max Planck Institute for Cell Physiology in Berlin, confirmed that the fundamental precondition for cancer is a lack of oxygen at the cellular level.

"We are all born knowing how to inhale and exhale correctly, but with today's technology, hurried schedules, and everyday stress, most of us have lost that ability. As a result, most of us 'under-breathe' in a dysfunctional way...You can have the heart and cardiovascular system of an elite athlete but the lungs and breathing muscles of a total couch potato."

— *Belisa Vranich, Psy.D.*
Breathe: 14 Days to Oxygenating, Recharging,
and Fueling Your Body and Brain

The rest of this chapter shares breathing techniques to help you optimize your oxygen intake and manage your stress through breathwork and meditation. Note that breathwork and meditation are not separate categories—breathwork is highly meditative, and meditation almost always uses breath as a focus. I've started with breathwork to get you used to the simple idea of conscious breathing. They are the most powerful stress busters around, and they're available to you all the time. So take a breath, and let's get started.

We've all been breathing since the moment we were born, but over the years, we have learned some poor subconscious habits that negatively affect our breathing efficiency. If we pay attention to our breathing and learn to breathe correctly, we can retrain our bodies to breathe the way nature intended—even when we're not aware of it. The U.S. Food and Drug Administration now recognizes breath training as a viable treatment for hypertension, and more than 1,000 studies have revealed that it is proven effective in relieving anxiety, depression, chronic fatigue, stress and tension, and other physical problems while simultaneously building energy and endurance and contributing to emotional mastery. Some yogis believe that we're given a set number of breaths in life—and we stop living when we use them up. The point being: we will even live longer if we learn to breathe more efficiently.

Meditation is like push-ups for your brain. When you practice controlled breathing during meditation, it can actually increase the size of your brain according to a 2005 Harvard study. Regular meditation practice boosts cortical thickness and may even slow age-related thinning of the frontal cortex for Boomers.

To begin conscious breathing, count your normal breaths per minute to determine your current breath frequency. Count a single inhale and exhale as one breath. Focus on taking slow, quiet, deep, and regular breaths. Try not to let your mind wander. If it does, just firmly refocus it on your breath and the sensation of the air moving through your nostrils. (This refocusing effort is the "push-up" of meditation—more on that soon.) Over time, your unconscious breathing will begin to mimic your conscious breathing, so you will enjoy the benefit of correct breathing all the time.

Most people in America take about 12 to 20 breaths per minute under normal circumstances, but under stress, you take even more. Over the years I've measured my breathing numerous times, and I usually take no more than 4 to 5 breaths per minute. If your breaths are in the 16-20 range, you are taking short, rapid, shallow breaths. This shallow breathing leaves lots of stale air in your lungs and can lead to greater stress.

THE RELAXING BREATH

One of the first exercises I learned is a "Relaxing Breath" exercise. It's almost ridiculously simple, but it makes all the difference in the world. This exercise is one of the best ways for people who are new to breathwork to experience the benefits of it right away. I started doing this exercise when I was dealing with the stresses of working on Wall Street, and it worked like a charm. I also use it for plane trips or if I'm having trouble getting to sleep, because it's an instant tranquilizer. You can do it lying down, sitting, or standing. If you can, close your eyes—

you want to have as few senses stimulated as possible—and follow these steps:

1. Exhale completely through your nose by drawing your stomach in, trying to pull your belly button to your spine, and releasing all the stale air from the bottom of your lungs.
2. Inhale completely through your nose by feeling your belly expand and rise through your rib cage and chest all the way to your clavicle.
3. Put your hand on your belly and silently count to four as you feel your belly rise as you breathe in; try to imagine the inhalation as a smooth wave of air flowing in and upward through your core.
4. Exhale completely through your nose, drawing your belly in as you count to at least eight.
5. Squeeze out the last bit of air by imagining you're pulling your belly button all the way back to your spine.
6. Begin again immediately with the next breath.
7. Repeat as many times as necessary until you feel calm.

Note that there are an infinite number of variations on this exercise. Your main objective is to keep your exhalation at least twice as long as your inhalation. As long as you maintain the longer exhalation, you achieve a relaxing effect—no matter how many seconds it takes. Take note of how you feel after you're done. If you're doing it properly, you should feel instantly more relaxed. You can do the Relaxing Breath several times a day, any time you feel the need for it. The more you do it, the more effective it becomes. Try doing it two or three times a day at first, then build up as needed.

THE ONE-MINUTE BREATH

Another favorite exercise of mine is what I call the "One-Minute Breath." Some yogis will tell you that this kind of slow breathing is a form of meditation. All I know is that it fills me with a simultaneous combination of energy and a profound sense of calm. Start by keeping your mouth lightly closed throughout the duration of the exercise, and follow these steps:

1. Inhale very slowly, very deeply through your nostrils into your belly, into your chest, and then up to your clavicle for a total of 20 seconds.
2. Hold your breath for 20 seconds.
3. Exhale slowly through your nostrils for a full 20 seconds.
4. Inhale immediately again on the next breath and repeat the exercise.
5. Continue 1-2 minutes at a time. As you continue practicing, go for longer and longer times.

I do 31 breaths in 31 minutes. When you're just starting out, I recommend that you begin with a much shorter count—even as short as five seconds per stage (five seconds per inhale, five seconds holding, and five seconds exhaling for a total of 15 seconds)—and slowly add seconds over time until you reach a one-minute cycle of 20 seconds inhale, 20 seconds holding your breath, and 20 seconds exhale.

An advanced form of the breath is 15 seconds inhaling, 15 seconds retaining the breath, 15 seconds exhaling, and 15 seconds holding the

A 2010 study published in the Journal of Alzheimer's Disease reported improved cognitive function in people with memory loss who practiced meditation for only 12 minutes per day over an eight-week period. Ultimately, those who practice meditation regularly, even for short periods of time, fare better on measures of associative learning, cognitive skills, mental health, and aging than those who don't practice meditation.

breath out. Do this for 31 to 33 minutes. Don't be afraid to get creative with this breathing technique. Try five seconds in, five seconds hold, and 10 seconds out. I find it very relaxing to inhale 15 seconds, hold 15 seconds, exhale 30 seconds. By practicing a variety of forms, you will increase your lung capacity. Just remember that the longer you exhale, the deeper relaxation you will achieve.

UJJAYI BREATHING

One way to slow your breathing down is to try ujjayi (ooh-jah-yee) breathing, which is a form of diaphragmatic breath used in Taoist and Yoga practices. Gently constrict your throat as you inhale and exhale through your nose. You should be able to hear the air passing through your throat, making an ocean-like sound. Keep your mouth closed. Yogis believe that this activates the energetic center of your throat, and the effect can be very relaxing. If you feel discomfort, stop, take a few breaths, and try again. Build up gradually by adding one second to each inhale and each exhale each day. Stop if you ever feel uncomfortable, as that is counterproductive.

BREATH OF FIRE

Another breathing technique that I recommend is the "Breath of Fire." It is slightly

According to Julie T. Lusk, the author of "Yoga Meditations," ujjayi breathing improves concentration and develops stamina and endurance. Additional benefits include alleviated pain from headaches, and reduction of sinus pressure, lessened phlegm, and strengthened nervous and digestive systems.

challenging to learn, but it is very satisfying once you master it. It is essentially the opposite of the One-Minute Breath, since instead of slowing down your breathing, you speed it up to 120-180 breaths per minute. The effect is highly

According to the Framingham Study, if you do nothing to improve your breathing techniques, you will by age 70 lose more than 70 percent of what you had at age 20. If you increase lung efficiency and prevent volume loss as you age, the longer your life will be.

energizing, as you'll feel a surge of energy course through your body. Here's what you do:

1. Put the tip of your tongue on the ridge above your upper teeth in the yogic position and close your mouth.
2. Keep your chest relaxed and high.
3. Begin breathing rapidly through your nose, expelling the air smoothly and continuously by bringing your belly button toward your spine each time.
4. Focus on your sharp exhalation, and your inhalation should become automatic.
5. Strive to equalize the length of inhalations and exhalations.

Note that both inhale and exhale should take the same amount of time. You're not breathing into your chest during this exercise—it's all in the stomach. Do this for just a few seconds when you start, aim for a rate of 120 breaths per minute at first. (Don't actually count all the way to 120. If you count your exhalations for five seconds—10 times in five seconds—you'll get a sense of how fast to breathe.) Focus on getting the technique right and note the surge of energy afterward. Gradually increase the number of breaths and how long you do this. Work up to 31 minutes or whatever feels right to you. Be sure to stop if you begin to feel dizzy, take some complete yogic breaths, and then try again. I do the breath of fire for three minutes before my one-minute breath meditation.

ALTERNATE NOSTRIL BREATHING

Another exercise that I learned when I first began to practice breathwork is called "Alternate Nostril Breathing," and I still do it now and then when I need calm energy. I always feel refreshed, my mood is improved, I think more clearly, and I feel more balanced after doing it.

1. Place the tip of your index finger of your dominant hand on the spot between your eyebrows.
2. Using your thumb, press one nostril closed and inhale through the opposite nostril.
3. Release your thumb and press down with your middle finger on the nostril through which you just inhaled; exhale through the nostril you just released.
4. Keeping your finger in place, breathe in through that same nostril that you just exhaled through.
5. Release your finger and press down with your thumb. Repeat the process, starting from step 2.

Basically, you switch nostrils at the end of each inhale (e.g., breathe in through the left nostril, close left, out through the right, in through the right, close the right nostril, out through the left). As you do this, make sure you are breathing slowly and gently but fully and deeply. Focus on how the air feels as it moves up and into your nostril and back out again through the other nostril. Pay attention to how different kinds of breathing can have different effects. For instance, a slow inhalation followed by a fast exhalation should give you energy. The opposite—a fast inhalation followed by a much slower exhalation—should have a relaxing effect. Manipulate your breathing depending on whether you want a stress buster or energy booster.

Try to practice daily in the morning before eating. If you can, practice outside in the cleanest air you can find. If you're in the city, stay inside. You don't want to breathe in a lot of highly polluted air. As you get better at doing this, you'll find that your breaths will get longer. Eventually, you'll want to take no more than five or six breaths per minute. But don't force them to be longer. Just let it happen over time. Note that you can also combine the pace of the Relaxing Breath with the Alternate Nostril Breathing. The more you practice, the more naturally your body will breathe effectively—and in doing so, you can create a shield against stress and anxiety.

"Breathing is the key that unlocks the whole catalog of advanced biological function and development. Is it any wonder that it is so central to every aspect of health? Breathing is the first place, not the last, one should look when fatigue, disease, or other evidence of disordered energy presents itself. Breathing is truly the body's most basic communication system."

—Dr. Sheldon Saul Hendler,
Oxygen Breakthrough

In *10 Percent Happier*, Dan Harris gives some of the simplest meditation instructions ever:

1. Sit comfortably…Whatever your position, you should keep your spine straight, but don't strain.

2. Feel your breath. Pick a spot: nose, belly, or chest. Really try to feel the in-breath and then the out-breath. [Try to breathe normally.]

3. This one is the key: every time you get lost in thought—which you will, thousands of times—gently return to the breath. I cannot stress strongly enough that forgiving yourself and starting over is the whole game. As my friend and meditation teacher Sharon Salzberg has written, "Beginning again and again is the actual practice, not a problem to overcome so that one day we can come to the 'real' meditation."

—*10 Percent Happier*, "Appendix: Instructions"

Simple, right? But how is this different from breathwork? On the level of basic physical activity, it's not: both exercises involve sitting comfortably and breathing. Step three, as Harris says, is the key: your goal is to achieve mental focus. Remember how I said meditation was like push-ups for your brain? Step three is the pushup. The work comes in constantly bringing your focus back to your breath. Like balancing on one foot, where you constantly adjust your muscles to stay centered, you will constantly adjust your mind during meditation, gently and repeatedly bringing it back to the center—in this case, your breath.

Most people give up on meditation because they think they can't focus. They don't understand that losing focus and bringing it back

Meditate every day.

You can choose among the many exercises suggested in this chapter, but be sure to do some form of meditation or breathwork for at least a few minutes every day. I have more lung capacity now, at 69, than I did at 20.

is the practice of meditation. It's an essential part of the process.

FOLLOWING YOUR BREATH MEDITATION

If you're ready to take conscious breathing to the next level, you can use breathwork as a form of a meditation. This involves focusing your mind entirely on the act of breathing and taking full complete breaths. To do this, lie down someplace comfortable or sit or even stand. In the beginning, place one palm down on your belly and the other on your chest. You do this to make sure you're breathing properly—your belly should rise first, then rise like a wave up the torso until finally your breath raises your chest slightly. As you get more advanced, you may want to have your hands by your sides or in your lap, with the tips of your thumbs touching the tips of your index fingers. Keep your mouth lightly closed, and follow these steps:

1. Begin by taking a few complete breaths.
2. Inhale and exhale slowly through your nose.
3. Focus on conscious but normal breathing—do not try to affect your breath in any way.
4. Feel your belly rise and fall.
5. Keep your mind focused on the sensation of the air flowing in and out through your nostrils. If your mind wanders, bring it back to your breath.

How long should you keep going? Harris writes, "No one has figured out the dosage question [How much do I have to meditate to get benefits?] yet. I don't have any evidence for this, but I think if you can manage five minutes, you'll start seeing changes in your own life, particularly as it relates to your level of emotional reactivity."

I suggest that you aim to meditate for 20 to 30 minutes, but I also suggest that you work up to that time. Try it for three minutes the first time, then increase the duration a little bit each day. This following of your breath is one of the simplest and most effective meditation practices available to us. Note how calm and rejuvenated you feel afterward. Sit quietly for a few minutes after your meditation ends and note how you feel. You should feel much more relaxed, although for some people it takes time and practice to gain that relaxation.

WALKING MEDITATION

Some people enjoy what's called a walking meditation. This is a great option for those who have trouble sitting still. Ideally, you'd do this outside, but it can be done inside as well. The idea is to coordinate the breath counts with your strides

1. Start your inhale and count the number of steps you take as you inhale.
2. Exhale and count the number of steps you take while exhaling.

When you start, you may take two steps on the inhale, then two steps on the exhale. But as you do this more, you may take four or five steps on the inhale, and as many as eight to ten steps on the exhale. Your pace will naturally slow down. You can even incorporate this into your daily routine, such as walking to the phone, walking to get the mail, etc. It can take some getting used to, but it is very meditative and a good mind-body focus exercise.

Progressive muscle relaxation is an important stress management technique that was developed in the early 1920s by Edmund Jackson, an American physician. Jackson's research revealed that muscle fibers tense up and shorten when we get anxious, triggering a variety of physical and psychological disorders. He developed Progressive Muscle Relaxation to release stress from muscle tension, alleviate anxiety, and provide a relaxing effect on the body and mind. The process is simple:

1. Begin by taking a couple of deep breaths.
2. Strongly flex a specific muscle—your bicep, for instance—and hold it tight, flexed for a few seconds.
3. Relax the muscle until it feels completely limp.
4. Focus your mind on what you're doing, which is going from one extreme to the other.
5. Repeat with every muscle of your body.

At the end of the process, you'll find that you're both relaxed and warmed up. This is a great technique to practice before bed to overcome sleeplessness. The American Academy of Sleep Medicine concluded in 1999 that progressive muscle relaxation was one of only three non-pharmacologic treatments demonstrated successful for the treatment of chronic insomnia. It can also be used any other time of day that you need to release a bit of built-up stress; for example, it was employed regularly by pilots during WWII, especially on their way to a mission.

You can do it one muscle at a time or two at a time (e.g., both biceps at once), or you can start with your toes and work up. Here's an example of possible timing:

1. Build your contraction to peak intensity for three-to-four seconds while you're inhaling fully and deeply.
2. When you reach the peak contraction, start exhaling through your lightly closed mouth for seven-to-twelve seconds, making an "sssssss" sound as you do, tensing that muscle and tightly holding the contraction.
3. Slowly release the tension for three-to-four seconds while you're inhaling and exhaling.
4. Relax completely with seven-to-ten deep breaths between muscles.
5. Move on to the next body part.

Another version of this exercise (which I described in chapter 13) is to flex all your muscles at once. I learned this exercise from John Peterson—he describes it in *The Isometric Power Revolution*. To do this, stand in a relaxed position with your arms at your sides and hands loose. While inhaling for three-to-four seconds, simultaneously start tensing all your muscles until you reach a peak of tension at the count of four, then exhale through your teeth, making an "sssssss" sound and counting to 12 seconds while holding that peak contraction. You'll feel an immediate surge of warmth. Then relax on the next inhalation and exhalation over the course of three-to-four seconds. Take three deep breaths, then repeat two or more times. If you do this three times a day, you'll feel the difference right away.

RESPECT YOUR BODY'S NATURAL LIMITS

Everyone has a finite amount of energy, and as a Boomer, you may be becoming especially aware of this. The reality is that the less you stress your body out, the more energy you will have to tackle daily life. So pace yourself, monitor your activities, and don't try to do everything at once to avoid Boomer burnout. One of the biggest mistakes we make in this day and age is to continually push ourselves past our natural limits, and as Boomers we often try to do activities at the rates we would have maintained when we were younger. Remember that it's especially important to be relaxed before you exercise, since a relaxed body is less likely to become an injured body. Sometimes it can take as little as taking three complete yogic breaths or doing a few minutes of meditation, alternate nostril breathing, or progressive muscle relaxation, or any of the other relaxation techniques I've described to get your body into the proper state for a workout.

If you are just beginning to exercise regularly or try out these new breathing techniques, make sure to build up slowly. I try to aim for an increase of 5 percent every week or two. Conscious breathing—slow, deep, quiet, and regular—will help us to slow down and take small breaks. I firmly believe that the success of

our training—whether body or mind—lies in how well and how quickly we recover between exercises.

"We breathe 20,000 times a day. That means we have 20,000 opportunities to feel better every day."

— Dr. Gay Hendricks,
The Breathing Box

An increasing number of studies are pointing out that meditation, breathwork, exercise, and other natural stress-management techniques are just as effective as, or even more effective than, modern antidepressants developed in the chemistry lab without the negative side effects of medication. Research from Harvard University has even demonstrated that meditation has the power to alter our brain structures and make them more resistant to memory loss and other brain diseases. Ultimately, however, the only way to really understand the powerful benefits of proper deep breathing and other stress-relief techniques is to try them yourself. You'll be amazed at how effective they are and how quickly you start to feel calmer, more energized, and more balanced.

AFTERWORD:
THE END OF AGING

As Boomers, for most of our lives we have accepted the idea that with age comes sickness, frailty, weakness, pain, and discomfort. That's the pattern we've seen in our parents and grandparents, and we have simply assumed that we will follow the same path. But we were wrong.

The longest-lived populations in the world show us that being healthy your whole life is natural. You don't have to be sick. You don't have to lose your youthful vigor. You can be vigorous in your 100s. You can live pain-free, with a sharp mind and great mobility. You won't have to become dependent on others, because you won't be sick and frail. You'll live an active life as a centenarian. Research and experience show us how to end "aging" as we know it. We will not only live longer, we will live healthier.

If you want to live a long and healthy life, this book gives you the roadmap. Good nutrition—whole-food, plant-based eating—and regular, well-rounded exercise combined with sleep, hydration, and stress management provides you with the tools your mind and body need. When given those tools, the body heals itself and prevents further damage.

Health, like love, or joy, or happiness, is one of life's greatest gifts. And of all these things, health is the one you can control the most. When you give yourself that gift, you enrich your life and the lives of all the people who care about and depend on you.

When I was 15 and my mother's health began to fail, I remember our many visits to the doctor. I remember looking around at the people in the waiting room, sick and miserable, and I decided that I would never let that happen to myself. I felt the same way as I watched my father's health fail. I watched him go from a tall, strong, strapping man to one who was stooped and frail from chemotherapy. I heard his voice change from youthful to frail and old. I don't want my children and grandchildren to see that happen to me.

I could talk about the benefits of this lifestyle all day, to anyone who will listen. But in the end, you must give this gift to yourself. It's not a quick-fix; it's a life-long practice that requires your daily choices to be healthy. The rewards, however, are well worth it.

The gift of health is very personal and meaningful to me. I wrote this book because I believe I have found the best path to longevity and vitality, and I want to share it with you.

From time to time, I come across people who have never heard about WFPB eating, and they say, "Oh, I could never do that." I respond, politely, by asking them the following questions:

- Would you rather live, look, and feel younger than your years, or die from an easily preventable disease years ahead of your true potential?

- Would you rather be sitting on the sidelines of life because you're too heavy and too tired, or have an abundance of energy and exuberance for living that never tires?
- Would you rather have diabetes and kidney disease that requires dialysis, or prevent either from ever happening to you?

By now, you've read this book and you understand the message: you have control over your health and your body, and your choices will shape your health destiny. Respect your body's need for proper nutrition, exercise, and sleep. If you give your body what it needs consistently, I believe you can live to 120 years old in excellent physical, mental, and emotional health.

It's your choice. You could begin right now. Go grab an apple, take a walk, try a new vegetable for your dinner salad. It's that simple.

APPENDICES

MORE THINGS YOU NEED TO KNOW

■■■

APPENDIX A

HOW TO COMBINE FOOD
FAMILIES

■ ■ ■

This appendix explains the details of how to combine
foods for the most efficient digestion. It breaks down the
specifics—for the overview of food combining
and why it can make a difference for you, please see
Chapter 10.

Every food is a little bit different, but in general you can follow the rules based on these categories of foods. The food families here include only whole, plant-based foods—by now you know that animal foods and refined foods shouldn't be part of your diet!

FAMILY A: FRUIT

1. The quickest digesting whole food is any variety of melon: watermelon, cantaloupe, galia, honeydew, and so on. Melon takes only about 20 minutes to digest (depending on how much you have; the more you eat, the longer it takes). They are especially great right after a workout, partly because they have such a high water content and also because you get a good amount of antioxidants during your post workout window.

2. Acid fruits: all citrus fruits, including oranges, grapefruits, lemons, limes, kiwis, pineapples, pomegranates, strawberries, raspberries, tangerines, tangelos, and tomatoes.

It is interesting to know that I have never had a person come to me who was ill or in difficulty from eating too many fruits and vegetables; the trouble lies mainly with eating too many starches or animal proteins."

—Bernard Jensen, DC, PhD,
   Blending Magic

3. Sub-acid fruits: apples, pears, peaches, plums, papayas, mangoes, some blueberries, blackberries, apricots, and cherries.

4. Sweet fruits and sun-dried fruits: bananas, dates (fresh and dried), figs (fresh and dried), raisins, grapes, persimmons, and cherimoya.

"Disease stems from deficiencies and a lack of understanding of Mother Nature's laws of health, plus the unwillingness to accept the obligation to keep the precious temple—the body—in order. This is accomplished by keeping it clean and well nourished. And of course providing necessary aids—such as rest, relaxation, positive thinking and plenty of exercise through hard work."

—Ann Wigmore,
   Why Suffer? How I Overcame Illness and Pain Naturally

FAMILY B. VEGETABLES

1. Leafy greens: kale, mustard greens, radish tops, spinach, Swiss chard (green and red), collard greens, green cabbage, bok choy.

2. Vegetable fruits: Peppers, tomatoes, cucumbers.

3. Other vegetables: radishes, onions, garlic.

4. Starchier vegetables: beets, carrots, turnips, sweet potatoes, yams.

FAMILY C. PROTEIN

Seeds and nuts (these are listed as protein, but they're also high in essential fatty acids).

FAMILY D. FATS

Avocado (also a protein), olives (try to get the unsalted kind), and vegetable oils (however, I don't use oils because they are fractured foods).

FASTEST TO SLOWEST DIGESTING COMBINATIONS

Vegetable juice (always alone)

Melons (always alone)

Fruit monomeals

Combining fruits within the same category with celery and green leafy vegetables in a blended salad

Combining fruits within same category, e.g., sub-acid with sub-acid; acid with acid

Combining fruits in adjoining category, e.g., acid with sub-acid; sub-acid with sweet

Leafy greens

Starchier vegetables

Vegetable combinations

Avocadoes with leafy greens and tomatoes (don't combine with protein)

Seeds and nuts together with other vegetables, such as tomatoes, leafy greens, and celery

Beans and vegetables

Beans and whole grains

RULES

You should always eat melon alone or with other melons. Whenever possible, eat one type of fruit at a time. If you want to combine them, you can combine fruits from the same category well (sweet fruits with other sweet fruits, or sub-acid with other sub-acid). Acid and sub-acid fruits combine fairly well, as do sub-acid and sweet fruits. Note that acid and sweet do not combine very well.

Fruits (except for melons, which need to be eaten alone) can also be combined with lettuce (and other leafy greens) and celery in a blended salad because those greens are neutral. Sweet fruits with lettuce and celery are an especially satisfying combination. Tomatoes combine very well with leafy greens and avocado.

It's a mistake to eat fruits for dessert because it will have to wait until the other food is digested and will therefore start to ferment and putrefy. That's why it's important to always eat fruit on an empty stomach.

Never combine an acid food with a starch food. If you eat an orange with a grain, the fruit will have to wait until the grain is digested. Also avoid eating nuts with grains because it slows digestion of both those foods.

Plan to eat one type of protein per meal. If you eat different protein sources at once (nuts and beans), digestion will suffer. Different enzymes are required to digest each one, so the body gets bogged down and confused. However, you can have a variety of nuts because they're close cousins.

Do not combine a fat with a protein. For example, avocadoes with nuts or seeds are not a great combination. This rule changes over time. For example, I can now have an avocado salad with ground flax seeds and/or hempseed sprinkled on top, but that's because I've been doing this for a long time and have a strong digestive system.

When your digestive strength increases, you can relax on the food-combining rules. However, if you consume whole grains, have them with leafy greens, never with seeds and nuts, no matter how strong your digestive system is.

APPENDIX B

SUPERFOODS

■■■

Here is a list of my favorite superfoods. These nutritional
powerhouses can enhance a raw plant-based diet.
You'll find the specific features of each one and ways to
consume them listed below. Many of these are also
excellent as part of an anti-radiation diet.

Hemp seed is, very simply, one of the most nutritious foods on Earth. It is a complete protein source that includes all the essential amino acids. You can get all the protein your body needs from this one seed. It is much better than animal protein and won't raise cholesterol levels since there is no saturated fat. It's the most easily digestible seed or nut, so it's not a drain on your energy. If you chew hemp seed thoroughly, it will just about dissolve into a liquid.

It contains enzyme-rich antioxidants, and it's an excellent source of essential fatty acids, all of which are monounsaturated fats. It contains a perfect balance of omega 3s, omega 6s, and omega 9s, which is good for your brain, cardiovascular system, joint lubrication, hormonal system, and more. It's much better than seafood, which is full of antibiotics (when farmed) or mercury and other heavy metals, pesticides, etc. (when caught wild).

"Maybe a person's time would be as well spent raising food as raising money to buy food."

— Frank A. Clark

Hemp seed is available shelled and unshelled. It has plenty of fiber when it has its shell, but shelled hemp seed is not quite as high in fiber. All hemp seeds sold in the United States are heat-sterilized as required by law.

This amazing seed is also vitamin and mineral rich. It's very high in vitamins B and E, calcium, magnesium, copper, zinc, and other minerals. It's one of the only nuts and seeds that contains chlorophyll, which explains the slightly green tinge. It has excellent anti-inflammatory properties, boosts immunity, detoxifies, and improves bone strength and blood health.

Please note that while some of these foods come powdered or in capsules, they are *whole foods, not* nutritional supplements.

It's excellent for workout recovery because of its intense mix of all three macronutrients (fats, protein, and carbohydrates). Have these about one to two hours after your post workout meal. You get the additional benefit of the synergistic effect of all of these nutrients working together.

The mild flavor of hemp seed makes it easy to incorporate into your diet. Consume 1 to 3 spoonfuls plain, add to salads and blended salads, or use in a dressing with celery and tomatoes.

Hemp seed does not need to be refrigerated until you open the package. Once you open the package, make sure that you get all the air out when you reseal it and keep it in refrigerator. Nutiva and Manitoba Harvest are two good options that come with expiration dates and resealable bags.

This blue-green algae was one of the first foods on Earth. It is a complete food source, and some people claim you can live on spirulina alone. It contains many essential fatty acids, including the rare fatty acid GLA (found in breast milk and essential for infant development), which improves health of your skin and hair and helps combat allergies. It contains a very bioavailable form of iron and it's one of the highest protein foods. The high protein content makes it excellent for athletic recovery.

Spirulina is loaded with antioxidants that provide protection against free radicals, lowering the risk of disease, reducing the effects of aging, and even helping prevent sunburn. Consuming it is a very effective way to build up your immune system. It contains almost a dozen carotenoids (powerful antioxidants that are linked with longevity), with far more beta-carotene than carrots. It's an excellent source of chlorophyll, is enzyme-rich, contains a full spectrum of minerals and vitamins (over 100 known nutrients), and contains sulfur, which will help you recover after workouts and is also a detoxifier.

The taste of spirulina can take some getting used to. Mix a spoonful into water, add it to

All whole vegetables, fruits, seeds, nuts, and beans are superfoods, in that they offer you excellent nutrition. The superfoods in this appendix are worth special mention because they pack so much nutritional value into a tiny package.

blended salads, or sprinkle it on salad. Another option is to add it to guacamole. Start slowly— just a teaspoon at first, then work your way up to 1 ounce.

This single-celled algae is a very popular health food in Japan, and it's one of Brendan Brazier's most highly praised superfoods. As Brazier says in *Thrive*, "I could write a whole book just on chlorella's amazing attributes and practical applications." Chlorella is one of the best sources of chlorophyll, which helps maintain an alkaline state and is essential for optimal health. It's very high in easily digestible, alkaline, complete protein as well as iron. It contains RNA, DNA, and CGF (Chlorella Growth Factor), all of which contribute to cell repair and renewal, so it's excellent for workout recovery.

In addition to being a great source of protein and iron, chlorella is high in antioxidants, so it strengthens the immune system and supports longevity. It's excellent for bone health as well as the health of the brain and nervous system.

Chlorella is a great all-around protective shield against environmental pollutants because it's very good at drawing out heavy metal contamination. It's especially good for detoxification, such as eliminating mercury or lead from your system. Take extra chlorella when you know that you're going to have X-rays taken because it is protective against radiation.

Not only does chlorella aid digestion and help assimilate nutrients from other foods, it also increases digestive strength. It speeds up growth of good bacteria in your digestive tract.

As a result, chlorella can also have a dramatic cleansing effect, so start slowly and give your body time to adapt. Brazier recommends 1.5 grams for anyone; he notes that he personally takes up to 15 grams when he's doing heavy training. Go slowly, and if you are on a low-iron diet for any reason, don't exceed 10 grams a day.

PISTACHIO NUTS

These nuts are the new almonds. They're rich in plant sterols, carotenoids, tocopherols, and arginine. Plant sterols provide a cholesterol-lowering benefit. All nuts have cholesterol-lowering benefits and other cardio-protective effects, but pistachios and pine nuts are highest.

Arginine is an amino acid involved in nitric oxide production, which regulates relaxation. Together they promote blood vessel and heart health and provide an abundance of nutrients. They decrease inflammation, increase antioxidant levels, and reduce oxidative stress.

MACA

Grown in mineral-rich volcanic soil at altitudes above 10,000 feet, this ancient Peruvian plant used to be consumed by Incan warriors before battle. Maca is said to increase strength and stamina and enhance libido and fertility.

Maca is a powerful adaptogen, which means that it can balance your body's hormones and help you adapt more efficiently to your

"Many of the major chronic diseases of modern industrialized societies, such as heart disease, hypertension, obesity, adult-onset diabetes, dental caries, and some types of cancer have a dietary basis."

— Timothy Johns, Ph.D.,
The Origins of Human Diet and Medicine

environment. For instance, it can help your body overcome the stress of a sudden change in altitude. It creates strong resistance to disease and normalizes functions in your body. It supports adrenal function and regeneration and reduces stress on adrenals, which also helps with immunity.

By reducing cortisol production, you increase serotonin (happy hormone) levels. Maca provides raw materials that the body needs to produce

338

serotonin, helping to reduce anxiety, stress, and depression.

Maca increases DHEA levels, which are known to help bone, muscle, and skin health, enhance the immune system, lower cholesterol, increase energy, and, reputedly, enhance your memory. It's also mineral rich, especially in magnesium, calcium, zinc, potassium, and iron, making it excellent for your general vitality and endurance.

Maca comes in powder form or capsules. Take anywhere from 2 to 4 capsules a day or add a spoonful of powder to blended salads. Your goal should be 6 to 7 grams per day. Take a break every so often (for instance, 1 day off every week, 1 week off every 6 weeks, and 1 month off every 6 months). This ensures that your body doesn't adapt to it and that it will continue to be effective.

PURE SYNERGY

This supplement contains over 60 ingredients, all of which come from nature. It contains a combination of superfoods, making it, in my opinion, the ultimate superfood. It has Chinese herbs, a dozen different algae, sea vegetables, Western herbs, mushrooms, roots, and more. Every single ingredient is powerful and deeply nourishing. It is, without a doubt, my favorite superfood of all time. It contains no fillers or preservatives. It gives your body what it needs for optimal performance.

Mitchell May, who developed Pure Synergy, had an accident that severely damaged his legs. They were fractured in 40 places, with all kinds of nerve and muscle damage, but he would not let the doctors amputate. As a result of Pure Synergy mixed in vegetable juice, he recovered the full use of his legs. It is said that he regenerated nerve, bone, and muscle tissue, which doctors had not thought possible.

Pure Synergy revitalizes and strengthens your immune system, improves endurance, and detoxifies. It contains RNA and DNA (like spirulina), sprouts of fruits, vegetables, grains (quinoa and millet sprouts, sprouts of many antioxidant-rich fruits), and enzymes. It's excellent for cell and muscle tissue repair, so it's great before or after a workout. It's loaded with antioxidants (it even contains royal jelly), protein, carbohydrates, and chlorophyll, so it's an excellent shield against all the stresses of modern-day life.

"Could cancer lose its grip on modern societies if they turned to a balanced vegetarian diet? The answer is 'yes,' according to two major reports, one by the World Cancer Research Fund and the other by the Committee on the Medical Aspects of Food and Nutrition Policy in the United Kingdom. The reports conclude that a diet rich in plant foods and the maintenance of a healthy body weight could annually prevent four million cases of cancer worldwide."

— Andreas Moritz, Natural News, 2009

339

It's a powerful detoxifier, so start slowly, with as little as 1/4 teaspoon and work up to a heaping tablespoon or two a day. Consume Pure Synergy on an empty stomach so that your body absorbs it quickly. You can consume it in powder or capsule form. In powder form, mix a heaping tablespoon with water until it dissolves. This will activate all the energy in it. You can also put it in vegetable juice or a smoothie. Once you activate it, you should drink it right away. I like the taste of it, but if you find it a bit strong, mix it with a bit of honey at first to make it more palatable. Once it's opened, keep it in the freezer to make it last longer. Capsules are a good option if you're traveling or just like to have them in convenient form. They're more expensive but contain the same ingredients.

GOJI BERRIES

These little raisin-sized berries are believed to enhance longevity, increase endurance, strength, sexual energy, and improve your immune system, among other things. They're a complete protein source, and they're vitamin and mineral rich (especially in zinc and selenium). Some Native American tribes, such as the Apache, consumed them. They are enormously rich in antioxidants (much higher than blueberries) as well as adaptogen, so they offer a natural way to get everything working better. They get the body to produce more Human Growth Hormone (HGH), which is part of why they're credited with increasing longevity. They affect levels of all hormones, and they're excellent for adrenals.

Consume 2 to 4 ounces a day. Eat them alone, toss into a blended salad, or add to trail mix or a salad.

> "If your wealth is a number, your health would be the leading '1' on a $1,000,000,000,000 ($1 trillion) jackpot. All the other zeroes represent your material wealth — a house, a car, your investments … etc. As you can see, without the "1" in front, it will just be $0,000,000,000,000 which is basically NOTHING. This is the same as your health. If you're NOT healthy, if you're getting sick all the time, all your riches do NOT matter."
>
> — Allan Inocente,
>   Rich Money Habits

AFA (APHANIZOMENON FLOS-AQUAE)

Also known as Klamath Lake blue-green algae, this phytoplankton is very rich in vitamins, minerals, and antioxidants. Loaded with B vitamins (anti-stress nutrients) and vitamin C, it's very high in chlorophyll. It contains long-chain omega 3s, which are the best kind because the body doesn't have to use extra energy to convert them. It also contains the fatty acids ALA and

DHA (as does fish oil, but AFA doesn't have heavy metal contamination). It offers a perfect balance of omega 3s, 6s, and 9s, which is important for long-term health. AFA is one of the most digestible forms of complete protein. It enhances mental focus, is high in beta-carotene, and is an excellent detoxifier, especially for heavy metals.

AFA does not taste especially good when mixed alone with water. It is one of the primary ingredients in Pure Synergy, however, so you can use that supplement as a source of AFA.

FLAX SEEDS

These seeds are extremely nutritious, and I use them interchangeably with hemp seeds (and sometimes both at the same time). They are high in fiber, both soluble and insoluble, so they're great for cleaning out your body. They're loaded with plant lignans, which are excellent for disease prevention and reputed to help with cancer recovery. They contain omega 3s, including ALA, and other essential fatty acids, which are great for an anti-inflammatory diet and help metabolize fat. Essential fatty acids are great for lowering your triglycerides, helping to prevent heart disease, and lowering blood pressure and cholesterol, especially LDLs.

Flax seeds are a good choice for men with enlarged prostates and women who want to prevent breast cancer. These potassium-rich seeds encourage smooth muscle contractions, which is especially important for Boomers. Finally, they're also a complete protein.

"If you are not your own doctor, you are a fool. Natural forces within us are the true healers of disease."

— Hippocrates

Do not buy preground flax seed. At worst, it will be rancid, and at best it will have lost too much of its nutritional punch. Grind it yourself in a coffee grinder or, preferably, a nut and seed grinder. Use flax seed immediately after grinding in blended salads or regular salads. I don't recommend using flax seed oil, a fractured food that could actually do more harm than good.

CAMU CAMU BERRIES

These berries grow in the Amazon rain forest, and they are the densest and most perfect form of antioxidant vitamin C we have found so far. They're especially beneficial for workout recovery because vitamin C helps with the formation of collagen, which is what connective tissue is made of. Healthy connective tissue means reduced stress on the body when you exercise. They offer an excellent source of potassium, calcium, phosphorus, and some B vitamins, making them good for the immune system and skin and for alleviating stress.

Camu camu berries can be consumed in either powder (mixed into a blended salad or water) or capsule form.

CHIA

This powerhouse of a seed is excellent ground up and sprinkled on salads or added to blended salads. It's loaded with iron (contains more than spinach), omega 3s (more than salmon), omega 6s, and fiber, as well as phytonutrients and antioxidants, including potassium (more than bananas), calcium, magnesium, selenium, and phosphorus. Finally, it is a complete and easily digestible form of protein.

TURMERIC

As you remember from Chapter 6, turmeric is one of my favorite superfoods. It contains inflammation-reducing phytonutrients that may reduce the risk of developing arthritis and Alzheimer's. When eaten after exercise, it reduces aches and pains and speeds recovery, so add some to your post-workout juice or blended salad.

"The truth is, Americans consume six to ten times as much protein as they need. That excess protein overworks the liver and kidneys, causing both these organs to become enlarged and injured ... One of the most time-honored approaches to healing the kidneys and liver, in fact, is to eat a low-protein diet, especially a diet low in animal proteins. When the protein content of the diet drops, kidneys are strengthened and very often healed."

—*John A. McDougall, M.D.,*
The McDougall Diet

APPENDIX C

FURTHER READING AND RESOURCES

■■■

While this book offers you a healthy dose of good advice, you may find yourself wanting more. Need a source for raw nuts and seeds? Check out the Resources section. Looking for more reading on meditation? Look under Stress Management in the list of books below.

| BOOKS

I read extensively, especially about health, nutrition, fitness, and overall well-being, and I have a sizeable library of books on these topics. Below you'll find some of my favorite titles on subjects I discuss in *The Ageless Boomer*.

GENERAL HEALTH AND LONGEVITY

Ragner, Peter. *How Long Do You Choose to Live? (A Question of a Lifetime)* (Roaring Lion Publishing, 2001).

Robbins, John, *Healthy at 100: The Scientifically Proven Secrets of the World's Healthiest and Longest-Lived Peoples* (Ballantine Books, 2007).

Weil, Andrew. *Why Our Health Matters: A Vision of Medicine That Can Transform Our Future* (Hudson Street Press, 2009).

"Often in this technological age where computers diagnose diseases and perform surgery, we tend to minimize natural therapies. It seems incredible that the simple act of drinking raw juices could turn around severe diseases, however I have seen it work in otherwise hopeless cases."

— Dr. Sandra Cabot,
Raw Juices Can Save Your Life

NUTRITION

"Besides agreeing with the aims of vegetarianism for aesthetic and moral reasons, it is my view that a vegetarian manner of living by its purely physical effect on the human temperament would most beneficially influence the lot of mankind."

— Albert Einstein,
Letter to Hermann Huth, 1930

Barnard, Neal, M.D. *Food for Life: How the New Four Food Groups Can Save Your Life* (Three Rivers Press, 1994).

Barnard, Neal, M.D. *Power Foods for the Brain: An Effective 3-Step Plan to Protect Your Mind and Strengthen Your Memory* (Grand Central Life & Style, 2013).

Bisci, Fred. *Your Healthy Journey: Discovering Your Body's Full Potential* (Bisci Lifestyle Books, 2009).

Brazier, Brendan. *Thrive: The Vegan Nutrition Guide to Optimal Performance in Sports and Life* (Da Capo Lifelong Books, 2008).

Brazier, Brendan. *Thrive Energy Cookbook: 150 Plant-Based Whole Food Recipes* (Da Capo Lifelong Books, 2014).

Cabot, Sandra. *Raw Juices Can Save Your Life: An A-Z Guide to Juicing* (SCB International, 2001).

Campbell, T. Colin and Thomas M. Campbell II. *The China Study: The Most Comprehensive Study of Nutrition Ever Conducted and the Startling Implications for Diet, Weight Loss, and Long-term Health* (BenBella Books, 2006).

Campbell, T. Colin, *Whole : Rethinking the Science of Nutrition* (BenBella Books, 2013).

Clement, Brian, and Theresa Foy Digeronimo. *Living Foods for Optimum Health* (Prima Lifestyles, 1996).

Cohen, Alissa. *Living on Live Food* (Cohen, 2004).

Cousens, Gabriel. *Conscious Eating* (North Atlantic Books, 2000).

Cousens, Gabriel. *Rainbow Green Live-Food Cuisine* (North Atlantic Books, 2003).

Davis Brenda, Vesanto Melina, and Rynn Berry. *Becoming Raw: The Essential Guide to Raw Vegan Diets* (Book Publishing Company, 2010).

Davis Brenda and Vesanto Melina. *Becoming Vegan: The Complete Reference to Plant-Based Nutrition* (Book Publishing Company, 2014).

Esselstyn, Caldwell. *Prevent and Reverse Heart Disease : The Revolutionary, Scientifically Proven, Nutrition-Based Cure* (Avery, 2007).

Esselstyn, Rip. *The Engine 2 Diet: The Texas Firefighter's 28-Day Save-Your-Life Plan that Lowers Cholesterol and Burns Away the Pounds* (Grand Central Life & Style, 2009).

Esselstyn, Rip. *My Beef with Meat: The Healthiest Argument for Eating a Plant-Strong Diet* (Grand Central Life & Style, 2013).

Fuhrman, Joel. *Eat for Health* (Gift of Health Press, 2012).

Fuhrman, Joel. *Eat to Live: The Amazing Nutrient-Rich Program for Fast and Sustained Weight Loss* (Little Brown, 2011).

Fuhrman, Joel. *The End of Diabetes: The Eat to Live Plan to Prevent and Reverse Diabetes* (HarperOne, 2012).

Fuhrman, Joel. *Super Immmunity: The Essential Nutrition Guide for Boosting Your Body's Defenses to Live Longer, Stronger, and Disease Free* (HarperOne, 2011).

Graham, Douglas. The 80/10/10 Diet (FoodnSport Press, 2006).

Meyerowitz, Steve. *Power Juices, Super Drinks: Quick, Delicious Recipes to Prevent & Reverse Disease* (Kensington, 2000).

Morris, Julie. *Superfood Smoothies: 100 Delicious, Energizing & Nutrient-dense Recipes* (Sterling, 2013).

Morris, Julie. *Superfood Juices: 100 Delicious, Energizing & Nutrient-dense Recipes* (Sterling, 2014).

Nison, Paul. *The Raw Life: Becoming Natural in an Unnatural World* (Three Forty Three Publications, 2000).

"Fasting is the oldest therapeutic method known to man. Throughout the long [history of medicine], fasting has been regarded as one of the most dependable curative and rejuvenative measures. Hippocrates, 'the Father of Medicine,' prescribed it. So did Galen, Paracelsus, and all the other great physicians. Paracelsus called fasting the 'greatest remedy; the physician within.'"

— Dr. Paavo Airola,
How to Keep Slim, Healthy, and Young with Juice Fasting

"It's bizarre that the produce manager is more important to my children's health than the pediatrician."

—Actress Meryl Streep,
"Food Trends for 2011," USAToday.com

Popper, Pam, and Glen Merzer. Food over Medicine: The Conversation That Could Save Your Life (BenBella Books, 2013).

Robinson, Jo. *Eating on the Wild Side: The Missing Link to Optimum Health* (Little, Brown and Company, 2013).

Schenck, Susan E. *The Live Food Factor: The Comprehensive Guide to the Ultimate Diet for Body, Mind, Spirit & Planet* (Awakenings Publications, 2009).

Shannon, Nomi. *The Raw Food Gourmet* (Books Alive, 1999).

Wolfe, David. *The Sunfood Diet Success System* (North Atlantic Books, 2008).

All books by Norman Walker.

STRESS MANAGEMENT

Goldstein, Joseph. *Insight Meditation: The Practice of Freedom* (Shambhala, 2003).

Harris, Dan. *10% Happier: How I Tamed the Voice in My Head, Reduced Stress Without Losing My Edge, and Found Self-Help That Actually Works-A True Story* (It Books, 2014).

Harp, David, *The Three-Minute Meditator: Reduce Stress. Control Fear. Diminish Anger. In Almost No Time at All. Anywhere. Anytime.* (Mind's I Press, 2008). This is the best book for beginners.

Kabat-Zinn, Jon. *Mindfulness for Beginners: Reclaiming the Present Moment-and Your Life* (Sounds True, 2011).

Salzberg, Sharon. *Real Happiness: The Power of Meditation: A 28-Day Program* (Workman Publishing Company, 2010).

Naht Hanh, Thich. *The Miracle of Mindfulness : An Introduction to the Practice of Meditation* (Beacon Press, 1999). A classic.

Weil, Andrew. *Spontaneous Happiness: A New Path to Emotional Well-Being* (Little, Brown and Company, 2011).

EXERCISE

Brazier, Brendan. *Thrive Fitness: The Vegan-Based Training Program for Maximum Strength, Health, and Fitness* (Da Capo Lifelong Books, 2009).

Carter, Al. *Rebound Exercise: The Ultimate Exercise for the New Millennium* (AuthorHouse, 2005).

Cooper, Kenneth, M.D., and Tyler Cooper, M.D. *Start Strong, Finish Strong: Prescriptions for a Lifetime of Great Health* (Avery, 2008).

Fenton, Mark. *The Complete Guide to Walking, New and Revised: For Health, Weight Loss, and Fitness* (Lyons Press, 2008).

Hitzmann, Sue. *The MELT Method: A Breakthrough Self-Treatment System to Eliminate Chronic Pain, Erase the Signs of Aging, and Feel Fantastic in Just 10 Minutes a Day!* (HarperOne, 2013).

Lauren, Mark. *You Are Your Own Gym : The Bible of Bodyweight Exercises* (Ballantine Books, 2011).

Metzl, Jordan, M.D., and Mike Zimmerman. *The Athlete's Book of Home Remedies The Athlete's Book of Home Remedies: 1,001 Doctor-Approved Health Fixes and Injury-Prevention Secrets for a Leaner, Fitter, More Athletic Body!* (Rodale Books, 2012).

Metzl, Jordan, M.D., and Andrew Heffernan. *The Exercise Cure: A Doctor's All-Natural, No-Pill Prescription for Better Health and Longer Life* (Rodale Books, 2013).

Morehouse, Laurence, and Leonard Gross. *Maximum Performance* (Simon and Schuster, 1977).

Peterson, John. *Isometric Power Revolution: Mastering the Secrets of Lifelong Strength, Health, and Youthful Vitality* (Bronze Bow, 2007).

Peterson, John, and Wendie Pett. *The Miracle Seven: 7 Amazing Exercises that Slim, Sculpt, and Build the Body in 20 Minutes a Day* (Bronze Bow, 2004).

Peterson, John. *Pushing Yourself to Power: The Ultimate Guide to Total Body Transformation* (Bronze Bow, 2003).

Peterson, John, and Rod Fisher. *Ultimate Push Ups for the Awesome Physique* (Bronze Bow, 2013).

Skup, Ted. *Death, Taxes & Push Ups: Confessions from "The Pusher"* (Abox Publishing, 2008).

Wharton, Jim and Phil. *The Whartons' Back Book* (Rodale Books, 2003).

SUNLIGHT AND VITAMIN D

Holick, Michael F., M.D., and Mark Jenkins. *The UV Advantage* (iBooks, 2013).

Holick, Michael F., M.D. *The Vitamin D Solution: A 3-Step Strategy to Cure Our Most Common Health Problems* (Plume, 2010).

| FILMS

Forks Over Knives: The Plant-Based Way to Health. Director: Lee Fulkerson. Producer: Brian Wendel. Featuring interviews with T. Colin Campbell, Ph.D., and Caldwell B. Esselstyn, Jr., M.D, (Monica Beach Media, 2011).

"The doctor of the future will give no medicine but will interest his patients in the care of the human frame, in diet and in the cause and prevention of disease."

— *Thomas Edison,*
    in newspaper accounts from 1902 and 1903

| RESOURCES

The internet is packed with information, both good and bad. The following sites are some of my most trusted sources for products and information.

TOOLS

Norwalk Juicer, www.norwalkjuicers.com

FOODS

Of course, your first choice for foods should be fresh, local, and organic whenever possible. When it's not possible or practical, however, the following online providers can help round out your pantry:

Bautista Family Organic Dates, www.7hotdates.com

The Date People, www.datepeople.net

Jaffee Brothers Organic Fruits & Nuts, www.organicfruitsandnuts.com

Living Tree Community Foods, www.livingtreecommunity.com

Seeds of Change, www.seedsofchange.com

Sun Food Nutrition, www.rawfood.com

Sun Organic Farm, www.sunorganicfarm.com

NUTRITION AND FITNESS

Monkey Bar Gymnasium, monkeybargym.com. Jon Hinds's site gives you plant-based meals and body-weight exercise workouts.

Thrive Forward, www.thriveforward.com. Brendan Brazier's site helps you plan your transition to whole-food, plant-based eating with a personalized program.

Transformetrics forums, www.transformetrics.com. John Peterson's site has discussions on every exercise subject, with special focus on slow-motion resistance exercise.

www.ingramcontent.com/pod-product-compliance
Lightning Source LLC
Chambersburg PA
CBHW080046280326
41934CB00014B/3233